ALLE · ZEIT · WACH · 1842

Economic and Medical Evaluation of Health Care Technologies

Edited by

A. J. Culyer and B. Horisberger

With 48 Figures

Springer-Verlag
Berlin Heidelberg New York Tokyo
1983

Professor A. J. Culyer
Department of Economics and Related Studies
University of York
Heslington, York Y01 5DD, England

Dr. B. Horisberger
Interdisziplinäres Forschungszentrum
für die Gesundheit St. Gallen
Rorschacher Straße 103 c
CH-9007 St. Gallen, Switzerland

Symposium April 1982, Wolfsberg, Switzerland

ISBN-13:978-3-642-69441-7 e-ISBN-13:978-3-642-69439-4
DOI: 10.1007/978-3-642-69439-4

2119/3140-543210

Preface

All too frequently, the largest effective barrier to interdisciplinary communication is jargon. The symposium whose proceedings appear in the following pages sought, of course, to eliminate unnecessary and obscurantist jargon; but it sought also to do something far more ambitious – to confront the *intellectual* issues that are attached to the use of the word "evaluation" in medicine and health services. To this end a carefully selected group of experts in medicine, epidemiology, and health economics was invited to present papers. They were selected for their reputations either as conceptualizers or as empirical evaluators, or – the rarest breed of expert – as both.

The context was to be empirical. Three procedures were selected that had been subject to evaluation but that posed rather different types of problem. The first was the treatment of renal failure by dialysis of various kinds. This has a relatively long history of evaluation, with a large literature, and particularly raises broad policy issues within the health services of Western societies as to – the size of programmes to be provided; the type, location, and mix of treatments; the selection of patients to receive treatment; and the measurement of the success of various strategies. The second was the treatment of duodenal ulcer by a new species of drug – the histamine H_2-receptor antagonists (specifically, cimetidine). This poses similar but also some rather different issues: its very newness involves the problem of making policy (as well as clinical) decisions before the results of long-term trials have been completed; its nature raises a host of interesting questions about the means of handling a comparison between a drug treatment that may be administered by physicians in the community health services and a surgical treatment that is administered in hospitals. The third was a diagnostic procedure – computerized axial tomography (CT) of the head. This is a spectacular example of high technology in medicine whose rapid diffusion, possibly rapid supersession by newer imaging techniques, and whose great expense, have all posed major policy problems. It also raises quite different questions from the other two technologies in that the immediate object of CT scanning is not improved treatment of, or outcome for, patients but improved diagnosis.

These three empirical contexts provide a rich diet of issues for those who care about evaluation. Ultimately, all evaluation is concerned with the question "is it *worthwhile* doing something?" The papers in this symposium all tackle in their various ways the different meanings that can be attached to "worthwhileness".

One sense of worthwhileness that is particularly used by clinicians seeks to answer questions of the sort: is diagnosis made more precise? is patient outcome improved? are adverse side effects or incidental risks to patients reduced? The framework for judging worthwhileness is couched essentially in terms of the beneficial and harmful effects on the patients receiving treatment. Another sense of worthwhileness, lying at the opposite end of a spectrum along which the level of aggregation increases, relates to questions of the sort: if there are net health benefits to patients from the use of a particular technology, are they sufficiently worth having at some particular scale of provision at the cost of, say, other health services not provided (or provided on a smaller scale)? Or, are the costs only to be measured in terms of, say, health services expenditure or general public expenditure or private expenditure, or should nonfinancial costs be taken into account? Where are facilities to be most appropriately located? Here the framework for judging worthwhileness is couched in terms of a wider set of advantages and disadvantages whose very diversity raises questions of how to make them commensurate (by using money measures?) and how to make major value judgements about evaluating the advantages and disadvantages to different types of person (e.g. patients, patients' families, potential patients, the public at large, the young, the old, those in employment, the unemployed, the retired, men, women, and so on). Between these two poles on the spectrum of aggregation lie a host of intermediate positions.

The papers in this volume are broadly divided into "micro" (or individual) and "macro" (or system-wide), corresponding to lesser and greater degrees of aggregation. However, as with all continua, the dividing line between "micro" and "macro" is essentially arbitrary. In addition to exploring the types of appraisal that seem appropriate at various levels of aggregation the papers were also selected so as to present alternative *disciplinary* perspectives. Just as there is no single correct *level* of appraisal (the appropriate level must clearly be determined by the question one seeks to answer or, ultimately, by the customer one envisages for an evaluative appraisal), there is no single correct discipline. Indeed, it rapidly becomes clear to anyone who cares to think about it that there are very few – if any – evaluative issues that can be satisfactorily resolved by using only one of the three disciplines (medicine, epidemiology, and economics) represented in the symposium. For example, in the most apparently medical of all questions of appraisal – is patient health improved? – it turns out that economists' notions of welfare and utility are essential building blocks in the measurement of changing health status. Conversely, in the most apparently economic of all questions of appraisal – is the benefit greater than the cost? – it turns out that medical and epidemiological understanding of the links between what is done and what happens to patients as a result is essential to the proper formulation of an appraisal. The relationship between the disciplines is thus interactive and symbiotic. Each is mutually indispensible.

To bring out these various levels of appraisal and analytical perspective the papers have been organized in the following way. Those in Part 1 are introductory. These papers set out the reasons why evaluation is important and explore the types of evaluation that have been (and should be) done. Two papers review the epidemiological and economic intellectual frameworks explicitly. The final paper in this section is an introduction to the three technologies that provide the empirical context for the subsequent discussion.

Parts 2, 3, and 4 deal with dialysis, cimetidine, and CT scanning, respectively. Each part is organized in the same way: the first two papers in each part relate to "micro" appraisal from a medical and an economic perspective; the second two relate to "macro" or "systems" appraisal, again from a medical and economic per-

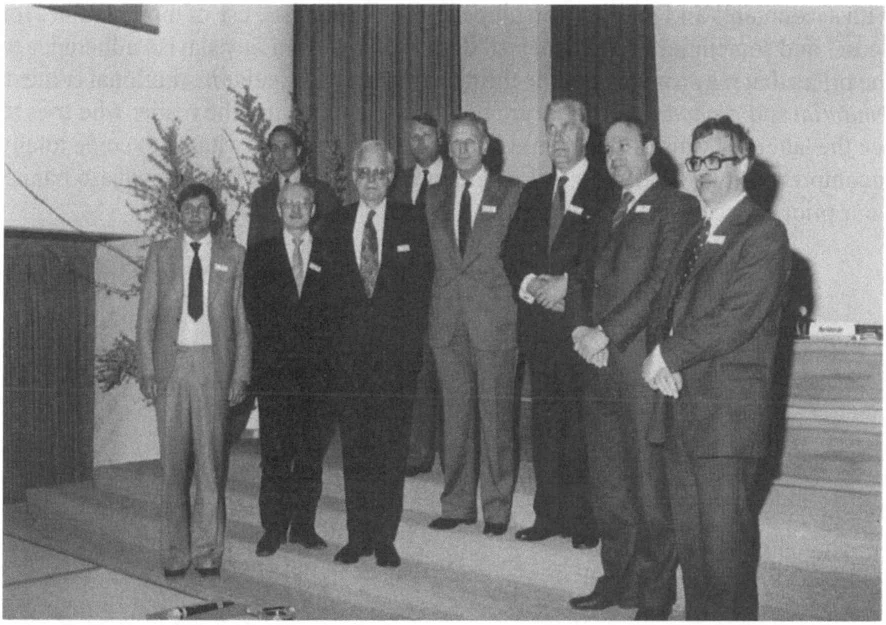

From left to right: B. Jönsson, M.L. Paterson, B. Horisberger, K.L. White, D. Sierp, U. Frey, L. Kaprio, H. Zöllner, A.J. Culyer

spective. Each paper is followed by a short discussion by someone from the other discipline.

Part 5 concludes the book with a general essay by the editors and – since *some* jargon is indispensible – with a glossary for easy reference. This can be used in conjunction with the index for those either seeking specific information or who want to follow an independent theme that the book itself does not use as an organizing principle. Part 5 also contains a very extensive reference section that we hope will be sufficient for those seeking to follow up their reading of this volume.

The editors had available to them some 500 pages of transcripted discussion from the workshops devoted to the examination of specific technologies and from plenary sessions. There was no space for any extended reporting of this material. Each paper, however, is followed by a very brief résumé of the discussion that followed it and, in the final paper, the editors have sought to draw out the principal threads of the discussions. We have had to be brutal in our judgement about what to exclude. We hope, nonetheless, that those who were present will detect *some* resemblance between their recollection of events and our summary version of them.

We believe that a double warning is appropriate if misunderstanding is to be avoided on the part of some of our readers. First, no one has a monopoly on the use of language. The same words are often used to mean different things. We have tried to standardize so that, at least in this book, there is a one-to-one correspondence between word (or phrase) and concept. If we have chosen a usage that is not yours, please be patient with us! Second, economists profoundly resent being identified with accountants and market-worshippers. The economists' use of money values for "cost" and sometimes even "benefits" does not flow from any slavish adherence to the prices that may (or may not) be thrown up in any particular institutional context. *Financial* and *economic* appraisal are not the same thing and the reader who tries to see the latter in terms of the former will find at least half of what is to come totally incomprehensible. So, if you feel prone to make this identification, please banish your prior expectation!

A. J. Culyer B. Horisberger

Acknowledgements

The first debt that the editors have is to the participants at the symposium at which the papers here were first presented and discussed in April 1982. While the debt is profound it is also, however, obvious to anyone who reads the following pages. Nevertheless, we want to make our gratitude plain to all those from so many disciplines, institutional affiliations, and countries whose courteous but intellectually uncompromising behaviour made the symposium the success it was. Particularly, we should record our thanks to the joint chairpersons of the workshops on each of the three technologies. Their tasks were arduous and delicate and the efficient and insightful way in which they reported their workshop discussions to the plenary sessions was exemplary. Those in the various chairs were: T. Scherstén (medical chair for the Dialysis Workshop), K. Davis (economic chair for the Dialysis Workshop); K. D. Bardhan (medical chair for the Cimetidine Workshop), A. Maynard (economic chair for the Cimetidine Workshop); H. Troupp (medical chair for the CT Scanning Workshop), D. Banta (economic chair for the CT Scanning Workshop).

Secondly, we owe a very much less visible – but no less profound – debt to Priska Eberle and her administrative and secretarial assistant Becky Brown. Without them, not only would the symposium not have worked but this book would never have appeared. The administrative chores were not only at the Swiss end in St. Gallen; Gail Shepherd (now Gibson) at the York end of the organization kept calm at times when the international shuffling of material began to resemble an aerial paper chase. Her typing and organizational skills, therefore, are no less appreciated than those of the St. Gallen team.

Thirdly, we owe a great debt to Smith Kline and French and particularly to Mort Paterson in Philadelphia and Dieter Sierp in Munich who funded the conference. Their behaviour has been a model of rectitude and seldom can industrial money have been less demanding of academic compromise: indeed no compromise whatever was demanded. That was a brave policy for a firm whose leading product was going to be, as it were, on trial. Fortunately, cimetidine came out of its intensive evaluative attention exceedingly well. Had it *not* done so, however, we have every confidence that the volume would have nonetheless appeared.

Fourthly, we owe a debt of gratitude to the European Office of the World Health Organization, whose technical assistance proved invaluable both at the scientific level and the more practical – but terribly important – level of "opening doors", widening our circle of contacts and helping with publicity – not just for the symposium, or even this book, but for the ideas about evaluation that both the symposium and the book contain.

Finally, to the other two members of the steering committee who jointly helped set up the symposium in its early days and cultivated it with their advice and support throughout, our heartfelt thanks: Bengt Jönsson and Herbert Zöllner need no particular publicity from us but it deserves to be known that their impact on this book is far more than could possibly be appreciated by reading any of its pages.

A. J. Culyer B. Horisberger

Contents

Part III: Cimetidine

Part IV: Computerized Tomography of the Head

Part V: Envoi

List of Participants

Prof. Dr. I. Hakki Ayhan
Dept. of Pharmacology
Medical Faculty of Ankara University
Sihhiye
Ankara, Turkey

Prof. Dr. D. J. Balaban
School of Public and Urban Policy
University of Pennsylvania
39th and Walnut Streets
Philadelphia, PA 19104, USA

Dr. David Banta
Assistant Director
for Health & Life Sciences
Office of Technology Assessment
U.S. Congress
Washington, DC 20510, USA

Ludwig Bapst, lic. oec.
Interdisciplinary Research
Centre for Public Health
Rorschacherstraße 103 c
CH-9007 St. Gallen, Switzerland

Dr. K. D. Bardhan
Rotherham District General Hospital
Moorgate Road
Oakwood
Rotherham R60 2UD, Great Britain

Prof. Jonas Bergström
Dept. of Renal Medicine
Huddinge University Hospital
S-141 86 Huddinge, Sweden

Prof. Dr. med. Fritz Beske
Institut
für Gesundheits-System-Forschung
Beselerallee 39/41
D-2300 Kiel 1,
Federal Republic of Germany

Prof. Jan E. Blanpain, M. D.
Department of Hospital Administration
and Medical Care Organisation
Vital Decosterstraat 102
B-3000 Leuven, Belgium

Dr. Bernard S. Bloom
Leonard Davis Institute
of Health Economics
University of Pennsylvania
Colonial Penn Center
Philadelphia, PA 190104, USA

Gerhard Brenner, Dipl.-Kfm.
Stv. Geschäftsführer
Zentralinstitut für die kassenärztliche
Versorgung
in der Bundesrepublik Deutschland
Haedenkampstraße 5
D-5000 Köln 41,
Federal Republic of Germany

Dr. R. Bulthuis
Senior Research Economist
Netherlands Economic Institute
Bergemeester Oudlaan 50
NL-3062 PA Rotterdam, Netherlands

Dr. A. Colombi
Leitender Arzt
Nierenstation, Medizinische Klinik
Kantonsspital Luzern
CH-6004 Luzern, Switzerland

Prof. Anthony J. Culyer
Dept. of Economics and
Related Studies
University of York
Heslington, York Y01 5DD,
Great Britain

Prof. Karen Davis, Ph. D.
Dept. of Health Services
Administration
School of Hygiene and Public Health
The Johns Hopkins University
615 North Wolfe Street
Baltimore, MD 21205, USA

Dr. James T. Doluisio
Dean
College of Pharmacy
The University of Texas at Austin
Austin, TX 78712, USA

Dr. M. Drummond
Health Services Management Centre
University of Birmingham
40 Edgbaston Park Road
Birmingham B15 2RT, Great Britain

Prof. W. van Eimeren
Director
Institute for Medical Informatics
and Health Services Research of
the GSF Research Centre (MEDIS)
Ingolstädter Landstraße 1
D-8042 Neuherberg,
Federal Republic of Germany

Harvey V. Fineberg, M. D., Ph. D.
Center for the Analysis
of Health Practices
Harvard School of Public Health
677 Huntington Avenue
Boston, MA 02115, USA

Dr. Ulrich Frey
Director
Swiss Federal Office of Public Health
Bollwerk 27
CH-3001 Bern, Switzerland

Prof. Shiro Fujino
Dept. of Economics
Chuo University
742-1, Higashinakano
Hachioji-Shi
Tokyo, 92-03, Japan

Urs Gessner, Dipl. Ing. ETH
Interdisciplinary Research
Centre for Public Health
Rorschacherstraße 103 c
CH-9007 St. Gallen, Switzerland

Dr. K. von Grebmer
Health Econ AG
Augustinergasse 21
CH-4051 Basel, Switzerland

Dr. Gunnar Griesewell
Referent für sozialökonomische Fragen
des Gesundheitswesens
Bundesarbeitsministerium
Rochusstraße 1
D-5300 Bonn 1,
Federal Republic of Germany

Jürgen Henning
Wissenschaftliches Institut
der Ortskrankenkassen (WIdO)
Bundesverband der Ortskrankenkassen
Postfach 200844
D-5300 Bonn 2,
Federal Republic of Germany

Dr. jur. Robert Van den Heuvel
President, National Association of
Christian Sick Funds
President, International Association
of Sick Funds
Rue de la Loi, 121
B-1040 Brussels, Belgium

Dr. med. Bruno Horisberger
Director
Interdisciplinary Research
Centre for Public Health
Rorschacherstraße 103 c
CH-9007 St. Gallen, Switzerland

Dr. James I. Hudson
National Organization for
Quality Assurance in Hospitals
P.O. Box 20064
Beneluxlaan 37
NL-3502 LB-Utrecht, Netherlands

Prof. Bengt Jönsson, Ph. D.
Dept. of Health & Society
Linköping University
S-581 83 Linköping, Sweden

Dr. Egon Jonsson
Senior Research Associate
Swedish Planning and Rationalization
Institute (SPRI)
Box 27310
S-10245 Stockholm, Sweden

Dr. L. Kaprio
Regional Director for Europe
World Health Organization
Regional Office for Europe
8, Scherfigsvej
DK-2100 Copenhagen Ø, Denmark

Dr. Peadar Kirke
Assistant to the Director
The Medico-Social Research Board
73 Lower Baggot Street
Dublin 2, Ireland

Prof. Jean François Lacronique
Ministere de la Santé et
de la Securité Sociale
Direction Generale de la Santé
8, Avenue de Ségur
F-75700 Paris 41, France

Prof. Dr. José Andresen Leitão
Rua Fernáo de Magalhães 11
P-1100 Lisboa, Portugal

Dr. rer. pol. Peter Lutz
Bundesamt für Sozialversicherung
Effingerstraße 33
CH-3003 Bern, Switzerland

Colin MacKay
Senior Lecturer in Surgery
Department of Surgery
Western Infirmary
Glasgow G11 6NT, Great Britain

David L. Martin
Consultant in Health Administration
Institutional & Professional Services
Health Services Directorate
Health and Welfare Canada
Health Services & Promotion Branch
Ottawa, Ontario K1A 1B4, Canada

Dr. Maurice Laurence Mashford
Reader in Clincal Pharmacology
University of Melbourne
Dept. of Medicine
St. Vincent's Hospital
Victoria Parade
Fitzroy
3065 Victoria, Australia

Prof. Alan K. Maynard
Dept. of Economics and
Related Studies
University of York
Heslington, York Y01 5DD,
Great Britain

Dr. Barbara J. McNeil
Associate Professor of Radiology
Harvard Medical School
Department of Radiology
721 Huntington Avenue
Boston, MA 02115, USA

Prof. André Meheus, M. D., D. P. H.,
Ph. D.
Epidemiology and Social Medicine
University of Antwerp (UIA)
Universiteitsplein 1
B-2610 Wilrijk, Belgium

Prof. Lechaim Naggan, M. D., D. P. H.
Head, Epidemiology and Health
Service
Evaluation Units
Ben-Gurion University of the Negev
P.O. Box 653
Beer Sheva 84120, Israel

Haruo Naito
Management and Control Dept.
Eisai Co., Ltd.
6-10, Koishikawa 4
Bunkyo-ku
Tokyo 112, Japan

Dr. Morton L. Paterson
Manager, Cost-Benefit Studies
Smith Kline & French Laboratories
1500 Spring Garden Street
P.O. Box 7929
Philadelphia, PA 19101, USA

Dr. Kjeld Møller Pedersen
Odense University
Insitute of Social Sciences
Campusvej 55
DK-5230 Odense M, Denmark

Prof. Dr. Martin Pfaff
Wissenschaftlicher Direktor
Internationales Institut für
empirische Sozialökonomie (inifes)
Haldenweg 23
D-8901 Stadtbergen-Leitershofen,
Federal Republic of Germany

Dr. Michael Philippe
Smith Kline
and French Laboratoires S.A.
Manager, Corporate Affairs Europe
Chaussee de la Hulpe 150
Boîte postale No 4
B-1170 Brussels, Belgium

David Pole
Department of Health
and Social Security
Friars House
157-168 Blackfriars Road
London SE1 8EU, Great Britain

Jean-Pierre Poullier
Principal Administrator
OECD, Organization for Economic
Cooperation and Development
2, Rue André-Pascal
F-75016 Paris, Cedex 16, France

Dr. N.T. Racoveanu
Chief Medical Officer
Radiation Medicine
World Health Organization
Avenue Appia
CH-1211 Geneva 27, Switzerland

Prof. Uwe Reinhardt
Woodrow Wilson School
of Public Affairs
Princeton University
Princeton, NJ 08540, USA

Dr. Paul-Albert Ruhr
Stv. Geschäftsführer
Bundesverband
der Pharmazeutischen Industrie
Karlstraße 21
D-6000 Frankfurt am Main 1,
Federal Republic of Germany

Dr. Ian Russell
Lecturer in Medical Statistics
Health Care Research Unit
University of Newcastle-upon-Tyne
21 Claremont Place
Newcastle-upon-Tyne, Great Britain

Prof. Frans F.H. Rutten
Professor of Health Economics
Rijksuniversiteit Limburg
Faculty of Medicine
Vijverdalseweg 1
P.O. Box 616
NL-6200 MD Maastricht, Netherlands

Simone Sandier
Directeur de Recherche
Directeur Adjoint
CREDOC
Division d'Economie Médicale
142, Rue du Chevaleret
F-75013 Paris, Cedex 13, France

Prof. T. Scherstén
Dept. of Surgery I
Sahlgrenska Sjukhuset
S-413 45 Göteborg, Sweden

Dr. Eberhard Schmitt
Klinik für Innere Medizin
Nierenstation
Wilhelm-Pieck Universität
DDR-2500 Rostock,
German Democratic Republic

Dr. Dieter Sierp
Manager, Health Economics
Smith Kline Dauelsberg GmbH & Co
Sapporobogen 6–8
Postfach 401642
D-8000 München 40,
Federal Republic of Germany

PD Dr. Amnon Sonnenberg
Medizinische Klinik &
Poliklinik, Klinik D
Gastroenterologische Ambulanz
Universität Düsseldorf
Moorenstraße 5
D-4000 Düsseldorf 1,
Federal Republic of Germany

Prof. Greg Stoddart
McMaster University
Dept. of Clinical Epidemiology
and Biostatistics
1200 Main Street West
Hamilton, Ontario, L8N 3Z5, Canada

David Taylor, BSc (Soc)
Deputy Director Office
of Health Economics
12 Whitehall
London SW1A 2DY, Great Britain

Prof. Dr. sc. pol. Manfred Timmermann
University of Konstanz
Weinbergstraße 13
CH-8280 Kreuzlingen, Switzerland

Prof. Henry Troupp
Chairman
Dept. of Neurosurgery
University Teaching Hospital
Topeliuksenkatu 5
SF-00260 Helsinki 26, Finland

Dr. Walter L. Trudeau
Associate Clinical Professor
Division of Gastroenterology
University of California
Davis Medical Center
4301 X Street
Sacramento, CA 95817, USA

Dr. Werner Ulrich
Abteilung
für wissenschaftliche Auswertung
Gesundheits- und Fürsorgedirektion
des Kantons Bern
Rathausgasse 1
CH-3011 Bern, Switzerland

Dr. Johannes O. Vang
Associate Professor of Surgery
Department of Surgery
Eksjö-Nässjo Hospitals
S-57500 Eksjö, Sweden

Dr. Hans Th. Waaler
The Norwegian Research Council for
Science and the Humanities
Unit for Health Services Research
Fr. Stangsgt 11/13
N-Oslo 2, Norway

Dr. Judith L. Wagner
Senior Research Associate
The Urban Institute
2100 M Street, N. W.;
Washington, DC 20037, USA

Dr. A. H. W. Wahba
Director, Development of
Comprehenisve Health Services
World Health Organization
Regional Office for Europe
8, Scherfigsvej
DK-2100 Copenhagen Ø, Denmark

Dr. Anders Walan
Department of Internal Medicine
Linköping University
Medical School
S-581 85 Linköping, Sweden

Prof. Burton A. Weisbrod
University of Wisconsin-Madison
Dept. of Economics
Social Science Building
1180 Observatory Drive
Madison, WI 53706, USA

Dr. Kerr L. White
Deputy Director for Health Sciences
The Rockefeller Foundation
1133 Avenue of the Americas
New York, NY 10036, USA

PD Dr. V. Wiggli
Institut für medizinische Radiologie
Universität Basel
Ch-4021 Basel, Switzerland

Prof. Alan Williams
Institute of Social and
Economic Research
University of York
Heslington, York Y01 5DD,
Great Britain

Dr. A. Wojtczak
Director
Research Planning
and Human Resources
World Health Organization
Regional Office for Europe
8, Scherfigsvej
DK-2100 Copenhagen Ø, Denmark

Dr. Herbert H. Zöllner
Regional Officer for Health Economics
World Health Organization
Regional Office for Europe
8, Scherfigsvej
DK-2100 Copenhagen Ø, Denmark

Welcoming Remarks

U. Frey

Director, Federal Office of Public Health, Switzerland

I am delighted to welcome you here to Wolfsberg on behalf of the Swiss Federal Department of the Interior and its head, Federal Councillor Hürlimann. I particularly wish to extend greetings to our foreign guests, but also to our Swiss colleagues and especially to the promoters and organizers of this event. I would like particularly to thank Dr. Horisberger, the Director of the Interdisciplinary Research Centre for Public Health in St. Gallen. He has once again managed to create the kind of atmosphere that is ideally suited for an international discusssion of the questions that cause deep concern to all of us involved in health politics and whose solution is causing us great difficulty at the moment. Credit and thanks are also due particularly to Professor Culyer of the University of York and to the Regional Office for Europe of the World Health Organization for their cooperation and support in preparing and holding the symposium.

I am particularly pleased to be able to welcome my friend Leo Kaprio here who is among us in his capacity as a regional director of the World Health Organization (WHO). I would like to thank him and his colleagues very heartily for the support lent by his regional office.

All industrialized and highly developed nations presently face the dilemma of technological progress in medicine on the one hand and of an impairment of the interpersonal relations between physician and patient on the other. Due to extraordinary advances in the biomedical and medico-technical sciences new diagnostic and therapeutic methods have been developed, incurable diseases have been cured, and lives have been saved. Such progress, however, often has to be paid for by a loss in terms of human warmth and by an exaggerated objectivization of the relationship between physician and patient. More and more technical devices, machines, and nonmedical assistants are being interposed between doctor and patient; direct contact between physician and patient is increasingly reduced, the consequence being feelings of increasing alienation and frustration by patients seeking help. This disastrous development is particularly a threat in hospitals, which in some places have degenerated into gigantic health factories.

This development must be stopped without holding up thereby healthy technological progress for the good of mankind. We must seek the golden mean. The human being must once again be returned to the centre and remain master of technology – not the other way around – otherwise the same thing will happen to us that Goethe's sorcerer's apprentice experienced, where he could not get rid of the spirits he had summoned. As far as research is concerned, this means that the practical side of research must be promoted more than in the past. This does not mean that the fundamental research should be reduced, but that alongside it the sociomedical, preventive, psychological, and psychiatric health sciences, which up to now have been poorly developed, must be advanced more strongly and that the health sciences and health services research must be promoted more than hitherto. As far as the training of physicians is concerned, a less theoretical and more practical new orientation towards the general medical requirements is absolutely necessary. The Swiss parliament has recently passed new examination requirements for physicians that come close to the above-mentioned needs.

Under these circumstances it is particularly creditable that this symposium is to concern itself with the economic and medical evaluation of medical technology, because only scientific evaluation of today's enormous technical possibilities can make it possible to choose rationally what is necessary in a medical sense and what is economically justifiable. In the final analysis, these investigations are an absolutely necessary aid to help those involved in health politics to make decisions.

Thus, I would like to wish every success to your symposium whose results will be awaited eagerly.

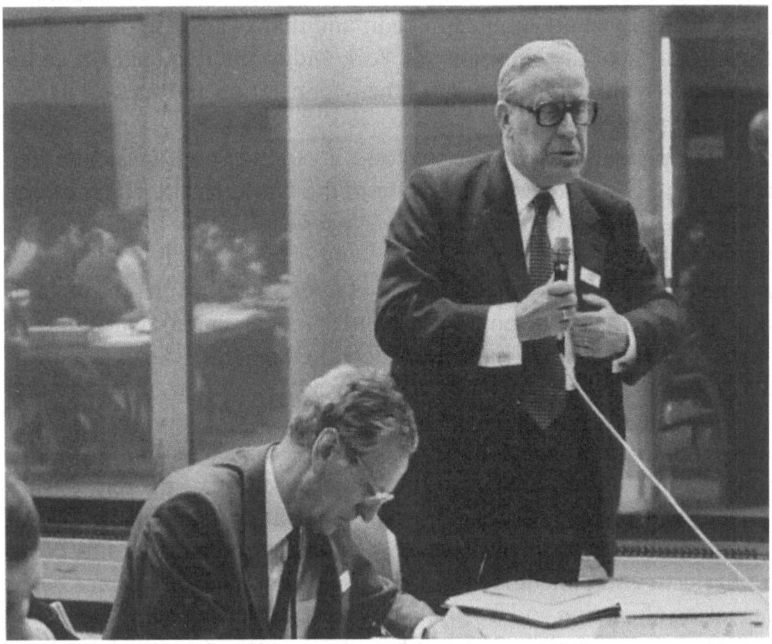

U. Frey and L. Kaprio

Opening Address

L. Kaprio

World Health Organization

The lack of vigorous economic growth during this decade will make it increasingly difficult for European countries to improve the health status of their populations and to avoid painful choices as to which health programmes to develop at the expense of others. A number of countries are now spending about one-tenth of their gross national product on health care, with a post-war growth of 1% or more per decade that has only recently been slowing down. In view of the numerous needs of societies, not only for health care but also for food, housing, education, energy, and other needs, it is most unlikely that governments will be willing and able to sustain further growth in the health services. Financial difficulties of social security systems have been aggravated by growing demands for unemployment benefits, food and other daily living subsidies, old-age pensions, as well as additional disease and disability benefits for those individuals who are most directly afflicted by economic instability.

The 30th World Health Assembly decided in May 1977 that the main social target of governments and the WHO during the coming decades should be the attainment by all citizens of the world of a level of health that will permit them to lead a socially and economically productive life by the year 2000. This historic resolution was followed in September 1978 by the Alma Ata declaration on primary health care, which was seen as the major key to attaining an acceptable level of health for all. Finally, in November 1979, the United Nations General Assembly called on their Member States and other United Nations bodies to support the WHO in this effort and requested that a global strategy be formulated. As Dr. Halfdan Mahler, Director General of the WHO, has said:

> Health for all *at bottom* is a political movement, in order to ensure that steps are now being taken which will permit a considerable improvement in the health of the populations of the world; the continuation of the present system and its strategies will probably mean, by contrast, a catastrophical situation within 20 years . . . If health for all meant medical repairs by doctors and nurses for everybody in the world for all existing ailments . . . it would certainly not be a realistic proposition. Nor does it mean that nobody will be sick or disabled. It means a different approach by which health is considered in broader context of its contribution to, and promotion by, social and economic development, so that all people will be able to lead socially and economically satisfying lives. It means that people will use better methods than they do now for preventing disease and disability, and better ways of growing up, growing old and dying gracefully.

The most painless way of attempting to achieve health for all in terms of the health care system would be to pour in extra resources in the hope of filling all the gaps, but this would not be economically feasible. Nor is it by any means certain that the present resources and skills would be redistributed in such a way as to meet the basic needs of many patients instead of providing highly technological services to relatively few. The technological imperative and the professional inclination to meet its challenge call for a fundamental revision of the health professional's code of ethics and basic attitudes.

In collaboration with its Member States, the WHO Regional Office for Europe has responded to this global challenge by drafting a regional strategy for attaining health for all by the year 2000, which was accepted and endorsed by the 30th Regional Committee. The strategy includes:

1. The promotion of life styles conducive to health and, more specifically: to develop awareness and provide opportunities for choice, to improve conditions that positively affect life styles and stimulate healthy behaviour, and to reduce exposure to self-imposed risks.
2. The reduction of preventable conditions and, more specifically: to reduce perinatal risks and improve maternal and child health, to reduce poverty, to reduce preventable communicable diseases, to reduce accidents and their consequences, to promote balanced nutrition and safe food, to reduce environmental risks, and to provide safe water and sanitation.
3. The re-orientation of the health care system to cover the whole population with comprehensive health care to the maximum degree possible for each country according to its stage of development and, more specifically: to provide equal access to appropriate health care, to provide special care for high-risk groups, to reduce the effects of chronic and degenerative diseases, and to improve cost-effectiveness and quality of services.

European indicators and targets are at present being developed for these strategies, and individual countries are making major efforts to develop their own national strategies for health for all, not, it may be added, in order to satisfy the WHO requirements but in order to prepare and stimulate a number of scenarios that will in the long run make the health services and related health measures more effective in spite of the absence of economic growth.

It is hard to see how these strategies can be implemented in the absence of technological progress and institutional change. This is most painfully evident in the case of the first two strategies, which are geared to make the life style and both the physical and social environment of us all more healthy. There has, by contrast, been a great deal of technological progress in reducing the effects of chronic and degenerative diseases, the diseases whose importance is likely to increase with the hectic pace of modern life and the aging of the population. Hardly a day goes by without today's sophisticated medical industry announcing the invention of new, often sensational, techniques; there is no end in sight to the technological progress of medicine. This allows more efficacious diagnosis and treatment of diseases that only a few years ago could hardly have been diagnosed, let alone treated.

A great deal of effort has gone into improving the technical quality of laboratory equipment, radiological technology, bioinstrumentation, pharmaceuticals, and medical appliances. This has made them safer, more reliable, and easier to operate and monitor, as well as making them more specific and sensitive in their diagnostic, therapeutic, or rehabilitative tasks. The performance of technical equipment is governed by the quality of both the hardware and the human operator, the latter being involved in several activities such as preparation, monitoring, and interpretation. Thus the reliability of results depends on the technical capability and accuracy of the device and, at the same time, on the skills and the diligence of the various persons engaged in the process. While the human factor is a technico-managerial question, the appropriateness of the instrument for the task required has to be assessed. The testing of instrument performance is at present rather limited, the main reason being the absence of international and national recommendations for evaluation. The necessity for coordinating attempts is universally recognized; such coordination would obviate unnecessary duplication of work, ensure optimal use of expert and financial resources, provide valuable information to potential users, and ensure comparable results. Because of the extensive availability of instruments and devices and the rapid introduction of new ones, certain guiding principles for assessment methodology and priority testing must be developed at national and international level.

In the present programme of the WHO Regional Office for Europe one project will develop and implement a health care technology assessment network by linking selected national institutes capable of ensuring technical, clinical, and economic assessments of new equipment and technologies. The main criteria for the choice of these institutes is their present capability in performing assessments. Whenever possible, evaluation of presently used and insufficiently assessed equipment will also be considered. These institutes will also be requested to engage in utilization studies at various levels of health care.

The third strategy demands, however, that the technologies have additional features besides technical quality: They have also to be effective, suitably oriented to the population (and therefore to primary health care), as well as economic. Here the picture is less optimistic. Some of the technologies are applied to medical conditions for which they are not indicated and may therefore even induce unnecessary iatrogenic effects; others are so sophisticated and costly that they are not accessible to all in need; others make the patients unnecessarily dependent on their use in hospital settings; there are some technologies that are quite costly but appear to improve diagnosis and therapy to no discernable degree in terms of health outcome; finally, there are many technologies that make the patient more dependent instead of independent of medical care in general. In addition, the supply of new medical technology is apt to create its own demand. It is often used in such a way that it does not replace traditional tests and procedures but rather "adds on" to their diagnostic and therapeutic powers.

The ethics of both physicians and nurses demand that everything, however marginal or illusory its benefits may turn out to be in the end, be done for the individual patients. In this attitude the professions have been supported by the public in their capacity as health care consumers; it is only recently that the public in their capacity as payers of tax and health insurance have been demanding more value for money. The move of the balance of care somewhat away from institutional and highly technological care, where it is now focused, towards primary health care – with its greater emphasis on prevention, earlier treatment, and earlier rehabilitation as well as on lay and self-care – will often serve to improve the cost-effectiveness of care. Let me emphasize that this does not merely mean shifting the burden from the institutional care sectors to families (in so far as it is families – and often the women of the families – that care for the sick, the elderly, and the disabled). Nor does it mean abolishing all so-called high technology. On the contrary, high technology is often of very great benefit to the patient and the only economically sensible way of making use of it may be to concentrate it in hospitals and other health institutions. Systematic multidisciplinary assessment of medical technology ought to help improve both the quality and rationality of technology-based health services.

In summary, technological progress in medicine has been a mixed blessing. There is a need for critical evaluation of both traditional and new technologies in order to help guide the health system towards more relevant research in the biomedical, clinical, and health services fields, the more appropriate use of health care technologies, better health care practice and delivery, and towards greater consumer responsibility. Within our Regional Office there are several programmes dealing with these questions, notably those in health economics and appropriate technology for health. As we are convinced that evaluation must be a multidisciplinary task, I am glad that this symposium has taken the challenge seriously and is reviewing technologies one step at a time in order to be able to focus more clearly on the evaluation process and methodology. The evaluation of three different medical technologies from the diagnostic, therapeutic, and rehabilitative fields will make the conclusions more relevant.

I would expect medical and economic evaluation to show that those health care strategies that are geared to the promotion of more healthy life styles, more healthy environments, and a more population-oriented health care system, are in fact both more effective and more cost-effective than traditional strategies. They will, unfortunately, not always be less costly. It would therefore be useful for the health sector to take a more active bargaining role vis-à-vis the other sectors of the economy and to show that health care and related health actions are not just a cost to the overall economy but also make a direct and sizable contribution towards overall productivity, employment, investment, and industrial innovation. The difficulties many countries experience in trying to close "unnecessary" hospitals adds to my point.

May I thank you for the opportunity you have given our Office in allowing us to assist in a technical capacity in the preparation and discussions of this meeting. I consider the scope of the meeting most relevant not only for Europe and other highly industrialized countries but also for developing and newly industrialized countries by bringing to their attention both the promises and pitfalls of modern medical technologies.

Part I

Overview

1 Evaluation and Medicine

K. L. White

The Rockefeller Foundation, New York

Numbers are the stuff of science. They are necessary but are rarely sufficient for many personal and political decisions about the credibility of both medical and economic claims, findings, recommendations, and generalizations. Numbers apart, however, there is little in any scientific endeavor that is value free. Indeed, the values of scientists are major determinants of the problems they choose to examine or the questions they choose to ask. In turn, these choices initiate the application of the scientific process. Values also influence the assumptions underlying the investigators' analytical or experimental designs and the conclusions they draw. In these respects, medicine and economics are alike in that both aspire to become more scientific by applying the laws of logic, the rules of evidence, and, to an increasing extent, the power of numbers to evaluate critically their hypotheses and improve their predictive powers. And it is predictability with respect to individual benefits and personal well-being as well as public policies and collective choices that we seek. As means to these ends, we use numbers to measure outcomes and attach relative values to the many complex issues that surround notions of health, disease, illness, and medicine.

If economics deals with the problems of resource allocation in the face of relative scarcity, politics must surely deal with these matters when resources are really scarce! In democracies, and even elsewhere, the diversity of value systems, as well as of individual and collective preferences, finds political expression in budgets and appropriations that are denominated in monetary units. Money then becomes a surrogate expression for more basic concerns such as those associated with personal and collective freedom, independence, well-being, health, security, and for energy distribution, particularly human energy, in the form of labor. Money expresses directly or indirectly the values we place on those more enduring, if intangible, qualities that so deeply affect the human condition.

This is not the place to dwell on the complexities and mysteries of the eternal verities that engage the efforts of philosophers and political scientists. It is the place, at the outset of this series of discussions, however, to emphasize that any critical discussion of medicine and its evaluation is confounded with untold complexities of definition, classification, measurement, and comparison, to say nothing of a vast array of ignorance. Such a discussion requires that we keep constantly in mind the underlying systems of belief, values, and prefererences that guide the medical establishment and are the stuff of philosophy, economics, and politics.

There is one who has preceded us in his concern for these many interrelated problems and issues. Sir William Petty was not only Professor of Anatomy at Oxford following medical training in the Netherlands and France, but he also conducted social and land-use surveys in Ireland, had a major hand in designing the public accounts and statistical systems of the day, was one of the original mercantilists, and was a Fellow of the Royal Society (Greenwood 1948). By many, he is regarded as one of the fathers of demography, health statistics, sociology, epidemiology and economics, and all this in the seventeenth century. He was, to boot, a medical statesman and a political leader of no mean account as he inveighed against inadequacies in contemporary social statistics and urged that greater attention be given to measuring the public benefits anticipated from increasing expenditures for the medical, welfare, and social services of the day. He pointed out that undue emphasis on counting the money disbursed without equal effort directed at assessing the outcomes of various good works made it impossible to compare the relative merits of alternate courses of action.

If matters are infinitely more complex three centuries later, our sources of data and our analytical tools are also more varied and powerful. Alas, what may not have advanced so far is our capacity for critical examination of the assumptions underlying our goals and objectives and the means of achieving them. Only in recent years has the nature and credibility of the evidence that informs individual and political choices and decisions in matters medical been examined seriously. It is still difficult, and at best, accompanied by much error, to predict who will benefit and who will fail to benefit, and by how much, from a particular intervention, and who has paid and how much for a set of health services. Evaluation and medicine are concerned with these matters and in this review I shall try to examine some of the fundamental problem and issues that need to be recognized, and usually accommodated, in discussions that surround them.

We start with the overt claim and the implicit presumption that the medical profession has skills and knowledge that some people believe will meet a need. Usually this is a perceived need to forestall or prevent premature death or functional impairment, to alleviate or ameliorate suffering or anxiety, or to enhance the individual's sense of well-being. On the face of it, the ensuing relationships seem to be based on a quaint set of expectations elaborated by the public and a questionable set of claims articulated by the medical establishment. At the core of the matter is the implication that a "doctor" can usually, if not always, participate in making a "patient" "better". At the next stage, both the public and the medical profession start believing that "doctors" are the primary arbiters of the public's health "needs" and what should be done about them.

With respect to the first proposition, there is much validity to it. In fact, it may be argued that, overall, the most important contribution of the medical establishment to the well-being of society is the glow of anticipation and hope generated by confidence in the healing and caring processes. These are the central features of the extremely powerful physician-patient relationship. Although medicine may refer to the "placebo" (Beecher 1955; Shapiro 1960) effect and industry to the "Hawthorne" (Röthlisberger and Dickson 1939; Levene and Cohen 1974) effect, the essential elements of both are faith, hope, and charity. The "placebo" effect is associated with the physician's conscious or unconscious efforts to make the patient "feel better". There is some evidence that it may be mediated through complex nervous and hormonal mechanisms that release compounds which modify the body's immune and other responses to external assaults and increase the individual's sense of well-being. Similar mechanisms may well be involved in related institutional experiences first described amost 50 years ago at the Western Electric Company's Hawthorne plant near Chicago. When the "company" was perceived by the employees as "caring" everyone felt better and production increased.

Estimates vary but overall it would appear that between 40% and 60% of the perceived benefits associated with the ministrations of the health professions are associated with various mixes of the "placebo" and "Hawthorne" effects. That is no mean contribution, particularly when referred to appropriately as tincture of "faith, hope, and charity." On the other hand, of the specific preventive, diagnostic, therapeutic, and restorative interventions employed by the medical establishment for, and on behalf of, patients, only about 10% to 20% are supported by scientific evidence as being more useful and beneficial than they are useless or even harmful for the purposes for which they are advocated. In the 1960s, a study conducted by all the general practitioners within a defined region of Wales showed that only 10% of their prescriptions were regarded as efficacious and specifically indicated for the conditions for which they were prescribed (Forsyth 1963). In a southeast Asian country, it is said that some 30000 different drugs and compounds are for sale, in the face of a list of 200 essential drugs recommended by the WHO.

I suggest then that we keep these two figures in mind – 50% improvement from the "caring" function and 15% improvement from the "curing" functions. The balance of 35% remains something of a mystery, a rather costly mystery, perhaps associated with such phenomena as waste, structural imbalances, or organizational rigidities in health care systems. However, there is no reason to accept these sets of figures as universal and I would urge their replacement with more accurate and precise measures that would inform future discussions.

So much for a gross view of societal "benefits" associated with the services provided by the medical or health care establishment. What about the "costs" to society of maintaining that establishment? The estimation of "costs" constitutes an equally complex quantitative exercise. Public expenditures from taxes and borrowings that flow through government agencies usually do not include private expenditures for health insurance or direct out-of-pocket payments. "Costs" for the economist also include "opportunity costs," that is, other benefits foregone either currently or in the future in order to obtain the benefit or service selected in the present. Time lost from work, travel expenses, care of one family member by another, or a vacation foregone to pay for a series of tests to tell you you did not have cancer; these are "opportunity costs." When the alleged benefits are in the future and the payment is required now or vice versa, either the costs or the benefits have to be "discounted" and economists argue about what the "correct" rate of discount should be. As a practical matter, central banks or taxing authorities increasingly tell us what it is. All of these and many sophisticated distinctions enter into the notion of net "cost" for a given benefit.

Again, let us consider orders of magnitude. Most Western industrialized countries spend from 6% to 10% of their annual gross national product or gross development product on their health care establishment. In the United States, this currently amounts to about US $ 250 billion or over US $ 1000 for every man, woman, and child in the country. The US federal budget for health and related services is the largest in the government; it beats defense by a considerable margin. The health care establishment is the second largest source of employment, and after energy costs and interest rates, the largest contributor to that country's inflation rate. Similar sets of relationships are to be found in many other countries.

Now this may be all to the good. It may be argued that a society in which such large numbers of people devote so much of their energies and funds to making their fellow citizens feel better must be headed in the right direction and that sooner or later everyone should enjoy a happier and even a trouble-free existence. Or it may be argued: "What is the value of a life saved." Is it the same for a 2-year-old child in India, a philosopher of 30 years in Philadelphia, a toolmaker of 40 years in Toulouse, an active architect of 70 years in Athens, and a widow of 80 years in Warsaw? Economists attach figures to lives saved, to years of life saved, or to days of work lost that are based on monetary estimates of increased productivity, taxes paid, and disability pensions saved. These estimates are used to offset other estimates of the costs of medical services to save the lives. Usually, these are done for specific diseases, such as kidney failure or coronary heart disease. But these are, at best, crude indicators and many argue that both sides of the equation should be corrected with measures of the quality of the lives saved expressed, for example, as "days of well-being" using a scale of, say, one to ten.

In their quest to improve the human condition and further the goals of social justice, the advocates for medicine, and especially curative medicine for individual patients, usually argue that no cost is too great and no effort too trivial in the endless task of postponing death, prolonging life, and easing pain. But the economist asks whether all the "costs," including the opportunity costs, are balanced against the measured value of some alleged benefit for a specific patient at the margin. In other words, is an increase of one unit of cost for one unit of benefit for the patient with the least chance of benefitting warranted? But who is the patient and who pays? Even more importantly, who decides which patient will benefit and who will pay and how much?

Consider the observation that each physician in the United States, Canada, and the United Kingdom seems to control annual outlays for patients that range in estimates from US $ 300000 to US $ 1 million. On what basis do these physicians make their choices? When the figure for the population becomes US $ 1000 and is rising, per person per year, the stakes become high and the debate ever more shrill. Who really wins and who really loses? Can we help to illuminate the debate by the judicious use of numbers and measurements?

Money is certainly one of the measures. But even with money, as I have tried to indicate above, it is important to define the concepts, assumptions, and entities to which the monetary terms are attached. Economic indicators in the fields of public finance, national economic welfare, and international trade, to take three examples, are improving. But they are far from perfect for purposes of prediction. A number of social indicators have been developed during the past two decades but little creative work on health indicators has been evident until recently. What is needed now is cooperation among economists, epidemiologists, health statisticians, and biomedical scientists in designing indicators that are of comparable reliability, validity, utility, and feasibility in the social and health sectors and in the economic sector.

Let me give some examples of concepts that require further clarification in order to achieve greater comparability.

1) "Perceived need" is a fundamental concept that merits greater attention than it is usually accorded. It involves the individual's expectation that information, services, and assistance can improve current functional capacity and well-being or avoid incapacity, disease, or pain. The collective expression of individual perceptions of the potential benefits anticipated from seeking medical care can be measured with some consistency (Kohn and White 1976). Indeed, perceived need is the single most important determinant of demand for and use of health services, but there are few national health information systems that regularly use such a measure.

2) Socially determined need is another important measure. Periodic redefinition of the socially unacceptable finds political expression in the provision of a variety of health and social services. For example, untreated venereal disease requires medical intervention to protect the health of the public, especially those at risk of being exposed to possible contagion. Legal sanctions may be invoked to ensure that the infected individual is indeed treated medically. Society may, for example, provide publically supported services for the mentally ill, especially when they are a danger to themselves or others. Family planning services and immunization against common communicable diseases are further examples of socially determined need.

3) Professionally defined need may, in part, be regarded as an aspect of socially determined need. Measures may be derived from direct examinations of the population or a sample of the population. Illustrations would include measurement of the prevalence of nutritional deficiency, anemia, high blood pressure, or parasites in the population. All of these conditions are relatively silent with respect to their manifestations insofar as they affect the individual's customary perceptions of personal health status.

4) Measures of "demand" for health services, particularly "expressed" and "effective" demand, in contrast to "potential" demand, reflect the actual pressures placed on a health care system. Where services are unavailable or the opportunity costs associated are high, as for example, those associated with loss of pay or transportation charges that cannot be afforded, there are deterrents to the tangible expression of potential demand. The presence of these deterrents will be reflected in differences for the entire population between potential demand, as estimated by measures of socially determined need, of professionally determined need, and of effective demand.

But not all expressed demand for medical care presented to physicians and hospitals is met. The medical professional may in fact control another aspect of the expression of need which precludes the acceptance or recognition of a patient's perceived needs. For example, some physicians regard certain types of emotional or social problems, or even early physical symptoms, as "trivial" or in some way unsuitable for medical attention. Implicitly or explicitly, they will reject the patient or refuse to respond to the presenting complaint. At other times, lack of personnel, drugs, or facilities restricts available care to those who are most seriously ill by a process of rapid assessment referred to as "triage." Similarly, by the use of waiting lists, a process of queuing, admission to a hospital for elective surgery really is controlled and much potential demand is precluded from becoming effective demand. Yet another device for controlling demand is through pricing. High charges for, say, elective cosmetic surgery, can successfully restrict effective demand.

5) The measurement of "use," or utilization as some call it, of medical care is a reflection of the actual consumption of services. Not all expressed demand, socially determined need, or professionally defined need is met. Some people tire of waiting in a physician's office and go home, others avoid or ignore opportunities for preventive immunizations. There are many barriers to acceptable, appropriate, and affordable care and the gaps between expressed demand and use may vary widely by social class, geography, and cultural patterns to name but a few of the more obvious constraints.

These then are five concepts that reflect levels of pressure on a health or medical care system. Each can be measured with a fair degree of precision through a combination of population-based household surveys and medical record surveys (White et al. 1977). Unfortunately, examples of coordinated health information systems that provide these estimates are few and far between (White 1980). Many health statistics systems provide data about the volume of attributes, events, or activities but few provide information about the number of persons with whom these measures are associated. For example, figures about the number of chronic conditions in a general population are less important than counts of the number of persons with chronic conditions. Similarly, counts of the number of visits to physicians may be less useful than counts of the number of persons with visits in, say, the course of a year. A frequency distribution of persons by numbers of visits per year would be even more useful. Or to take another specific example, it may be possible to obtain counts of the numbers of visits made by nurses to homebound patients with heart failure but it may not be possible to get counts of the number of persons with heart failure who are in fact visited.

In the broader sense, from a policy standpoint at the macrolevel, measures should be available of perceived need, preferably stratified by measures of severity, urgency, and anxiety, of socially determined need, of professionally defined need, of expressed demand, and of use. These should be calculated as rates, preferably standardized by statistical manipulations to remove the effects of different age and sex distributions among populations or subsets of general populations. The rates should apply to geopolitical jurisdictions for which financial budgets are prepared. So much then for several macromeasures of pressures on the system. They can be used to compare changes associated with the provision of health services in relation to financial measures at similar levels of population aggregation or geopolitical jurisdictions.

Health status as a global indicator is really a combination of perceived need, professionally defined need, and socially determined need, preferably measured so that duplications are avoided. As a composite measure, it can be used as the initial baseline for purposes of evaluating a health care system. After a period during which a determined amount of money is expended, health status can be measured again to determine the net impact of the money spent on that population's health. The health status of the population at a specified time can be used both as a guide for planning future expenditures and organizing efforts to improve or sustain health and for measuring the benefits, outcomes, and impact of a health care system and its costs on the population served.

Unfortunately, many traditional health indicators such as standardized mortality rates, proportional mortality rates, infant mortality rates, and life expectancy figures are too imprecise to measure short-term (i. e., 1 or 2 years) fluctuations. Perhaps of greater importance, for most jurisdictions, it is not possible to detect associations between money expended on medical care and improvements in the presently used measures of health status. Although it is possible that positive associations do not exist, it seems more probable that our measures are too crude.

But equally crude are many of the monetary measures. Not only is there a need to distinguish the many elements that constitute the flow of funds through a health care system, i. e., those through ministries of health, social security organizations, private and public insurance schemes and sickness funds, philanthropy and private payments, but it is also important to determine for what purposes the payments are made. One classification would include such categories as payments for physician's services of different types, for X-rays and diagnostic tests, for drugs, hospital services, ancillary services, and custodial services, for preventive services, and for prosthetic and other devices and aids. Another classification would emphasize expenditures for different types of research, such as fundamental and applied research. Still another would classify expenditures by levels of care such as primary health care, basic medical care (using the WHO terminology), secondary or consultant care, and tertiary or subspecialty care. Perhaps the most important classification, however, would distinguish between capital expenditures and operating costs, including fixed and variable costs. Little attention is paid to the implications of new capital expenditures for facilities, and for ever more complex and expensive equipment, and the continuing operating costs that flow from the use of these new resources. Similarly, the costs of depreciation (which is largely unfunded in most settings), as well as the costs of redundancy, obsolescence, and replacement should be included in any analysis that purports to assess total costs and benefits.

The health care field is replete with unanticipated financial perturbations flowing from investment decisions whose long-range implications are ignored. Two of these, renal dialysis and computed axial tomographic (CT) scanners, will be discussed in detail in the course of these deliberations. Cost or profit centers of the types used in industry and commerce are virtually unknown in health care systems and it is usually impossible, under most budgeting and accounting systems now in use, to relate revenues and expenses to specific services. To relate the output or products of those services with measures of benefit or outcome for individuals or communities, as we have noted above, is of equal or greater difficulty.

In summary, an evaluation of the impact of medical efforts at the macrolevel involves diverse arrays of fairly distinct concepts and of complex measurement problems on both the expenditure or cost side and on the outcome or benefit side. There is a need to define and refine with increasing precision both the concepts and the measurements on both sides of the equation.

Let me turn now to the microlevel and another set of problems that have a direct bearing on our capacity to evaluate medicine and medical services. The first is the concept of "efficacy." It is concerned with the capacity of a medical intervention, be it a drug, vaccine, surgical operation, a bit of advice, an X-ray, or a diagnostic test, to do what its proponents claim it will do. Analytical and experimental designs for assessing efficacy are concerned essentially with distinguishing the benefits associated with the "placebo" and Hawthorne effects from the intrinsic favorable or unfavorable outcomes and from the accompanying errors and variations associated with the measurement process itself. This is no easy task but in the past 30 years increasingly sophisticated methods have been evolved for the conduct of such studies.

The most important of these is the randomized control trial (RCT). It includes the designation of a universe of patients, or possibly people without overt or perceived health problems, who fully understand the nature of the proposed study, including any associated risks, hazards, and costs, and who agree to participate in the study. The critical aspect of the study then involves the assignment of patients to experimental and control groups in accordance with a set of predetermined rules not under the control of the patients, or the physicians, or other health prefessionals managing the patients. The process of "randomization" is the feature of RCTs that distinguishes this approach to measuring "efficacy" from the use of anecdotes or testimonials from enthusiastic physicians or the derivation of conclusions from haphazardly collected series of patients with unbounded faith in a renowned institution or its staff to do them good (Hill 1952). A universe of patients randomized into two groups, experimental and control, and given similar forms of intervention consisting of identical tablets, one with an active ingredient and the other with inert substances, would be a simple example of an RCT.

The problems become more complicated when two modes of treatment are involved say, one medical and the other surgical, or when, for example, one eye of a series of diabetic patients is treated with a laser beam designed to control hemorrhages and the other eye is not. More complicated designs include before and after studies, crossover studies in which the experimental and control groups are reversed at some stage, and studies that involve comparison groups which are only assessed at the beginning and end of the study. The latter design is used to separate the benefits associated with the Hawthorne effect, from external circumstances or the passage of time, from those associated with the "placebo" effect and from those stemming from specific intervention (Chalmers 1981).

There are many problems associated with the proper conduct of prospective studies of "efficacy." Ethical issues are important. In many instances it should be asked whether an RCT should not start with the first patient regarded as eligible for some new form of intervention. If the advocate hopes or expects that the new drug or procedure will be more efficacious or beneficial than others currently in vogue or that it will accomplish the same result with fewer side effects, less risk, or at lower cost than present methods, or is more beneficial than doing nothing, it would be regarded by some as unethical not to start an RCT. Problems arise when the enthusiastic clinician is unaware of the need to distinguish the benefits associated with a specific intervention from the "placebo" and Hawthorne effects.

There are, however, other ways of assessing "efficacy." They include retrospective or case-control studies, which involve matching patients who have received a specific treatment or intervention with a second group of patients that has as many characteristics as possible in common with the first group except that it has not been exposed to the treatment. In general, such studies are better suited to the detection of factors in disease causality than to studies of efficacy when they are only marginally helpful. Occasionally, there are examples of a new drug for a disease which was heretofore universally fatal. If the first patient to be treated is cured, there is no need for an RCT. An example would be the initial use of streptomycin years ago for tuberculous meningitis in infants. Such events are the exception, however. There are other quasiexperimental studies in which comparison between discrete and even isolated populations or subsets of populations or groups of patients permit limited inferences to be made, but these are not usually conclusive.

Neither the complexity nor the costs of conducting a sound RCT should be minimized. Some of these require large numbers of patients, a long time for completion, or both, in order to detect a statistically significant and a clinically important effect. These elements tend to become important when the benefits anticipated are modest or marginal or when the conditions under study are rare in the populations. Although the process is tedious and the costs great, it may be asked in the face of the plethora of drugs, equipment, and procedures now in use or advocated from many quarters, and their attendant costs, whether in fact most societies can afford not to insist on evidence from RCTs before accepting any new medical intervention. Many would argue that most unevaluated interventions in contemporary use should be subjected to critical evaluation but that it would pose almost unsurmountable practical and political problems. For the long run, one may ask whether in spite of the difficulties, the direct costs and even the opportunity costs that could accrue to those randomized into the control group, each individual is not better off by living in a society with a system of RCTs for assessing all new medical interventions than in a society without such a system. The costs to society of a rigorous system for assessing efficacy will be great, but what are the costs of not doing so? I do not think we know.

The next problem is concerned with measurement of benefits or outcomes that accrue to individuals as a direct consequence of a specific medical intervention. Again, measurement is fraught with variations and errors made by those who do the observing and make the actual measurements. Problems of validity, accuracy, and reliability must be confronted. Validity is concerned with the extent to which the phenomenon or attribute measured actually reflects the process or state of affairs it purports to describe. This is particularly true when a proxy measure such as a symptom is used to indicate the presence or absence of underlying pathology. Accuracy is concerned with the quality of the observation or measurement. Reliability is concerned with the reproducibility of the observation by the same observer on repeated occasions or by different observers assessing the same phenomenon. The problems are relatively simple where weights, volumes, or dimensions are concerned, slightly less complicated when biological, chemical, or physical properties are measured, considerably more complicated when physician's observations or perceptions are employed, and especially difficult when subjective symptoms, functional capacity, behavior, of feeling states reported by the patient are involved. Nevertheless, the measurement sciences have made considerable progress even in the latter areas. Preferences can be rank-ordered, feelings can be scaled, and discrete activities can be counted. A variety of techniques developed by behavioral scientists, particularly experimental psychologists and social scientists, are used increasingly to measure benefits (Freeman and Rossi 1981).

We turn now to the assessment of "effectiveness." Having established that a given intervention is relatively more efficacious than doing nothing or than interventions currently available, it is important to establish the extent to which the new intervention can be made available to all those in a defined population who might be expected to benefit from it. Eventually, this involves an assessment of medical or health services and their associated institutions, personnel, organizations, and systems as well as the procedures and interventions they use. It is quite possible to have a demonstrably efficacious intervention that is not effectively provided to all who could benefit. Measles vaccine is clearly efficacious but there are large populations of children who never receive it because of an ineffective medical care system. The principles of design for purposes of evaluating "effectiveness" are similar but not identical to those employed for studies of "efficacy," although the former task is more difficult. Here the investigator tends to randomize groups of people rather than individuals and these groups may include entire geopolitical jurisdictions such as villages or counties or they may include institutions such as hospitals or health centers. Crossover designs, before and after studies, and quasiexperimental designs may be employed.

Unfortunately, the terminology used in evaluation is often confusing. The terms "efficacy" and "effectiveness" are sometimes used interchangeably and in other service systems the distinction between what is done or used and how it is used is less important than in medicine. For example, in an aircraft, each subsystem as well as the entire system is usually subjected to critical evaluation and the influences of the placebo and Hawthorne effects are absent.

Measures of "efficiency" are concerned with whether or not the desirable level of effectiveness is achieved with the most prudent or optimal mix of resources. A remarkably "effective" service can be highly inefficient. The ideal arrangement would be an optimally "efficient" and "effective" health care system employing only "efficacious" interventions in a caring and compassionate fashion. "Efficiency" is again concerned with monetary units as they reflect human energy inputs to the system.

We come now to a consideration of two of the most important concepts in the evaluation of medicine – cost-benefit analysis (CBA), or more properly benefit-cost analysis, and cost-effectiveness analysis (CEA). We all use the type of thinking embodied in these two approaches toward evaluation much of the time and usually without disciplined thought. For example, we ask casually: "Is it worth the candle?"; "Does the perceived benefit to me justify the effort, sacrifice, or cost to me?" The economist's opportunity costs enter the equation and a choice is implied. The range of studies that fall under these two rubrics is great. On the one hand, it may be and it customarily has been in the past a matter of so-called intuitive judgment for an administrator or clinician to weigh what information there is available about the purported benefits and monetary costs associated with a particular intervention or a service and make a decision. On the other hand, large-scale computer-based studies using epidemiological and other data can provide the material for much more elaborate and sophisticated studies although the logic and the thought process should be similar. It is important to bear in mind that it is the essential features of the analytic process that require emphasis rather than the methods by which the data are manipulated.In essence, how does all the available evidence about direct and indirect costs, capital and operating costs, replacement and obsolescence costs, out-of-pocket and opportunity costs compare with our best estimates of all the positive and negative outcomes, all the benefits, direct and indirect, individual and collective, now and discounted into the future?

There is really a continuum of analytical methods for measuring or estimating the two essential elements that form the basis for the final CBA or CEA assessments. The impetus for assessments will also determine the methods used. For example, there may be evidence that the benefits or outcomes of two procedures are the same. In that case, the task is to determine which of the two is less costly, including all the elements of cost enumerated above. Risks or hazards associated with one or other procedure might also involve costs that need to be considered. A classic example is the treatment of varicose veins by surgery or by injection. The net benefits were the same, but the injection method cost less in monetary terms and therefore was favored in the final decision (Piachaud and Weddell 1972). In this instance, the net benefits were similar. Another type of analysis would start with the goal of a defined benefit, say a reduction of all road traffic accidents by 25%. Estimates would be made of the optimum cost for achieving this level of benefit and might include enforcement of seat-belt use, reduction in highway speed limits, enforced "breatholator" or blood alcohol tests, or speed governors on automobiles. Costs in this case would include political opportunity costs and many perturbations and indirect implications of choosing any one method or a combination of several methods.

In general, the principle distinction between a CBA and CEA lies in the way the benefits are measured or valued. This in turn influences the methods employed for the evaluation itself and often the complexity and extent of the analysis. In a CBA where the benefits are dissimilar, the costs are usually assessed and expressed in monetary units and the "values" or relative worth of the benefits being compared are also expressed to the extent possible in monetary units. The ratios between the costs and the benefits for the two types of enterprises can then be compared, e.g., a smoking-cessation campaign for teenagers versus a pneumonia-immunization program for all those over 65 years of age. In this case, a clinical trial of the efficacy of the maneuvers to be used and an assessment of the effectiveness of the service systems to provide the interventions would enter into the analysis. The final assessment would have to be expressed in monetary units.

On the other hand, CEA does not express the benefits in monetary terms as a rule but usually in some measure of the duration or quality of life, functional capacity, sense of fulfillment, or well-being. Years of life gained, days of work saved, or increases in the number of persons capable of independent living are the types of measures employed. It is estimates of the costs of attaining these objectives that are used in the analysis. Where the objectives can be clearly defined and the measures are adequate, it is possible to compare the relative direct and opportunity costs of attaining the specified objectives. To a large extent, the distinctions between CEA and CBA are arbitrary. For the most part, they help to distinguish a process of analysis and a way of ordering the information about a problem. They encourage critical thinking with respect to the evidence about a particular intervention or service and the extent to which it will accomplish what its proponents claim for it. There would be few, if any, examples where a CBA or CEA alone would serve as the single or even the most important consideration in a decision to accept or reject a new intervention, to start, stop, or modify a health service. The major contribution of these analyses is heuristic and it would be naive to think otherwise (Office of Technology Assessment 1980).

Indeed, the nature of the dialogue between clinicians, epidemiologists, and economists will vary with the question being asked or the problem being addressed. There are, however, several generic principles which it may be helpful to bear in mind:

1) The *problem* needs to be defined clearly. What is the direction of association and the strength of the association between the *intervention* under analysis or study and the predicted outcome, benefit, or change in health status?

2) The *objectives* need to be stated clearly. To what extent can or does the intervention under analysis or study achieve the objectives specified? What *alternative interventions* or strategies are there for achieving the same objectives?

3) The *benefits* or *effects* (both favorable and unfavorable) associated with the intervention need to be identified and assessed and, to the extent possible, measured. What measures are to be used? What errors and biases are associated with the measurement process? Are benefits of effects, including savings from other interventions or procedures avoided or superceded, being compared or valued in the same units? Can these be expressed in monetary units?

4) The *costs* of all types, including the *opportunity costs* and the *indirect costs* associated with the intervention, need to be identified, *valued* and, when possible, expressed in monetary units.

5) Are the *benefits, effects,* and *costs individual* or *private* or are they *collective* or *social,* or a mixture? The several viewpoints need to be distinguished and the implications considered in the analysis. Who gains or loses and who pays will determine the social or political value attached to one or other part of a CBA or CEA.

6) All future *costs* as well as future *benefits* and *effects* need to be *discounted* to their present value in accordance with equitable discount rates prevailing at the time and place of the analysis.

7) Possible *imponderables, unknowns,* and *uncertainties,* both favorable and unfavorable, should be analyzed to estimate the extent of their possible influence on the results of the analysis. Again, an attempt should be made to attach a value, or a range of values, to these potential influences.

8) *Ethical, cultural,* and *social values* and *preferences* need to be identified and "valued" where possible. This is at once probably the most difficult and the most important aspect of any CBA or CEA. There are indeed "fates worse than death" and it is possible to scale and rank preferences for outcomes associated with different forms of functional incapacity (Rosser and Kind 1978).

These eight steps describe a process of analysis that emphasizes clarity of thought and comprehensiveness of viewpoint rather than precision of measurement. The latter is but a means toward an end. Given the present state of the art, it is probably preferable to consider all, or as many as possible, elements that enter into an evaluative process and to establish a cost-benefit ratio based on best estimates or even pseudoquantification of only those elements that can be readily expressed in monetary units. The use of the latter is simply one way to emphasize clarity and precision. The process is far from perfect or ideal but with wider application and more critical discussions of the results, better methods will evolve. In summary, it is better to be roughly right than precisely wrong!

Turning now to some broader implications of the role of evaluation with respect to a medical care or health care system in a society, we come to even more difficult terrain. For example, we may consider the broad social and human costs of premature death, disease, disability, and even discomfort or pain. What toll do these take on the productivity and sense of well-being of the entire community? Again, efforts can be made to cost the burden of illness in a society (Black and Pole 1975; Rice et al. 1976). The overall costs of maintaining a health care establishment can only be estimated in a gross fashion. However, with increasing insistence, politicians, particularly those in the developing world, ask whether investments in education, agriculture, nutrition, jobs, clean water, and transport may not do as much or more for society, particularly one with scant usable resources, than can the development of ever more elaborate and costly medical care systems, especially those focused on curative medicine. This type of evaluation of medicine's role in the social fabric puts pressure on the advocates of more, different, or allegedly improved health care interventions to make their points with clarity and precision. Authoritarian pronouncements and explanations based on the experiences of individual clinicians need to be replaced with objectively designed studies and the presentation of facts, preferably with numbers attached. In one sense, CBAs and CEAs are concerned less with the facts themselves than with the "facts about the facts." It is the critical review of the evidence that is at the heart of the process of evaluation in medicine. In the second and perhaps more political sense, CBE and CBA are concerned with who decides and who receives what and on what basis and who pays.

What we are to explore in the balance of this conference is the structure for more critical and constructive deliberations among economists, epidemiologists, and clinicians as they examine the problems of evaluating medicine and health services. The same process should be encouraged in academia, industry, and governments. Indeed, the whole process should be imbedded in the thinking of all scientists whether working at the fundamental or applied levels, by all policy analysts concerned with government support for both research and service activities, and for all those concerned with setting priorities, allocating resources, and organizing health services. It is no less important for industrialists considering their strategies for research, development, marketing, and postmarketing surveillance in relation to the burden of illness in the populations they serve.

If doing good, being kind, and organizing science and technology to improve the health status of society are worthy goals, it does not seem unreasonable to try for increasing precision in our evaluation of their impact. Medicine may expect that both its supporters and its critics will require much more of this type of thinking in the next century than has been forthcoming in the three centuries since William Petty first discussed such endeavors in a treatise he called "Political Arithmetic." That is really what evaluation in medicine is all about.

2 Medical Evaluation of Health Care Technologies

D. J. Balaban and N. I. Goldfarb

Thomas Jefferson University

Introduction

This paper describes different approaches and technologies used in the evaluation of health care technology. It is intended as an introduction for physicians, economists, and others without formal training in evaluation research, epidemiology, or biostatistics. We will try to develop the concepts and methods with a minimum of jargon and without going into great technical detail. Some examples of specific technology assessments are used to illustrate methodological points.

Exploring methods of evaluation is a formidable task. At the outset one must recognize that the methods are not independent of the reasons for the evaluation, the sponsor of the evaluation, type of evaluation, or the backgrounds of the evaluators. The multidisciplinary approach to health evaluation on the part of epidemiologists, biostatisticians, and social scientists including psychologists, decision scientists, and sociologists, has taken on the formal title of "evaluation research." A similar effort on the part of an essentially similar group of academic disciplines, health services researchers is often referred to as "quality of care assessment." Both the substance and theoretical framework of these approaches are closely related to technology assessment. Technology assessment introduces new dimensions (and more economists) to evaluation methodology but is by and large not a special case. The formal title of any of these approaches to evaluation is not important; what is important is the definition of questions and the methodologies employed in seeking answers. Unfortunately, each academic discipline spends considerable time developing its own methods intended to separate fact from fiction and to discover the "truth." In evaluation of health care the problem is intensified. Evaluation efforts are routinely influenced by the disciplinary or professional tendency to reward those who remain closest to the fold and punish those who do not.

Although technology-related studies can be very narrowly defined based on disciplinary research (Arnstein 1977), Coates (1974) has emphasized the broad scope of technology assessment:

> Technology assessment is a class of Policy Studies which systematically examines the effects on society that may occur when a technology is introduced, established or modified with special emphasis on those consequences that are unintentional, indirect or delayed ... Comprehensive impact or assessment studies are a class of holistic studies which attempt in some sense to embrace everything that is important with regard to technology ... One characteristic of holistic thinking is that we do not know how to do it routinely; secondly, it al-

most certainly cannot be done routinely; and thirdly, it is not a scientific or an engineering or a disciplinary enterprise. It is essentially an art form.

The point is that technology assessments must be multidisciplinary. In a recent review of the contributions of social sciences and health services research to public policy, Bice (1980) states that: "Although the field draws upon knowledge from biomedical and epidemiological research, and upon experience in clinical medicine and health care administration, its theoretical and methodological bases are drawn largely from the social sciences."

We are reluctant actually to define technology. Others have been less timid. Altman and Blendon (1979) distinguish three categories of technology as:

1) Those that require large capital expenditures to purchase, such as the computed tomographic (CT) scanner;
2) Those with high personnel costs, such as renal dialysis;
3) Those that do not require large capital expenditures or high costs of attendant personnel but have potential for enormous utilization because of the large number of providers who have ready access to them, such as common laboratory tests or certain drugs.

Rosenthal's (1979) categorization of technology interventions is a convenient grouping, especially for the "hard technologies":

1) Diagnostic, such as CT scanner, fetal monitor, computerized electrocardiography, or automated clinical labs;
2) Survival, such as intensive care unit, cardiopulmonary resuscitation, or iron lung;
3) Illness management, such as renal dialysis or pacemaker;
4) Cure, such as hip joint replacement or organ transplantation;
5) Prevention, such as pediatric orthopedic repair, diet control for phenylketonuria, or vaccines for immunization; and
6) System management, such as medical information systems or telemedicine.

Other "soft technologies" such as drugs and diagnostic tests will fit the scheme as well. Actually, any intervention will; in the broadest sense, what is not technology? Fineberg and Hiatt (1979) state that technology "... refers to the wide range of equipment, devices, drugs, and procedures employed in the care of patients ... including the capital and human investments that establish the capability for medical practices as well as the practices themselves."

One major reason to evaluate health care technology is to minimize society's exposure to harmful or unsafe practices and to maximize exposure to beneficial ones. The dramatic escalation of health care costs, accompanied by the realization that health resources are limited (Hiatt 1975), has made the importance of sound technology evaluation techniques increasingly clear. Researchers, administrators, and legislators at all levels have intensified and redirected their efforts at cost control. Cost-cutting is most useful when it is the by-product of a reevaluation of a program's success in achieving goals. Issues involved in evaluating the economics of medical care, such as through cost-benefit analysis or cost-effectiveness analysis, are of great interest and importance, and will be considered in detail in separate papers in this volume. These evaluations concern resource consumption and resource allocation, such as by setting dollar values for nondollar benefits, costs versus charges for services, discount rates, and the various models of health care organization which place primary emphasis on economic issues.

Framework for Evaluation

How can medical technology be assessed? One broad category, research evaluation, asks the question "does it make a difference in what happens?" A second category, technical evaluation, is summarized by the query "does it administratively work the way it is supposed to?" Most formal evaluation in health care is technical, the US government's direct evaluation of providers and institutions being one example. Physicians and other health providers are licensed (sometimes relicensed) by states, and certified by professional organizations. Institutions are accredited by professional associations. These accreditations or evaluations are required by the government in order for the institution to be eligible for federal reimbursement of certain patient care programs. The evaluations require following certain procedures for patient admission and discharge and periodic formal review of patient care, as documented in the hospital record. Standards, or minimum levels of performance, are required for approved institutions. The evaluation of hospitals demanded by government agencies is essentially the same as that required by the industry, through the Joint Commission for the Accreditation of Hospitals (JCAH). These programs, intended to regulate and control the quality of health care, are productive if the health services provided are in fact related to improved health of the population or reduced cost.

Economic factors are a primary motivation for the US government's involvement in the evaluation of health care; however, the public benefit value of government involvement is questioned. There is widespread agreement that the Professional Standards Review Organization (PSROs) were intended more to control costs than to improve the health of society. It appears that neither has been accomplished (Lohr et al. 1981) and the program is likely to be abandoned.

Drucker (1974) distinguishes efficiency (doing things right) from effectiveness (doing the right thing). Cochrane (1972) and many others have emphasized that effectiveness and efficiency should be the primary goals of programs providing services. Effectiveness concerns the adequacy of delivery of a treatment to members of a population that could benefit, i.e., how many potentially treatable patients are successfully treated. Effectiveness assumes the application of an efficacious treatment. Efficacy is distinguished from effectiveness. An efficacious treatment is one that has been demonstrated to influence favorably the outcome of disease in an ideal situation in a population capable of benefit. The concept of efficiency refers to the amount of resources consumed in delivering a given level of care and/or achieving a given outcome. Measurement of efficiency and effectiveness is an expensive and tedious task. One may categorically state that a program that identifies and effectively treats 90% of hypertensives in a community at a cost of $ 50 per patient is clearly superior to a program in a similar community providing the same treatment to only 75% of the hypertensives at a cost of $ 150 per patient. However, the similarity of communities (or comparison groups) is often an unsupportable assumption and the costs are not clearly identifiable. Moreover, the effectiveness of treatment for hypertension may be judged simply by using a blood pressure measuring device. However, for many chronic diseases, there are no clear-cut measurements for judging the effectiveness of treatment.

Feinberg's formulation for evaluating the CT scanner is generally useful for technology assessment. It is primarily related to how efficacy and effectiveness of an outcome are defined and thus is an important first step in understanding the importance of what is being measured as an outcome. The nosology distinguishes between measured changes in resolution or accuracy, measured changes in diagnostic acumen, measured changes in diagnostic approaches, measured changes in therapeutic strategies, and measured changes in patient outcome – all as separable and identifiable endpoints:

1) Technical capability. Does the device perform reliably and deliver accurate information?
2) Diagnostic accuracy. Does use of the device permit accurate diagnoses to be made?
3) Diagnostic impact. Does use of the device replace other diagnostic procedures, including surgical exploration and biopsy?
4) Therapeutic impact. Do results obtained from the device affect planning and delivery of therapy?
5) Patient outcome. Does use of the device contribute to improved health of the patient?

Another problem in assessing the efficacy and effectiveness of health care technology is determining the appropriate situation and proper target populations. The distinction to be made is that there may be general agreement about the efficacy of a particular technological intervention, but the intervention may be much more broadly used than can be supported by the efficacy studies and thus appears to be less effective. For example, cimetidine (to be considered in depth at this symposium) is used clinically far more than the clinical trial evidence supports. Little control of drug prescription can be exerted over providers except through reimbursement mechanisms; for example, government-funded payment for the health care of the indigent and elderly (through Medicaid and Medicare) can be denied. This is an awkward and inefficient tactic for control of behavior and while it has been successful, it can simply result in changes in what is reported to reimbursers.

The majority of provider activities for health care and the bulk of organizational behavior patterns and arrangements are currently neither formally nor rigorously evaluated. This is especially true of care provided in doctors' offices or hospital clinics for ambulatory patients. Individual physicians and the medical establishment in general view government involvement in medical care and evaluation of common practice as a nuisance and as nonproductive.

To the office-based clinician whose primary concern is treating patients, evaluation means obtaining a medical history, performing a physical examination, making a diagnosis, and instituting appropriate treatment. The emphasis is not on policies or populations, but on individuals. Slater (1971) describes as the "technologic imperative" the concern of providers with giving the best available care to all patients without regard to cost. There is reason to believe that the socialization of providers that leads to dedicated concern for individual patients is in part responsible for the difficulty in reconciling policy and population studies of health and disease with clinical practice (Mechanic 1968; Friedson 1970). Murphy (1978) and Feinstein (1978) draw attention to the limited use of probability theory or Bayesian approaches in clinical medicine. This may relate in part to the fact that probability theory is inherently based on consideration of populations and scientific sampling rather than individuals and in part to the fact that the marginal benefit to individual providers or patients is not great, and the marginal benefit to society is not visible.

Reiser (1978) has eloquently traced the history of physicians' use of medical innovations and techniques. He points out how diagnostic judgements based on "subjective" physician observations and patient reports have become supplanted by "hard data" based on "objective" laboratory procedures and mechanical and electronic devices. He associates the concomitant emphasis on specialty medicine and hospital care with use of technology.

A conceptual model described by Donabedian (1969) for evaluating quality-of-care has gained widespread acceptance. The evaluation schema distinguishes between measures of the process, the structure, and the outcome of care. Process measures are activities performed as part of patient care, related to:

1) Screening;
2) Diagnosis, including clinical workup, patterns of disease classification, and support for diagnosis; and
3) Treatment, including use of drugs, surgery, referral pattern, and coordination and continuity of care.

Measures of structure relate to the setting or background in which the process occurs, such as facilities, equipment, financial arrangements, information systems, and organizational characteristics such as staffing and administration. Accreditation and certification criteria used by the JCAH, as well as by academic institutions and state licensing boards that provide diplomas, certificates, and licenses are based on the fulfilment of explicit standards (structural measures).

Outcome measures, intended to assess the end results of care, have been recognized for many years as the ultimate measures of a program's worth (Nightingale 1859; Codman 1914; Brook 1977). But even when a decision to use outcome measures has been made, one must select which outcome should be measured and the source of data for assessment. Some organize outcome into the five "D's", defining health outcomes as death, disability, disease, discomfort, and dissatisfaction (White 1963). Mortality and morbidity are roughly equivalent to death and disease. Starfield (1973) defines outcomes emphasizing positive aspects, such as longevity, activity, comfort, satisfaction, absence of disease, potential for activity, and resilience. A positive aspect of health outcomes is also embraced by the World Health Organization, which defines "health" as a positive state of physical, social, and emotional well-being. In the recently completed Health Insurance Study undertaken by the Rand Corporation in 1974 for the US Department of Health and Human Services (DHHS, previously DHEW), "health" is defined as a positive state with specific dimensions of social, mental, and physical health outcomes. Physical status is dissected into physiological (organ) health and physical (organism) health, and includes assessment of social and physical activity or mobility, disease conditions, symptoms, and disability. Mental health is defined in terms of anxiety, depression, and emotional or behavioral control. Improved health perceptions are also included as positive health outcome measures.

Given the provider and institutional disincentive to evaluate, it should not be surprising that evaluative studies that look at outcomes of care and costs of care (or efficacy, efficiency, and effectiveness) have not been very common. A review of cost-benefit analysis (CBA) and cost-effectiveness analysis (CEA) studies in the 1970s demonstrates the limited number (Office of Technology Assessment 1980). With such a limited number of studies it would seem particularly important that those undertaken are well done. This is frequently not the case. The issues that must be attended to in performing an evaluative study are quite different from the methods used in bench research.

Riecken (1977) has identified four "principal components" or categories of interest in performing evaluation research. These components, not intended to be mutually exclusive, but equally appropriate for medical evaluation of health care technology, include:

1) Ethical/legal – issues dealing with protection of the study population from invasion of privacy, adverse effects, and improper use of information (breaches in confidentiality). Also of concern are the legal matters related to informed consent and the authority of an agency to conduct experiments with human subjects.

2) Administrative/managerial – including in this component are issues related to the day-to-day operations of a study, including implementing the design in the real world (field), insuring that the data are appropriately collected and of high quality, and documenting modifications from the ideal specifications.

3) Political/social – issues here deal with power, whether it be the power to permit an evaluative study to take place, to influence the direction or conclusions of the study, or to implement policies based on results of the study.

4) Scientific/technical – the concerns with research strategies, study design, and measurement traditionally receive the greatest amount of attention from researchers. These specific technical issues will be discussed in the remainder of this paper.

Study Design

The primary scientific issue relates to making comparisons between groups. One wishes to separate the effect of a particular intervention from population characteristics (extraneous variables or factors which may be linked with a response). An intervention may be considered to be any type of maneuver done, it is hoped, to benefit the patient. Interventions may be drugs, procedures, devices, or organizational arrangements for health care delivery. Level of prevention is one way of categorizing interventions. Primary interventions are those activities that prevent disease, secondary interventions are activities that enable early diagnosis and treatment, and tertiary interventions are those directed at rehabilitations and limitation of disability. Another way to categorize interventions is from the easily defined (e.g., drugs) to the complex (e.g., system care such as the Health Maintenance Organization). Evaluative designs appropriate for the former may be appropriate but insufficient for the latter. Various research designs may be used to assess interventions.

Case Reports – Anecdotal Studies

Anecdotes or case reports are descriptions of cases or events of interest to whoever prepared the report. The report may be accurate, reliable, and important, although we usually can not be certain. The report is judged by how well it fits beliefs, prejudices (including respect for the reporter or investigator), a previously constructed logical framework, or related factual evidence. The problem is in determining whether the report is representative, and whether a causal relationship can be inferred. The primary issue here has to do with sampling. Case reports or anecdotes do not sample a defined population, although some case reports sample a convenient group such as a clinic or hospital. One usually does not know if any scientific sampling plan was followed, and "unless inference can be generalized beyond the data at hand, a study is of little value to others" (Houston 1972). A report may be based on a selected few; one cannot determine the prevalence from the report. The danger of bias or systemic error is great. There is no way to tell if the report applies to 10%, 50%, or 90% of a reference population.

A murder is most interesting to the media if it occurs once a year or if an important person is the victim. However, in neither case would it represent a problem for the police or for society. Similarly, the initial case reports of acute renal failure with cimetidine were difficult to interpret. Was renal failure really associated with use of cimetidine? How often did it occur? Only when reports were accompanied by provocative, prospective investigation (rechallenge dose) was an important, but probably rare, adverse effect unequivocally established (Rudnick et al. 1982). Many technologies as well as therapies and adverse reactions begin as case reports. A new drug, device, or procedure is developed and reported. Frequently, the reports lead to widespread use before definitive evaluation is considered or undertaken, and the intervention becomes well established before evaluation can establish its appropriate usage. CT scanning (Banta et al. 1918), coronary care units (Mather et al. 1976), and many surgical procedures including coronary artery bypass grafts are prominent examples.

Case-control – Retrospective Studies

The case-control or retrospective study is the most commonly used epidemiological design. It is intended to overcome many of the limitations of the case report. The cases may be exactly those reported in the case report – what is added in this design is a comparison group. The selection of the comparison group is a critical feature in case-control design (Miettinen 1970; Cole 1972; Greenland et al. 1981; Sartwell et al. 1969; Feinstein 1978; Hayden et al. 1982; Schlesselman et al. 1982). In theory, the controls are as alike as possible to the cases except for the absence of disease (or factor of interest). Obtaining an appropriate comparison group may present difficulties and also may introduce various types of bias or systematic error (Feinstein 1977). In a classic case-control study relating lung cancer to smoking, Doll and Hill (1950) compared the smoking histories of lung cancer patients with control patients selected from the same hospital during a similar period, matched for neighborhood, age, and sex. In another classic case-control study, Sartwell et al. (1963) compared female patients with thrombophlebitis to controls matched for multiple characteristics, including age, number of pregnancies, and marital status. He was able to demonstrate that oral contraceptives increased the risk of thrombophlebitis for some women. Obviously, the more characteristics that must be matched between cases and controls, the larger the pool of control patients that must be available. The advantage of the case-control method design is that it can be carried out relatively quickly and cheaply. It is particularly suitable for studying rare events. The disadvantages are that one can never be certain that the comparison group (or groups) is truly "just like" the cases (unbiased). Nor can it be guaranteed that recall of exposures or events is not selectively different in each group (Berkson's bias). A last disadvantage is that laboratory measures and other descriptive information not collected at the time of suspected exposure can not be obtained. Technology assessment using case-control methods is a feasible and appropriate technique for hospital-based technology if the existing data can answer the research questions posed. The problem is that most of the questions related to technology assessment are not answerable using hospital records.

Cohort – Prospective Studies

The prospective study design is also called a cohort, panel, longitudinal, or natural history study. It is essentially a randomized clinical trial without randomization. The investigator does not determine who becomes exposed to an intervention. Groups of individuals are compared based on whether they possess certain characteristics (such as renal disease) or are exposed to a particular factor (such as CT scan). Hammond and Horn (1966) conducted a prospective study of smoking in the 1950s in which several million individuals were identified and followed for many years. Smokers and nonsmokers were compared for incidence of lung cancer, chronic obstructive pulmonary disease, and cardiovascular disease. The results of that study were an important impetus for the Surgeon General's Report on Smoking. The Framingham Study (Dawber et al. 1972) and similar studies at Tecumseh and in Evans County, Georgia are examples of prospective-longitudinal studies that have yielded important clinical information on the natural history of disease and the association between various risk factors (exposures) and disease. Belloc and Breslow's (1973) well-publicized longitudinal study in Alameda County used the same design to demonstrate an association between life-style and longevity.

The advantage of prospective studies is that incidence and prevalence rates can be calculated for diseases or events in the study population. Independent and combined effects of risk factors on a particular disease can be studied and different effects of a risk factor or exposure can be examined. The relative risk is a computation of the probability of an event or disease given exposure compared with the probability of that event without exposure. The disadvantages of the prospective design are that it takes a long time to obtain results, the cost is high, and it is administratively difficult to maintain longterm contact with subjects.

The historical prospective study is not burdened by some of the disadvantages mentioned above. This design examines historically defined exposure groups. A population is required on whom data was previously collected. Subgroups with particular characteristics or suspected risk factors can be studied for development of disease or adverse effect. Follow-up studies can be conducted quite rapidly to relate exposures (or risk factors) to subsequent events. Pfaffenberger has published numerous studies relating physical examination, medical history, and physical activity data collected during the 1930s on college students at the University of Pennsylvania and at Harvard University to various chronic diseases. For example, a follow-up study (Thorne et al. 1968) conducted in the 1960s on these former students related myocardial disease to various factors (exercise, smoking) reported or observed in the 1930s. It is theoretically possible to obtain good estimates of adverse effects associated with environmental factors or drug usage in this manner. In practice such studies are uncommon.

Randomized Clinical Trials

The randomized clinical trial (RCT) is the standard design for assessing health care interventions. It is a powerful design and its use has been encouraged as the least costly way to examine controversial treatments. The history of RCTs has been frequently reviewed (Byar et al. 1976; Hart 1972; Lambert 1978; Armitage 1972) and clinical trials have been dated to Biblical times, the Middle Ages, and the Renaissance. The essential ingredient in a randomized clinical trial is random allocation of patients to an intervention. The patient cannot choose the intervention and therefore by chance extraneous patient characteristics will have equal opportunity of being in any treatment group. Treatment groups may be two, treatment and control (nontreatment), or more, such as various levels of treatment or various different treatments. The problems are logistic rather than scientific. One major problem is sample size or power; frequently, the conclusion is that an intervention did not make a difference when in reality the intervention did not make a large enough difference to be detectable. One of many rules of thumb in clinical trials is that a difference of 20% between treatment and control groups should be detectable.

Undertaking a randomized clinical trial is always an ambitious venture. There are literally hundreds of conceptual and practical details that must be attended to if one expects to complete the study and obtain meaningful results. Specific details of design are of interest to epidemiologists and statisticians. There is particular emphasis on calculation of power and assurance of blindness. Problems of patient enrollment, data collection, and processing are less exciting but are probably more often the real reason why clinical trials do not achieve the results intended. Numerous investigators concerned with the theory and practice of clinical trials recognize that many RCTs have design or implementation problems that give them little chance of establishing usable evidence (Chalmers 1974; Green and Lewis 1979). From a public policy standpoint – one which considers the ethical issues, use of resources, and scientific progress – a clinical trial is worthwhile only when it is completed with conclusive results. Clinical trials should not be discouraged but should be organized so that they can be afforded the best chance to be completed with meaningful results that could potentially influence policy. Evidence may not suffice – but it is a good start.

Physicians are sold (often oversold) on RCTs. Britton Harris, Dean Emeritus of the University of Pennsylvania's School of Public and Urban Policy, recently asked if we could randomize the stars. Astronomers have learned a great deal about the universe without randomization. One cannot always employ randomized designs. Designs other than randomization can achieve almost the same degree of certainty in separating differences in populations from the effects of an intervention. These so-called quasi-experimental designs (Campbell 1969) can be used like more traditional epidemiological designs to evaluate technology. When randomization is impossible, interventions can be assessed and comparisons made in ways that minimize bias (internal validity) and maximize generalizability (external validity). A rich literature relating to use of designs for evaluation of health and social programs has developed (Riecken and Boruch 1974; Freeman 1974).

Measuring Benefit

Measuring benefits in studies of chronic disease is a different matter from measuring benefits in acute disease. By definition, acute disease means a patient recovers (with or without a lingering deficit) or dies. If deaths are averted, deficits are avoided or minimized or recovery is hastened, the benefit is clear. Measuring benefit in chronic disease is more difficult. Positive change in health status or health outcome has received increasing attention in the past 10 years (Balaban et al. 1980; Brook 1977; Fries and Spitz 1980; Chen and Bush 1979; Katz et al. 1963; Bush et al. 1981; Bergner et al. 1976) as chronic conditions account for greater consumption of health care resources. The ultimate endpoint in Feinberg's nosology (see above), patient outcome, is of most interest to the public. However, there is not general agreement on what constitutes an improved patient outcome, and there are numerous conceptual and technical considerations.

How one chooses to measure patient outcome and how well one measures it are perhaps more important to the scientific merit of a study and in particular to the policy and administrative decisions which follow. An issue to examine is the relationship between a measured physiological change and a measured change in a patient's functional ability and behavior. The individual physician should want to achieve the best possible response for each patient. However, the primary concern is with the disease process (physiology). If the patient is not improving, an alternative course of action (which will ultimately include reconsideration of diagnoses and, perhaps, psychotherapy) will be undertaken.The primary impetus is to achieve a more normal physiological response. This is intended to be descriptive rather than judgemental. The problem is that many patients with chronic diseases lack an understanding of their disease or there are sociopersonal or work factors that act as disincentives for improvement in function (sometimes even with an apparently good physiological response). It can be argued, therefore, that an apparent positive physiological response is only one aspect of patient benefit.

Judging benefit for an individual or a population (particularly when treatment groups are randomly assigned to different therapies) should include measured changes in physiological response related to disease, as well as changes in patient functional outcomes, such as disability, satisfaction with the result, level of pain, and general well-being. The patient outcomes of mortality and morbidity are inadequate bases for evaluation of many interventions; the intervention will not result in a change in death rate or disease rate. Similarly, in judging benefits in chronic disease, the benefit expected is not deaths averted but improved function. Since chronic diseases account for an ever increasing portion of health care utilization and expenditures, we must face the problem. How can we quantify health or the quality of life?

An intervention may be thought of as having potential effects on the quantity and quality of life. The quantity of life is measured by mortality or death rate. Historically, death rates have been used as the indicator of choice. The selection of death as an endpoint makes the researcher's life simpler. The event is usually unambiguous, adjustments can be made for population differences and the timing of the event is, in Western countries, easily determined. Recently, a national death index has been introduced in the United States, which will make it much easier to obtain follow-up data for mortality studies. For longevity studies on cancer and coronary artery disease, the quantity of life, if not the sole measure of outcome, is clearly a meaningful one.

The quality of life is measured in numerous ways and is influenced by numerous factors other than disease, such as personal life-style, interactions with the health care system, and treatment. It was for cancer patients that the famed chemotherapist Karnofsky and Burchenal (1946) developed the Karnofsky scale to assess nonfatal outcomes in cancer. That scale, which rates disability in ten-point increments and without sharply defined categories, continues to be used in cancer studies.

Another traditional health status scale in wide use was developed by Katz to measure the functional status of elderly and chronically ill patients. Katz has been conducting natural history studies and randomized trials of therapies for chronic disease patients for many years. The Katz et al. (1963) Activities of Daily Living (ADL) is an ordinal scale of activities which includes dressing, toileting, transferring, bathing, feeding, and continence. The ordered values are based on the return of biological function found in independent studies of patient recovery. ADL has taken on a more general meaning (and has come to be used as a generic term) in clinical studies. There are now dozens of ADL-like scales in use. Most of these scales have not undergone careful assessment for reliability and validity (Donaldson and Wegner 1973). Katz's scale is not disease-specific but Fries et al. (1980) have developed an expanded ADL that is set specifically for arthritis patients.

New questions arise when we consider different measures of the quality of life or improved health status. Even when a population is adjusted or standardized the outcome measures are difficult to compare. Can the results of studies employing different endpoints be compared? First, the distinction between an index and an indicator must be made clear. An indicator is a single measure often used as a basis for inferences. These inferences may turn out to be misleading. An index is formed either from the adding together of multiple endpoints or from the adding together of multiple endpoints after such endpoints have been weighted in some fashion. Such a composite measure provides a summation of results in individuals and in populations. It allows us to compare populations that have been treated differently. One difficulty lies in the setting of weights. Preferences or weights for the components of the index are also called utility functions, multipliers, social value scores, and coefficients. The issue is how to combine the different components. If components are simply added to devise a total score, the implicit assumption is that each component is equally important. Investigators from various fields are investigating methods for assigning weights to components and procedures for validation and adjustment for different populations (Kahnemann and Tversky 1982; Torrance et al. 1972; Bush et al. 1981; Kaplan et al. 1979). For purposes of policy and for the assessment of most technologies, a global (as opposed to a disease-specific) measure is required. Disease-specific measures are expensive to develop and have limited usefulness in technology assessment and policy. Global measures are expensive as well; but the developing and validating of global measures are finite tasks and are transferrable. Even so, we should encourage the development of rigorous disease-specific measures for prevalent chronic conditions.

There are many other technical points concerning health status indices, that although not commented on in this paper are nevertheless very important to those interested in this field (Bice and Bernstein 1977; Sackett and Chambers 1977; Balinsky and Berger 1975; Chen and Bush 1979). The National Clearing House for Health Status Indices is published periodically by the National Center for Health Statistics in the US Department of Health and Human Services. It is a useful reference source of current literature in the field.

A health status index should be appropriate for a wide range of conditions and age-groups. In addition, it should be easy to administer, brief, sensitive to changes in health status, reliable, valid, acceptable to patients, and interpretable by the public, clinicians, and decision markers. No index meets all of these criteria. However, several indices can be considered as appropriate endpoints for health care evaluation. Such acceptable indices are capable of: (1) detecting improvement in individual patients; and (2) enabling comparisons between groups with different sociodemographic characteristics and diseases. Health status indices can be based on aggregate population data related to mortality and morbidity (including restricted activity). Chiang's "H," (1965) Sullivan's "Life Free of Disability" (1971), and Chen's "G's" (1976) are examples of indices designed to express in single numerical scores information regarding mortality and morbidity.

Chiang's index distinguishes three states – death, alive with activity limitation, and alive with no activity limitation. Levels of disability are not incorporated and the resulting numbers are not related to expressions of policy. Sullivan's index of "Expected Life Free of Disability" incorporates time by using life table methods, in particular disability strata. Numerical expessions using national data are developed; however, the index is not applicable for policy decisions related to specific interventions. Chen's G's are disease specific and compare death and disability in a target population with a reference population. The measures may be used to aggregate disease-specific data on large populations but again are not intended or appropriate for evaluating specific interventions or programs.

There are indices of health status that incorporate different levels of functional status. Some are disease-specific, some are global. Few, however, have been sufficiently studied such that the quantitative expression of health statistics has meaning for evaluative studies. There are several, however, that have received the most recognition by policy makers and academics. The index developed by Bush and colleagues has had numerous iterations and name changes. The current name is the

Quality of Well Being (QWB). This index is based on function states of mobility, social activity, and physical activity. The levels of function in these three activity areas are combined with a score from a problem/symptom complex in arriving at a final function level. The data are based on 4–8 days of reported performance (rather than capacity). The weights for different levels of function are empirically defined by a survey of different population-groups and are explicit social preferences. The index has been used in populations of different age composition with various health conditions. Bush and his associates (Kaplan et al. 1976) have devoted considerable attention to validity issues. The QWB, in at least one report, correlates highly with other independent measures of functional ability and disease. We have administered the QWB periodically on several hundred patients to evaluate a multidisciplinary treatment program (Balaban et al. 1980) and are using it currently to evaluate a new treatment procedure and traditional rehabilitation for stroke patients. It is being used in at least one drug study. The Sickness Impact Profile (SIP) developed by Bergner et al. (1975, 1981), is a comprehensive measure of dysfunction in12 areas of activity, using 136 items. The weights developed by successive interval methods are reportedly stable in various populations. Like the QWB, the SIP is being used in randomized clinical trials.

One can easily judge the length of health status measures and quickly determine their acceptability to patients. The acceptance of a health status measure by clinicians and by policy makers is more difficult to predict. This issue will be discussed subsequently. The primary scientific issues concern the reliability and the validity of a health status measure.

Reliability

Reliability has been used interchangeably with repeatability, constancy, reproducability, and precision. Some investigators distinguish between different types of reliability. The conceptual notion is the extent to which the same measures give the same results on repeated applications. When a particular measure varies at two points in time or when the same measure (instrument or test) done by different observers gives different results, it is not reliable. A measure cannot be valid if it is not reliable. It can, of course, be reliable without being valid.

The reliability of the instruments must be formally tested. Problems of measuring reliability and validity are well recognized but usually not dealt with in an optimal fashion. The problem is more than a theoretical one. Practically, it means that the "noise" or variability in the measures thereby decreases the power of the measures, making it more difficult, or impossible, to determine if a particular intervention really has an effect.

Validity

Validity refers to truth. The more valid a measure, the more closely it resembles the true state of nature. Validity is defined somewhat differently by epidemiologists and social scientists. An epidemiologist defines validity in terms of sensitivity and specificity. A sensitive test or measure is able to identify correctly as positive all those who truly have a disease or condition. The specificity of a test is its ability to identify as negative all individuals who truly do not have a disease or condition. Both are expressed as percentages. False-positives are positive by the test but do not have the disease. For a given level of sensitivity and specificity, the ratio of false-positives to false-negatives is determined by the prevalence of the disease. For example, Neuhauser and Lewicki's (1975) provocative simulation study of screening for colon cancer demonstrates how an inexpensive and yet sensitive test can lead to extremely high costs of identifying all cases of a disease.

Validity is categorized by social scientists according to the manner of assessment. There are many different concepts and terms for validating instruments, all intended to help in deciding how well attributes not directly measurable are quantified. Face and content validity refer to procedures that assess whether a measure appears to measure what is supposed to be measured. Content validity considers whether all pertinent attributes are included in the measure. There is no comparison made to a standard. Concurrent and predictive validity are based on the correlation between one measure and another at a particular point in time. Predictive validity concerns the extent to which a particular measure predicts an event.

Data Requirements

Choosing an appropriate design is important for evaluation, but dealing well with data from collection to analysis is an equally important ingredient, particularly in randomized clinical trials. It is essential that the appropriate data be collected at the appropriate times. Data may be primary – collected for a particular study – or secondary – collected for another purpose but useful in a particular study. It may be collected by observation or by report. Reports may be test results or direct statements from subjects to an interviewer, either in person, over the telephone, or via questionnaires through the mail.

In every study, there needs to be a model or explicit theory detailing why each factor (structure, process, or outcome) is important, how the factor will be measured, and how it will be used in the analysis. Very frequently, data that would be helpful or required for classification are collected using scales that make it impossible to sort or reclassify patients. Scaled measures of a subject's life-style, demography, social situation, emotional status, functional ability, and medical history have been developed that are associated with response to disease and recovery. Unfortunately, routine hospital records for inpatients and office or clinic records for outpatients do not contain the appropriate information or are incomplete or inaccurate.

Spitzer et al. (1975) separated "health care trials" from ordinary clinical trials based on the intervention and the collection of information on nonclinical variables. They distinguish between "health care trials", which go beyond strictly disease-oriented investigations, as "patient care trials" by examining sociopersonal as well as physiological characteristics and "health services trials" as those used to study nonconventional therapies. By assessing the effects of sociopersonal determinants, along with diagnostic grouping and other clinical measures of interest, characteristics operating selectively or similarly in patients with different diagnoses can be identified. The more important characteristics or predictors can be used to develop a scale classifying patients with chronic illness into meaningful subgroups that increase the statistical likelihood of demonstrating the effects of an intervention. A second reason for collecting baseline sociopersonal data is the opportunity they afford to isolate factors or attributes that characterize responsive subgroups and therefore allow interventions to be targeted efficiently.

Discussion

Evaluators believe the best decisions are made when appropriate facts or information are available (and therefore often require collection of primary data). Evaluators also recognize that appropriate information or facts are not sufficient to ensure that good decisions will be made. Many other factors come into play and criteria for decisions are usually not explicit. The perspective or values of the decision-maker may be based on experience (judgmement), political expediency, economics, or logic and will influence the use and interpretation of evidence.

Relman (1980) suggests that consensus panels (expert judgement) brought together by the US National Institute of Health (NIH) to review evidence, and develop a consensus opinion are successful in influencing behavior. He suggests that physicians have modified and will modify further their practices given appropriate information through appropriate channels. This point is contested by some (Lambert 1978; McKinlay and McKinlay 1977; Chalmers 1975, 1981). Chalmers suggests that physician behavior has not been influenced in some cases in spite of clinical trials that question the efficacy of their therapies. He noted, in 1975, that sales of oral hypoglycemia agents had continued to rise since 1970 in spite of the UGDP studies indicating that the agents may be associated with increased cardiac death rates. (However, since 1975 the use of oral hypoglycemia agents has fallen dramatically.) Another example is the use of diethylstilbesterol (DES) by pregnant women. In spite of six studies in the early 1950s showing the treatment to be totally ineffective, the use of DES continues in certain high-risk pregnancies (Heinonen 1973). Radical surgery for breast cancer continues to be performed at rates hardly supportable from the evidence, and Reiser (1978) has compelling comments on the use of technologies and procedures by physicians despite evidence of inefficacy.

Behavior is difficult to change, whether it be a certain type of behavior (e.g., smoking or drinking) or behavior by certain types (clinicians or academics). It may be that once a reasonable amount of evidence is established, better and faster implementation of policy changes will be achieved by behavioral modification techniques rather than by additional studies.

It may be easy for the comprehensive approach to assessment and the strong public interest emphasis to be usurped by special interest groups. This is especially true in view of the continued discussion of the impact of evaluation studies. Relman (1980, 1982) while supporting NIH concensus groups has also in two New England Journal of Medicine editorials called for the establishment of a national institute for health care evaluation on the premise that new information is required for intelligent decision-making – something that will not emerge from NIH research. Schroeder and Showstack (1977) observed that the compartmentalized nature of NIH with many separate institutes and disciplinary study sections and its protechnology bias would not lead one to expect it to be a fertile area for producing evaluation studies.

There are structural disincentives to evaluation in academe associated with disciplinary boundaries and also referred to the modest rewards for tackling problems that are complex, difficult to solve, applied, and long-term. Bunker et al. (1982) recently made specific proposals for an Institute for Health Care Evaluation, which would generate cost-effectiveness data with a strong emphasis on measurement of outcomes of therapeutic interventions. Four major objectives are proposed: "establishment of a uniform data base, systematic identification of issues for its agenda, generation of new data and analyses, and dissemination of information to carriers, professionals, and consumers."

It will be quite a feat if the door continues to be open for evaluation of health practices. Hospital utilization review committees, Professional Standards Review Organizations, and academic researchers have barely begun to evaluate health practices and policies. And now, methods accepted by the medical and health industry stakeholders for controlling the economic consequences of expensive and unproven devices and techniques are being applied to previously accepted procedures and organizational arrangements for health care delivery.

If technology assessment is itself a technology, and if Blendon's observation on the natural history of the public's interest in particular technologies waxing and waning are correct, then conferences such as this could signal the beginning of the end for technology assessment! It is to be hoped that evaluation and technology assessment is a special case, and that the attention of researchers, journal editors, legislators, and the public is maintained. The methods for technology assessment are being refined. If interest in evaluative studies is maintained, technology use as well as health care practices and policies that are in the public interest may be based increasingly on evidence rather than a priori logic or self-interest. We believe that true efficiency requires demonstrated effectiveness. And, although there is evidence to support this conclusion, it is predominantly an article of faith.

3 Discussion of Paper by Balaban and Goldfarb

U. E. Reinhardt

Princeton University

Introduction

In essence, the evaluation of a health care technology is addressed to the following three questions:

a) Does the application of the technology achieve the intended outcome?
b) If the answer to (a) is yes, can the benefits associated with the intended outcome justify the costs incurred in the application of the technology?
c) If the answer to (b) is yes, does the application of the technology result in the *minimum* resource cost required to achieve the intended outcome or, alternatively, does it result in the *maximum* benefit attainable with a given resource expenditure?

If the answer to the first to these questions is yes, then the technology is judged to be *efficacious* or, as some authors would have it, *effective* (according to Webster's Dictionary, the terms "efficacious" and "effective" are synonyms). If the answer to the third question is yes, the technology can be judged *efficient*. A "yes" to the second question, of course, merely signals that the technology is *not inefficient*. It may still be the least efficient of several alternative technologies.

If it were perfectly clear just what is meant by "the technology," if the "outcome" could be unambiguously identified and accurately measured, if it were possible to control accurately for all factors (other than the application of the technology) that may influence the observed "outcome" and, finally, if the "costs" of and "benefits" from the application of "the technology" could be properly identified and accurately measured, then the evaluation of a health care technology would be child's play. One could entrust it to a high school student. If some of these conditions are not met, more advanced training needs to be brought to the task. And if some of these conditions cannot possibly be met, the matter is turned over to teams of PhDs and MDs who alone have the authority to enunciate truths they cannot possibly know. As the paper by Balaban and Goldfarb and the following piece by Williams clearly demonstrate, the evaluation of health care technology typically falls into the domain of PhDs and MDs.

Balaban and Goldfarb confine their discussion almost exclusively to question (a) above. They address strictly the issues involved in the *medical evaluation* of health care technology. Williams, on the other hand, focuses primarily on questions (b) and (c) with only passing reference to question (a). The full complexity of the overall evaluation problem can thus be appreciated fully only if the two papers are read in tandem.

In what follows, however, I shall confine myself mainly to Balaban and Goldfarb's paper. In the next section, I shall summarize what I believe to be the authors' main points and provide intermittent commentary on these points. In the concluding section, I shall offer some additional observations not directly limited to specific points in the paper but to the subject matter in general.

Summary of the Paper

The authors' paper represents, in the main, a logically structured review of the several steps involved in the medical evaluation of a health care technology, and of the several facets of each step. The discussion begins, appropriately, with some thoughts on the definition of "health care technology" and "technology assessment." It is quickly discovered that these terms mean different things to different people. Some authors define the term "technology" in its very broadest sense, that is, as the organized application of human and nonhuman resources toward particular ends. Included in this definition would be, as Williams puts it, any new or existing arrangements of beds or medical staff, any new or existing drug, and so on. Other authors endow the term "technology" with a much narrower interpretation, requiring either that it be costly (Williams), involve sophisticated procedures or equipment, or that it be "new." Disputes over the intrinsic merits of one or the other perspective are usually fruitless. All one can reasonably ask of individual researchers – and of the readers of volumes such as this – is that they state clearly at the outset the particular interpretation they impose on the term.

There is similar diversity in the interpretation of the terms "assessment" or "evaluation." The diversity emerges from the compass and time dimension one associates with the term "outcome." As Balaban and Goldfarb point out, some authors adopt a holistic perspective – indeed, so holistic as to raise (or lower?) the act of "assessment" from the level of scientific inquiry to an art form. Less ambitious souls are content to confine their contribution to the domain in which scientific inquiry can yield fruit. This approach imposes a narrower compass on the definition of "outcome," although not an arbitrary one: measured and evaluated are those dimensions that are, *ex ante,* tractable by the scientific method. Although inherently limited, the scientific, nonholistic approach can be quite productive and well worth its cost. It becomes inadequate only in the hands of those policymakers who assign a zero weight to the intangible dimensions of "outcome" that cannot be scientifically evaluated. The blame rests on the user rather than on the producer of limited scientific research.

The authors next comment on the framework adopted for technology evaluation. As I understand them, they mean by "framework" the basic question one seeks to answer with technology evaluation. They distinguish between what they call *research evaluation,* which is addressed to the question whether the technology "makes a difference" to the outcome, and *technical evaluation,* which is addressed to the question whether the administrative process surrounding the application of a technology conforms to expectations or official rules. The authors assert that most technology evaluation in the United States is of the second variety. Actually, one wonders whether the second variety deserves the label "technology evaluation" at all. It is nothing other than a mere administrative audit.

In their section on the "Framework for Evaluation" the authors also seek to define the terms "efficacy," "effectiveness," and "efficiency." "Efficacy" is defined as the ability of a technology to influence the "outcome" favorably. "Effectiveness" is said to refer to the extent to which the health care system applies an efficacious technology to all members of society who might potentially benefit from it. The term, as used by the authors, appears to pertain to a system's performance. Finally, "efficiency" is said to "refer to the amount of resources consumed in delivering a given level of care and/or achieving a given outcome." It is my impression that most authors would not share Balaban and Goldfarb's distinction between, "efficacy" and "effectiveness" but treat them as synonyms, as Webster's Dictionary would have us do. The authors' definition of the term "efficiency" is vaguely correct. The economist's more precise definition has already been given above in connection with question (c) in the introduction to this discussion.

After exploring what questions an evaluation study should answer and what criteria it should adopt, the authors turn their attention to the *design* of evaluation studies, by which they mean the approach used to gather data and to draw inferences from it. Among these approaches are anecdotes, retrospective case-control studies, cohort-prospective studies and, finally, randomized clinical studies.

Purists may be shocked to see anecdotes elevated to the rank of study design. As McKinlay (1981) points out in his "Seven Stages in the Career of a Medical Innovation," however, many medical innovations are widely diffused primarily on the basis of anecdotes (or "case studies" as they are sometimes more felicitously called). Indeed, the typical patient probably has no idea about the extent to which modern medical practice relies on completely unreliable data, or even mere habit, hunches, or beliefs. An interesting excercise, for example, would be to submit a, say, French or West German fee schedule and utilization profile to a Delphi panel of, say, British or American physicians, and to have the latter identify procedures whose application they consider wasteful or even harmful. I would expect that list to be lengthy. The audit could, of course, be reversed, and one would expect a similarly lengthy list, albeit with different items. The point of the exercise would be to highlight the rather shaky and often completely unscientific empirical foundation on which day-to-day medical practice still rests.

As Balaban and Goldfarb point out, the randomized clinical trial (RCT) is generally recognized as the scientifically most rigorous approach to technology evaluation. The basic idea underlying the RCT is so straightforward that one may wonder why medicine has so belatedly discovered it. The reason, one suspects, is not some form of mental limitation on the part of physicians, but rather the severe limits ethical considerations must put on inquiries of this sort. After all, can a physician who strongly believes intervention X to be superior to intervention Y randomly assign, in good conscience, half of his patients to X and the other half to Y? In their discussion of RCTs, Balaban and Goldfarb stress the purely technical difficulties of undertaking RCTs – the problem of sample size, measurement, the power of the test, and so on. It would seem to me that these problems pale next to the ethical problems raised by RCTs. In the face of these problems, one might question the authors' contention that physicians have been oversold on the potential of RCTs.

Next to the often vexing ethical questions raided by evaluation research ranks the difficulty of measuring changes in "outcome." Balaban and Goldfarb review these problems in their section on "Measurement," and also in the sections on "Reliability," "Validity," and "Data Collection." At first blush, it may be thought that technology is most easily solved when the costs of applying a technology consist exclusively of measurable nonhuman resources and when the outcome can be measured by "lives saved." A moment's thought dispels that notion. First, because one cannot save lives but only years of life, the analyst must assess the quality of the saved life-years. Second, because the quality of life can be measured only by multidimensional indices, the analyst typically faces the problem of converting the multidimensional index into a one-dimensional overall index. Implicit in any such conversion is a set of relative weights (indicators of relative importance) for the individual outcome dimensions. Balaban and Goldfarb discuss this problem in passing, but are not, in my view, sufficiently critical of the questionable weights that are frequently used in practice (e.g., the mere arithmetic summation of the numerical scores assigned to individual outcome dimensions). The fact is that whenever the problem of relative weights in this context is approached by researchers, they tread on treacherous ground and more often than not leave the realm of objective, scientific inquiry. As Balaban and Goldfarb mention, the construction of overall outcome indices involves one in the task of identifying the preference functions of individuals or of the "representative" member of groups of individuals. Economists have long wrestled with these problems, but even the Nobel Laureates among them have registered little headway in this area. Thus, long before the evaluation of health care technology proceeds into a full-fledged cost-benefit analysis, the task can easily degenerate into a veritable "Mission Impossible."

A particularly vexing problem, not specifically addressed by Balaban and Goldfarb, arises when both the costs and the benefits associated with a technology consist primarily of human life-years. For example, one can imagine a technology composed of a diagnostic test and a particular intervention indicated by a positive test result. Suppose now that intervention on the basis of a true-positive yields, on average, additional life-years, but that intervention based on false-positives results in the early death of at least some perfectly health patients. One occasionally comes across studies in which the net impact of such a technology is measured simply by "net additional life-years." But the life-years saved and those sacrificed belong to different human beings. Widespread application of the technology thus redistributes, so to speak, life-years. It is not clear how one should view redistributions of this sort. The problem is made more difficult still by the possibility that society may not view man-made and God-made death symmetrically – that is, that people in general can cope more easily with the potentially avoidable loss of life-years resulting from an illness than they can with the early, iatrogenic death of a perfectly healthy person.

Some General Observations

The paper by Balaban and Goldfarb and, indeed, this entire conference leads one to wonder: (1) why the evaluation of health care technology should be of concern to public policymakers; and (2) why, in the face of that long-standing concern, this particular line of inquiry is still in its infancy.

It could be argued that in instances where patients pay the full cost of the application of a technology at the point of consumption, the medical and economic evaluation of that technology is no one's but the patients' and their physicians' business. Some economists – perhaps Milton Friedman and his disciples – may well take this position. Health care providers and the industrial producers of health care technology, for example, the Health Industry Manufacturers Association in the United States, seem comfortable with this position as well, as can be inferred from their attacks on publicly funded efforts in technology evaluation. For example, both the American Medical Association and the Health Industry Manufacturers Association in the United States successfully used their influence with the US Congress to close the Health Care Technology Center of the US Department of Health and Human Services in 1981.

Those who take the opposite view – that the evaluation of health care technology falls into the domain of the public sector regardless of the source of payment – do so on the premises (1) that the individual consumer is ill-equipped to undertake the requisite evaluation, and (2) that evaluations offered by physicians and/or the industrial producers of health care technology cannot be trusted, because both groups are subject to a severe conflict of economic interest. There is clearly something to this point of view.

In their paper, Balaban and Goldfarb assert that:

> One may categorically state that a program that identifies and effectively treats 90% of hypertensives in a community at a cost of $ 50 per patient is clearly superior to a program in a similar community providing the same treatment to only 75% of the hypertensives at a cost of $ 150 per patient.

To longtime students of the health care sector – certainly that in the United States, but elsewhere as well – this assertion betrays a charming innocence. Do the authors really believe that, say, physicians in an overdoctored area would invariably prefer efficient programs to inefficient ones? To think about this question, it is helpful to recall the old tautology that one person's (the patient's) health care expenditure is another person's (the provider's) health care income, or, to put it another way, that inefficiency from one person's point of view may spell income maintenance from the viewpoint of another. One need not be a card-carrying cynic but only a cognisciento of human nature to appreciate that under certain circumstances, health care providers (and/or the industrial producers of health care technology) would have no problem at all with the second (high-cost) program mentioned by the authors. Indeed, I see in that possibility one reason for these groups' seemingly instinctive aversion to publicly funded health care evaluation, which answers in part the second question raised above, namely, why despite its importance, health care evaluation is still in its infancy.

A further reason for the suspicion with which health care providers seem to view publicy funded evaluation of health care technology may reside in a concern over the potential intrusion of government into medical practice. This concern may or may not be legitimate. The concern strikes me as not legitimate when the public sector uses technology evaluation merely to help it determine which treatments it will or will not pay for with public funds. Several years ago, for example, the Canadian province of Saskatchewan decided, after careful study, that it would no longer compensate physicians under the province's medical care plan for certain types of hysterectomies. Although physicians may have viewed this decision as an unwarranted intrusion into the practice of medicine, it was in fact a purely financial decision. No one had proposed to stop mutually consenting physicians and patients from performing the hysterectomy of their choice.

The concern of providers – and of the manufacturers of health care technology – *is* legitimate when technology evaluation leads to the imposition of a public preference function on medical treatments for which the individual patient is willing to pay. Let us consider once more a technology whose application will, on average, add life-years to patients with a certain disease, but which may also lead to iatrogenic death of perfectly healthy patients identified with a false-positive. Public policymakers may quite properly decide that, in view of the inherent risk of the technology, its application should not be financed out of public funds. To reach this decision, they should, ideally, have applied the degree of risk aversion they believe to be representative for the population at risk. The degree of risk aversion, however, is apt to vary considerably among individuals within a nation (and even more so among nations). A gamble public policymakers assume is not worth taking may well look attractive to less risk-averse individuals in society. The question then arises whether the public policymakers' risk aversion (preference function) should override that of individuals willing to pay for the gamble they are willing to take – that is, whether the technology should be outlawed altogether. This is a troublesome question. The question is most easily answered (in the affirmative) in societies in which the distribution of health care must, above all, obey the so-called principle of solidarity. In the United States, on the other hand, where an egalitarian distribution of health care is not officially espoused, one might well wish to let self-paying patients gamble as they see fit.

The preceding observations have particular relevance to international trade in health care technology. Americans, for example, occasionally flagellate themselves over the export of health care technologies (equipment or pharmaceuticals) deemed too risky at home. There may be combinations of political contexts and commercial practices that lead to indefensible sales abroad. On the other hand, one should not reject out of hand the possibility that individuals in other nations weigh the actuarial benefits and costs associated with particular technologies differently than would the representative American (or European) – that is, that societies elsewhere might well be willing to take gambles we reject at home.

In sum, then, the evaluation of health care technology is at its most useful when it furnishes the appropriate decision-maker in health care with information on the odds inherent in the application of the technology. Just who the "appropriate" decision-maker is depends in good part on who pays for the application of the technology. It may be a public policymaker or, alternatively, the patient and his/her physician. Technology evaluation can lead to abuse when it becomes the vehicle for the imposition of a centrally directed preference function on individual consumers at home and abroad. In the conclusion of their paper, Balaban and Goldfarb express their hope that the attention of researchers, legislators, and the public in evaluative work be sustained in the future. Sustained success will be more likely if the research community jealously watches the use to which its efforts are ultimately put in the policy arena.

4 The Role of Economics in the Evaluation of Health Care Technologies

A. Williams

University of York

What Is the Problem?

An electronic fetal monitor was developed in the mid-to late-1960s in the US. It was proposed for high-risk pregnancies. It undoubtedly had some dramatic successes in high-risk pregnancies and was used in major medical centres. [But] ... once something has had some success in one group of patients there is an inevitable tendency to use it with other patients. The definition of the patient group becomes fuzzy and may be eventually applied to all patients in that particular category. Fetal monitoring was expanded and expanded so that it is probably now used in almost every delivery in the US for the women who come in in time to have the machine hooked up. But controversy followed ... Women objected to being interfered with to this extent. So one of the advocates of the procedure decided to do a controlled clinical trial to prove that it worked. The results showed no benefit, much to his surprise. That opened up the question all over again, and questions that should have been asked 10 years earlier were asked for the first time. It did not appear to benefit every woman. Then, over a period of about a year, many of the advocates backed off from that position and went back to their earlier position that it is of benefit to high-risk women in terms of mortality. But again clinical trials and other analyses seem to show that even this is questionable. Then there is a great deal of talk about prevention of mental retardation and cerebral palsy via use of the fetal monitor. However, some very good epidemiological analyses of the causes of mental retardation and cerebral

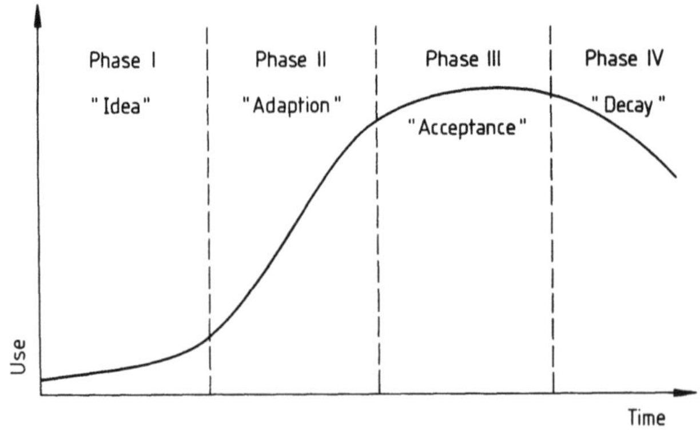

Fig. 4.1. Product life-cycle curve for medical technology

> palsy indicate that this appears not to be the case. Finally the most recent assertion is that the electronic fetal monitor is for efficiency; that we can't provide the nursing care but that this is an adequate replacement for the nurse (Banta 1979).

This theme, with appropriate contextual variations, seems to reflect so common an experience that it has become encapsulated in a standard scheme to represent the "product life-cycle curve for medical technology" (Neuhauser 1979; see also, Russell 1979; Stocking and Morrison 1978) (Fig. 4.1).
Neuhauser epitomises each phase as follows:

> *The idea period.* Hundreds of new ideas occur all of the time. Only a fraction of these are actually pursued, and a fraction of these go into production or use. If the producer or innovator is required to pay for the careful, costly evaluation it is likely that fewer ideas will be turned into use ... A new procedure changes with time ... If evaluation is undertaken too soon these improvements will not be accounted for. At the end of Stage I the producing company has invested a lot of money and has yet to see the return on this investment. At this point articles are appearing in the medical literature. These articles are likely to be wildly enthusiastic but often based on faulty research design and inadequate evidence.
> *Adaptation.* At the end of Stage I or at the beginning of Stage II the careful evaluative trials may have been started. These may be randomised trials with several years of follow up ... In Stage II there is growing acceptance. Sometimes this is by trial and error ...
> *Acceptance.* Use has levelled off. Perhaps at this point the results of randomised trials are reported ... and ... the results are far less favourable than the initial enthusiastic reports. However, now hospitals have invested in equipment and doctors have learned these new skills and the climate has changed. These reported studies may be ignored or attacked with hostility. Unless the study shows clearly harmful results they may have very little effect on changing medical behaviour. ... However, to delay adaptation until the trial results are available may be a political impossibility or, in the case of beneficial procedure, result in some patients being deprived of benefit.
> *Decay.* Eventually the technology falls out of use. This may be easy if it is being replaced by something new, and very difficult if there is nothing to replace it.

Among the important general principles Neuhauser derives from this analysis is that: "The 'burden of proof' ... is important in the assessment of medical technology. The burden of proof in Phase I is on the innovator. In Phase III it is on the investigator who criticises the accepted practice"; thus "evaluation can be done too soon and too late".

I, therefore, take the problem facing *economic* evaluation of health care technology to be to determine the optimum height, shape, and timing of Neuhauser's "product life-cycle curve" *from the point of view of a health care system.* This last phrase is of vital importance, because this particular viewpoint is to be differentiated from that of (a) the scientists who invented the technology, (b) the commercial interests which seek to make a profit out of it, (c) the practitioners who seek to add it to their armamentarium, and (d) the patients who may benefit from it. Not even the impact on the latter category is to be seen as the 'touchstone' by which the optimum is to be determined, especially in a health care system that is financed to any significant degree by taxation of one kind or another. A favourable effect on patients is a necessary but unfortunately not a *sufficient* condition for the optimum level of utilization of a new technology within a health care system to be positive (I am excluding from consideration here the use of these technologies within a research context, which raises different, but equally intractable, problems of evaluation).

Some Ground Clearing

In a complex field of interdisciplinary endeavour it behoves us all to be careful about our jargon, and I hope that the reader will bear with me if I devote a few pages of this paper to defining certain key concepts, thereby removing in advance (I hope) some potential misunderstandings which experience has taught me have a better than even chance of obscuring our vision. I intend to work my way remorselessly through the key words in my title ("economics", "evaluation", and "technology" – only "health care" am I taking for granted!) and then I am going to distinguish different types of evaluation, stressing the differences between medical, financial, and economic, finally coming to some subdivisions within the latter category. Only then will we be in a position to tackle the substantive problems before us.

It is convenient for the flow of the discussion to dispose of the meaning of "technology" first. It is tempting to include any innovation in the practice of health care delivery, be it a different arrangement of beds (or patients) in a ward, a different division of labour among staff, a change in the location of treatment, a new surgical procedure, a new drug, a new piece of diagnostic or monitoring equipment, a new prosthetic device, or even improved heating or ventilating systems in a hospital. Indeed, one could strike out "innovation", "different", "new", or "improved" in the foregoing sentence, and include all existing ones too. In principle there is no reason to exclude from our remit *any* "technique" bearing on health care delivery but it seems more appropriate to this occasion to limit ourselves to those with two particular properties: firstly, that if or when widely used they are (or will be) "very costly" (a phrase I do not propose to define further at this stage), *and* secondly, that there are strong professional or commercial pressures on those managing health care systems to adopt them at a rate that is faster than their "natural" inclinations would have generated. Thus my presupposed "client" for the evaluation studies I am going to discuss shortly, is the health care system's management, acting on the English Common Law doctrine of *caveat emptor* (let the buyer beware), and seeking to establish what rate of investment (including zero) is in the best interests of the community it serves.

To understand the role that economics might play, we need some common understanding about what economics is. Elsewhere (Williams 1979) I have gone on at some length about the distinctions between economics as a "topic" and economics as a "discipline". The "topic" of economics has a its subject matter everything to do with "the economy" in general (inflation, unemployment, the balance of payments, productivity, etc), and for some people, therefore, economic evaluation means extending evaluation to take into account "economic' variables, such as effects on employment, or earnings, or prices, or public expenditure, etc. Economics is certainly about those things, but that is not *all* that it is about, and although this interpretation does have important implications concerning the proper scope of evaluation in the present context, it is nevertheless *not* my central theme in this paper. My central theme concerns economics as a "discipline", i.e. as a systematic body of knowledge with its own distinctive concepts and modes of thinking. I shall argue that it is these concepts and modes of thinking that need to be harnessed in a more sustained manner to the problems before us and especially those to be found in that branch of economics concerned with allocative efficiency (of which more anon).

I take "evaluation" to be synonymous with evaluative research and, on the distinction between evaluative and non-evaluative research, I take my text from Suchman (1967) who writes:

> Evaluative research is a specific form of applied research whose primary goal is not the discovery of knowledge but rather a testing of the application of knowledge ... In contrast, non-evaluative research, while it may have practical implications, is primarily aimed at increasing knowledge rather than manipulation or action ... A corollary of this distinction between understanding versus manipulation relates to contrasting degrees of abstraction versus specificity. Basic research aims at the formulation of theoretical generalisations or abstract predictions, while applied research stresses action in a highly specified situation involving concrete forecasts ... As one moves from the theoretical study to the evaluative study, the number of variables over which one has control decreases appreciably, while the number of contingent factors increases ... This is a major reason why so many evaluation studies appear repetitive – one can never be sure that a programme which works in one situation will work in another. To the extent that evaluative research can focus upon the general variables underlying a specific programme and test the effect of these variables rather than the effectiveness of the programme as a whole, it may hope to produce findings of greater general significance.

Note that Suchman is writing about evaluation in general, not particularly about economics, though much later in the book (in a passage concerning the role of operations research!) he writes (Suchman 1967, pp 145–146):

> One component of evaluative research that is often neglected ... is the cost of a programme. Few programme can be justified at any cost ... Competition among service programmes sets the stage for a public demand for evaluation of results in terms of required resources ...... In using these cost criteria however, one must keep in mind the social aspects of such financial evaluation. As Flagle (1963) cautions: "The construction of a table or scale of utilities, although cast in terms of economics, is essentially a psychological experiment involving social values".

Thus *all* evaluation studies need to be interpreted carefully with respect to the time and place at which they were conducted, the options that were considered, the range of factors that were taken into account, the criteria of success/failure that were adopted, and how these were measured (and weighed one against another). A "definitive" evaluation is likely to be as elusive as an "ultimate" truth, and this is intrinsically so for *all* types of evaluation, economic or non-economic, a thought which brings me naturally to my next topic.

The principal kind of non-economic evaluation on our agenda at this meeting is variously referred to as medical, clinical, or epidemiological. For my purposes any differences between them are unimportant because they all seek to answer the question "will technology X improve the health of the patients?". To answer that question involves a careful specification of: (a) the alternatives (to answer the supplementary question" compared with what?"), (b) the patients (i. e. the condition to be treated and all other significant personal or social variables), and (c) the precise nature of all the concurrent activities associated with the use of technology X. Still more, it requires some definition of what is meant by the patient's health, how we know when it has improved, and what measurements are used to establish this, over whatever time horizon is taken to be appropriate for the investigation. It is a tough assignment, and it is no wonder that a great deal of such evaluation is inconclusive or downright misleading because of weaknesses in research design or data collection and analysis.

Two of these common weaknesses in medical evaluation are particularly important for the subsequent discussion of economic evaluation, and for that reason alone warrant further discussion here. They concern the measurement of health and the time horizon. The measurement of health is a vast topic, worth a conference of its own (see, for instance, Holland et al. 1979; Culyer 1978; Culyer 1983), however I wish here to make a few simple but important points. First, that clinical trials frequently concentrate on very narrow technical indicators (such as blood pressure, or tumour size, or presence or absence of some other biochemical abnormality), or upon some variant of change in life expectancy (such as case fatality, survival rates at some arbitrary future time, etc). More complex measures such as relief of pain, date of discharge (length of stay), date of return to work, or other effect upon normal activities will more rarely be included, and effects on relationships with others are still more unusual. Thus a treatment may be declared "successful" by some narrow test, yet it might cause a patient's marriage to break up, or even lead to a patient's suicide, and would clearly be judged "unsuccessful" by these broader criteria. I would describe these phenomena as cases where the *costs* of treatment (in health terms) outweigh their *benefits* (in health terms), i. e. where the treatment is not in the best interests of the patient (or the patient's family). This calls for an extension of clinical trials beyond the scope called for by *safety* regulations, which are typically concerned with clinical side effects of an equally narrow nature to the dimensions in which the benefits were measured (e. g. reductions in blood pressure are associated with, say, increased risk of pulmonary embolism). But, in the general case, whenever multiple criteria are used (narrow or otherwise), some valuation process is inevitably entailed in weighing one against another, i. e. in weighing "costs" (in health terms) against "benefits" (in health terms) and this process itself is of key interest to the economist and important grist to his mill.

The other important element in medical evaluation in which economists should show a great interest is the time horizon of the study. Two potential sources of trouble lurk here. The first is the tendency of such trials to operate on a crude "before" versus "after" basis, which obscures what happened "during". Thus a trial might show the patient better off *1 year later*, without specifying what the patient's health state was like *during* the year-long "therapeutic process" (and especially how much worse it might have been compared with the no-treatment option), and after experiencing the treatment patients might actually declare that it was not worth it (the cure is worse than the disease). The second trouble spot is the endpoint itself, since there is no natural terminating point for sequelae (not even the death of the patient if direct or indirect effects on others are significant). Thus there is always residual doubt and a natural tendency to weigh proximate effects more heavily than remote ones (other things being equal). The lessons for economic evaluation are that it is essential to ensure a full identification of *all* the implications of a technology, before, during, and after its use and to attempt to get the *timing* of each change accurately established (and monitored), and not just whether or not it occurs sometime or other. This applies both to the changes in health and to the changes in resource use.

For the rest of this paper I shall assume that, within its intrinsic limits and the usual limits of time and resources, the medical evaluation of any particular technology has been well done, but that it will not have concerned itself with any costs or benefits other than those upon health. Thus the stage is set for some kind of economic evaluation. Here our first problem is the common confusion between finance and economics due to the ambiguity in ordinary speech of the term "cost". At a superficial level, the question "what will it cost?" is readily answered by specifying the price of the product in question, i.e. the amount of money that will have to be handed over to the supplier to induce him to part with it. This is rarely the end of the story, however. Shopping itself costs money (e.g. in terms of transport) but it also costs *time*, both in the act of purchasing and collecting but also in gaining information, making decisions, organising the "use" of the purchase, etc. Some products occupy space, incur running costs, need repair and maintenance, take time to learn how to use, etc. Anyone who thinks that the cost of motoring begins and ends with buying a car has a shock in store! It is therefore important to rephrase the question "what will it cost?" much more carefully if unambiguous answers are (even in principle) to be attainable. One such rephrasing would be "how much of my money will I have to part with over the relevant time period?" This might be the relevant question for a budget-holder whose receipts are unaffected by the purchase, and who did not care about the non-pecuniary costs falling on him or about any costs falling on anybody else. If a purchase affects receipts as well as outgoings, then the net effect on the budget holder needs to be estimated, not just the expenditure effects. But even then we would still only have a *financial* appraisal, not an *economic* appraisal. To move to this higher plane of awareness the initial question would have to be rephrased "what valuable things will I have to sacrifice over the relevant time period?". The notion "valuable things sacrificed" is much broader than money, including time and any other resource which has value, whether having to be bought or not (e.g. something which you already have, but are willing to redeploy to this new use, like space). This notion of "opportunity-cost" (the value of a resource in its best alternative use) as the relevant notion is what distinguishes an economic appraisal from a financial one (and there is no necessary presumption that a resource will be correctly valued in opportunity-cost terms by the price that is paid for it, though fortunately the two do frequently coincide in broad terms).

Within the realm of economic appraisal (e.g. Drummond 1980, 1981 a) it is common to distinguish between cost-effectiveness analysis (CEA) and cost-benefit analysis (CBA). Within the context of this paper the difference is best seen in terms of the treatment of health in the analysis. If the effects on health are left in terms such as blood pressure, mortality risk, or even quality-adjusted-life-years, but the effects on resources are valued in money terms, then we are operating within the realm of CEA (the hallmark of which is that "costs" and "effects" are non-commensurable). Thus the necessity to value health in money terms (or money in health terms!) is avoided, but at the "cost" of being unable to offer any guidance as to whether *any* of the evaluated options should be accepted or not (because CEA can only tell you which of them is *more* cost-effective, not whether the effect is worth the cost!). In principle, CBA enables one to go to this last stage, but it forces the analysis to be explicit about the valuation of benefits, a matter which is left to the (implicit) judgement of the decision-maker in CEA.

Economic Evaluation in General

In order not to have to face too many difficulties at once, I shall initially assume that a cost-effectiveness framework is adequate for our purposes and that we have at our disposal medical evaluations that have used measures of effectiveness that are appropriate for our purposes (the frequency with which this last condition is *not* met is a strong argument for economists playing a role in the setting up of medical evaluations, counterbalancing the advantages of clinicians playing a role in economic evaluation!). I shall also ignore here general problems of research design not peculiar to the economic dimension (e.g. the specification of options, controls, study size, etc). I therefore assume that we know the likely distribution of benefits amongst a defined class of patients, and that we know how many such patients there are likely to be in the population served. (I am only too keenly aware how heroic these assumptions are, but I will come back to them later).

The broad format for a CEA is now simple, namely: *Effectiveness* is measured by a change in some index of health (e.g. quality-adjusted-life-expectancy); *Cost* is measured by the net value of the changes in resource availability occasioned by the technology under appraisal, and, in the case of mutually exclusive options, the preferred one will be that with the lowest ratio of cost to effect. If more than one option could be adopted, then it will normally be useful for the decision-maker also to know the *incremental cost* of improving effectiveness, as one moves from the most cost-effective to the least (especially if the most cost-effective option is limited in scope for any reason). Further complications arise if there is a special constraint on one or other of the resource inputs, making for large discontinuities in resource availability (e.g. the use of a particular site). These complications over "rationing" and "lumpiness" can be handled (with difficulty!), but would take us well beyond the scope of this paper. For present purposes I shall assume that comparative cost-effectiveness ratios are a satisfactory indicator.

The next important decision of principle is – what costs are to count? The managers of the health care system may decide that it is only a narrow range of costs that is to be considered, viz. changes in those resources for which they are directly responsible, e.g. land, buildings, staff, supplies, assigned for use by the service itself. They may, however, be under an obligation to take into account effects on related services, e.g. upon other social services, upon the social security system, upon other public bodies such as local governments, or even upon voluntary bodies (and charities). They may also feel that it is their duty to take account of all resource effects falling upon the population they serve, so that they will be concerned with effects on patients' time, patients' earnings, or other resource consequences for patients or their relatives and friends, etc. There may even be an obligation placed upon them by the government to consider rather broader economic considerations, such as effects on employment (local or national), on the balance of payments, though in my view these issues are best handled at a level other than that of the managers of a health care system. Even so, the appraisal might need to be designed to include such variables, if only for subsequent negotiating purposes. Thus the range of resource consequences considered has to be appropriate to the particular decision framework, and will differ from one to another (cf. Suchman's comments above on p. 41).

But there are nevertheless some general rules that are important whatever the range of variables included. Firstly, that true resource costs must be separated clearly from "transfer payments". A transfer payment is a cash payment *not* reflecting any offer of a real resource in the opposite direction. Thus a wage payment establishes a claim on labour supply (which is a *real* resource), whereas a pension payment establishes no such claim (there is no quid pro quo, so it is a transfer payment). Thus sickness benefits and other social security payments are "transfers", which merely *redistribute* the consequences of *real resource* changes (so that the loss of output and income occasioned by illness is redistributed so that part of it is borne by the sick person and part by the taxpayers via the social security system), and to count *both* the loss of output from sickness absence *and* the compensating/redistributing transfer payments would be to count the same phenomenon twice, as it manifests itself in different guises. Thus it is advantageous to keep a "real resource account" separate from a "transfers account", because both may be interesting to policy makers (the former for efficiency, the latter for equity reasons). The other general point about the real resource costs is that irrevocable *past* resource commitments can never be a relevant consideration in an economic evaluation, since they will be the same whatever future course of action is chosen. Thus the commonly heard assertion that "having gone this far we must go on" is quite specious (good money after bad?), as is the argument that we must include the recouping of those "sunk" costs amongst the costs of any option that they helped to facilitate.

We come now to the central issue of resource valuation, remembering that this should, in principle, reflect the value of any used resource in its (sacrificed) alternative use, or the value of any released resource in its (facilitated) alternative use. If the resource in question can be bought and sold freely in a perfectly functioning market, then the "price" of that resource can be taken to represent *both* of these values, providing that the changes in the volume of resource availability occasioned by the options under investigation are so small in relation to the total availability of the resource that they will not themselves affect the price. This is a point to which I will return later. Meanwhile, let us consider what has to be done in those cases where the market is not functioning perfectly. Possible reasons for considering "adjustment" of market prices on these grounds are: (a) the existence of subsidies or indirect taxes on the resource, which mean that its true costs are, respectively, higher or lower than its market price; (b) monopolistic elements in the market, which imply that even at the margin the price charged for the resource will be higher than its cost; (c) not all costs incurred in supplying the resource may have to be met by the vendor, hence the price charged understates its true costs (e.g. if the production of the good generates uncompensated air or water pollution, or if in supplying it congestion is generated in the transport system, which falls on others). Any or all of these "efficiency" adjustments may be necessary in a particular study, or it may be demonstrated by prima facie argument that they are of such small quantitative significance it is justifiable to accept market prices as a good approximation for the true value of the resource. It is a judgment that will frequently be valid, but which needs arguing in each case. In labour markets there are special problems when skills are so specific that alternative use values are really very low or when unemployment in general is so high that it can genuinely be argued that if not used in the project the resource would not be used at all, hence its alternative use value is zero. This can be a valid argument, especially in the short run, but it is less likely to be the case over a time horizon within which retraining becomes possible, or within which some turnover of labour might be expected as people withdraw from the labour force and are replaced by (more versatile) newcomers.

But even "adjusted" market prices may be rejected on the grounds *either* that people are not the best judges of their own welfare (and hence market prices generated, to some extent at least, by consumer choice are not "reliable") *or* that the distribution of purchasing power is ethically unacceptable (hence market prices, which are partly influenced by it, are also ethically unacceptable). If the economic evaluation is to encompass these views about the valuation of resources, then the way forward lies along one or more of the following routes: (a) to conduct experiments in which people who are held to be "good judges" of other people's welfare establish relative valuations, and to test these for consistency and consensus; (b) to cast some "responsible" person (or persons) in the role of the Delphic oracle to declare what the relevant values are to be (an obvious role for paternalistic politicians and philosopher kings); (c) to set up market simulations in which purchasing power is equalized (or whatever other distribution is held to be ethically acceptable) and then see what relative valuations emerge from this. This is controversial territory in which one school of thought holds that to go beyond efficiency-based adjustments of market prices is to go outside the proper scope of welfare economics, and hence both professionally foolhardy and politically dangerous, while the other school argues that since people do hold such views about valuation it is better for economists to help sort them out than leave such valuations unanalysed. All agree that whatever basis of valuation is adopted, it must be made explicit. My own views are set out in Sugden and Williams (1978). For an opposing view see Mishan (1981).

Having identified and valued all the relevant resource changes in one way or another, we must now turn to the problems of timing and time horizons. Since a given quantity of a particular resource may have a different value according to *when* it is used (or released), we must consider the problem of intertemporal valuation. Here there are two phenomena to be distinguished – inflation and "pure" discounting. There are two ways of handling the effects of inflation, *either* make all the valuation estimates on a "constant price" basis (e.g. 1984 prices) adjusting only for expected *relative* price changes through time, *or* estimate a fresh set of valuations each year, incorporating any expectations about changes in the *general* price level as well as specific changes in *relative* prices. But if the *former* approach is adopted, the discount rate, to be used in the phase to be described next, must be an inflation-free rate, whilst if the latter approach is used the relevant discount rate is one that incorporates inflationary expectations. What must *not* happen (but sometimes does) is to work with "constant prices" and then use as the discount rate a market rate of interest that has a lot of inflationary expectations in it! The "pure" discount rate is there to reduce to a common (present) value, the value of resources at different points in time, where the differences in value are due *not* to inflation but to either of the following phenomena: (1) the fact that resources used (or released) earlier in time could be reinvested to produce returns elsewhere, hence releasing resources early is more valuable than releasing them later, and, conversely, using them earlier is more costly than using them later; (2) people generally prefer early to late gratification of their wishes, hence expect greater "returns" if they are to be induced to set aside resources for their own later use (or, a fortiori, for the use of later generations!), an observation which also leads to the use of a discounting procedure. There is much dispute amongst economists as to whether either, both, or neither of these observations justifies discounting, and if so what the actual appropriate discount rate should be. However the majority view seems to be that a positive discount rate of up to 5% is generally justifiable (with which I agree) and that this is based on the view that this is the range within which long-term productivity growth lies in most economies (a basis I personally do not accept!). However, the issue can be avoided in most practical studies by discounting at a range of alternative rates from 0% to 5% just to see if it makes any significant difference to the preferred option and then ask the policy-makers to worry about it if it does!

This brings me to my final general point about cost-effectiveness studies, namely, the treatment of uncertainty. There are some common devices in use here that need to be treated with the utmost suspicion. The first of these is to adjust for uncertainty by taking a very short time horizon (the "pay-back period"). This is acceptable *if* what we face is the expectation that everything will go as planned for a (short) period but then the project might totally collapse (e.g. fall down, get blown up, or be confiscated by a hostile power). This does not seem to be a very realistic scenario in most cases, it being more likely that things will go awry more gradually, possibly at an increasing rate as time progresses. This is what lies behind my next bête noire, which deals with uncertainty by a "risk premium" to the discount rate. This has the effect of giving relatively more weight to proximate elements and relatively less to more distant ones, but its weakness is that it will treat all items at a particular point in time as *equally* susceptible to such risks, which is again unlikely to be the case. A better approach is to ask the "experts" what is the range of alternative assumptions that prudence dictates should be considered as possible for the elements that enter the appraisal, so that we can see how sensitive the outcome is to such variations. This is even better, of course, if such a sensitivity analysis can be buttressed by explicit judgments of the probability distribution associated with each of the uncertain variables. The *very* ambitious analyst might go to the ultimate stage, and attempt to check the degree of risk aversion of the decision-maker and then estimate certainty equivalent valuations, but I personally would rest content with sensitivity analyses, with some gentle probing on possible probability distributions.

My last point in this section concerns the move from CEA to CBA and the problem of valuing health care *benefits*. This merely raises once more all the valuation problems discussed above on pp. 45 ff., but in a rather more highly charged atmosphere. First of all, the "market price" valuation method has frequently been applied to benefit measurement in a context in which the value of health is taken to be solely its value as a means of earning money (the "lifetime earnings", or "productivity", or "human capital" approach). This is unfortunate, because whilst effects on productivity are undoubtedly relevant, they are certainly not the *only* relevant "value" outcome, and may not even be the most important. However, finding a satisfactory way of valuing health per se (i.e. other than as an instrument for earning money) raises sharply issues such as the proper role of the distribution of income and wealth in influencing such valuations, whether people's own valuations can be reliably elicited, and even if they could whether they are a proper basis for *social* policy in this field, or finally, whether this is not essentially a political judgement, which is the responsibility of the legitimate political authority. I have views of my own on these issues (Williams 1974, 1981) and they cannot really be escaped even by resort to CEA, because at the end of the day, even if the analyst has shied off and left the health effects unvalued, the decision to accept (or not accept) one of the options *implies* such a valuation, however unwitting it may be.

Some Special Problems with New Technologies

The special problems posed by new technology for the conduct of economic evaluation are caused by the conflicting demands of pervasive uncertainty and political urgency, which together generate the dilemma mentioned at the outset, namely, that economic evaluation can be done too soon or too late, so we need to think carefully about the "right" time to do it. Uncertainty diminishes with the passage of time, hence the advantages of waiting. But in the meantime some decisions may have to be taken anyway and these may prove to be pre-emptive so that the subsequent analysis, however thorough and polished, becomes a mere footnote for history. So what useful role is there for economic or indeed any other kind of evaluation in this treacherous territory? Let us seek appropriate responses to three particular sources of difficulty in turn: (a) the absence of conclusive medical evaluation; (b) feedback from the decision itself to the assumptions on which the analysis informing the decision is to be based; (c) technology in state of flux.

Hitherto I have explicitly been assuming that we had at our disposal an appropriate body of medical evidence concerning effectiveness. This is unlikely to be the case, especially if we are considering *early* economic evaluation. It might be thought that in the absence of medical evidence on effectiveness, no economic evaluation is possible, but this is not so. Just as it may be useful (but not conclusive) to do a medical evaluation without any economics, so it may be useful (but not conclusive) to do an economic evaluation without any effectiveness measures. For instance, if it is clear that technology X is going to cost 100 times what technology Y costs, this may be sufficient for immediate purposes because it may be quite evident to everyone that X cannot possibly be 100 times as effective as Y, so cannot be a cost-effective alternative. Similarly, it may be evident that X is probably somewhat more effective than Y, though how much more so is not clear. If an economic evaluation showed X to be less costly than Y, then we would not need a more accurate medical evaluation to decide to prefer X to Y, whereas we would need one if it turned out that X were "somewhat more" expensive than Y. Since fairly crude economic evaluation, aimed at establishing broad orders of magnitude from desk-based guesstimates, is a relatively cheap and speedy activity, I am surprised that it is not more frequently used in these initial stages to keep a sense of proportion about the wilder claims for cost-effectiveness, often based on poor identification of relevant costs and rather dubious valuation practices, which could readily be spotted by a competent economic analyst.

The feedback problem is not so readily disposed of, but I suspect that it could be handled adequately by appropriate sensitivity analysis, buttressed by some astute political negotiation! The archetypal assertion that we are now considering is that if the new technology is adopted quickly and on a large scale its costs will come down rapidly, whereas if it remains for years at a prototype stage or at restricted experimental levels of utilization, then costs will remain high. It should not be difficult to work out how low costs would have to fall to generate a change in the preferred option (noting, however, that *other* associated costs may *rise* if a lot more resources need to be drawn in), but the difficult judgement is how likely this is to happen. There may be some advantage in testing out the likelihood that fixed price "bulk purchase" agreements can be negotiated, as part of the evaluative process itself, and not to accept such estimates of cost reductions as a basis for decisionmaking unless firm commitments can be obtained from suppliers. This is especially important where such a decision would leave the system dependent on one supplier and not able easily to switch to an alternative if the estimates proved wrong. "Vulnerability" (defined as the cost of putting things right if things do not go according to plan) is an important subject for sensitivity analysis in a highly uncertain world populated by risk-averse people and organizations.

This is even more true of the continuously evolving nature of some technologies, and the consequent tendency for any substantial evaluation to be outdated by the time it is completed. Here I will assume that by careful technical assessment we have distinguished genuine evolutionary change from specious product differentiation. My response then would be that up-dating the economic aspects is likely to be rather easier than updating the medical evaluation, since so much of the work could be done on the "quick and dirty" basis outlined on p. 48. It also seems to be a case where *crude* economic evaluation should be associated with strict limits on the rate of adoption of the technology, the pattern of introduction being designed to generate knowledge for the next round as well as to generate immediate health benefits. In this context it may be justifiable to adopt a deliberately varied pattern of introduction as part of the field evaluation process itself and *not* to aim at "definitive" outcomes but "provisional" ones with relatively short time horizons, which are designed to inform successive negotiations or policy reviews. In the flux of uncertainty about the rate of technological advance, pre-commitment to any one technology is to be minimized, even though a "premium" has usually to be paid for such "insurance" in the form of "wasteful" spreading of one's portfolio of assets. Thus the analysis of risks in the sensitivity analysis should be used to guide the system away from concentration on a narrow range of options, *all* of which are vulnerable to an adverse movement in the *same* uncertain variable.

Against this background my final point will come as no surprise. It is that in this context the objective of economic evaluation should not be to decide what is the best technology to adopt, for in the presence of pervasive uncertainty that oversimplifies the problem. Rather, the objective is to explore the likely implications of variations in the scale and timing of the replacement of one technology by another. Moreover, since this sort of decision is best made on a provisional basis that commits the system as little as possible, it is essentially a search for a *robust next step*, i. e. guidance on what we should do *now* so as to be in the best position to exploit whatever are the most likely (but still uncertain) developments that will constitute the options before us when we next have to make a decision. Thus economic evaluation, presented in summary form as a decision tree (Raiffa 1968) seems to me to be the most promising way to clarify thought in this confusing territory.

To structure a decision as a "tree" involves being careful and explicit about the way in which possibilities are specified, probabilities are attached to contingencies, and choices are made in a sequence that works back from multifarious end-points (in future), each of which has a "payoff" (positive or negative) and a probability of achievement (partly the result of chance, partly of choice). This focusses our attention on the choice we have to make now, which inevitably turns out to be a choice between rival "lotteries" (i. e. between one "package" of risky outcomes and another). In simple cases this is easy to see but in the more complex real world, it is often incredibly difficult just to *structure* the problem correctly, let alone collect the economic data on costs and benefits and form a judgement about probabilities.

A problem that has characteristics similar to those we are interested in is described and analysed in detail in the Appendix to this paper. It has a moderate degree of complexity and I defy anyone to "spot" the solution simply by looking at the description of the problem. Needless to say, the "answer" is sensitive to the payoffs, the probabilities, the problem structure, *and* the decision rule employed, but the important point it is designed to illustrate is that to know what to do *now*, one needs to think ahead as far as one can, though in a contingent manner. But this does not imply that one has to have a "plan" in the sense of a firm intention to do this now, that next year, and then that the year after. Facing a world that is in a state of flux, one avoids commitment as far as possible and makes those decisions one has to make in the light of all the information one can bring to bear (with the possibilities for recontracting built into one's analysis). This will not prevent us from making "mistakes" (in the sense that with *hindsight* we may later see that there was something better we could have done) but it will enable us to *adapt* more readily to changing circumstances, so that our "mistakes" should not prove fatal!

Appendix: An Economic Decision Model Applied to Investment in Medical Technology

The Problem

There is pressure to invest in a new medical technology, to which the following data relates:

1) The machine being offered now (period 0) costs £ 1 million to buy and instal, and its running costs are £ 0.5 million in the 1st year, £ 0.6 million in the 2nd year, £ 0.8 million in the 3rd year, and £ 1.0 million in the 4th year. The machine has an expected physical life of 4 years, and running at optimum capacity it generates benefits of 1 000 quality-adjusted-life-years (QALYs) per annum.

2) There is a slight chance that medical practice will change in such a way to make this machine (and its rivals) totally redundant within this 4-year period. The (incremental) probabilities of this happening by the beginning of each year are as follows: 0.01, 0.03, 0.09 and 0.27.

3) It is much more likely that the present technology will be improved, with much more compact and economical machines becoming available shortly, reducing both the setting-up and running costs but generating the same benefits. There are known to be two rival developments being pursued by other firms, one of which (A) would generate a 20% reduction in both setting-up and running costs compared with the machine currently on offer, and the other (B) a 50% reduction. The (incremental) probabilities of each of these being available in each of the first 3 years are as given in Table 4.1.

4) The firm supplying the current machine claims to be able to meet the rivals' claims by upgrading existing machines (these machines, unlike A and B, are subject to import licences, and when you have bought one, only upgrading is possible). Independent estimates suggest that there is a 50 : 50 chance that for an additional expenditure of £ 0.4 million it will be possible to obtain running cost reductions of the following order (benefits unchanged): year 1 10%, year 2 20%, year 3 30%. For technical reasons, a machine can only be upgraded once, but if the original machine is

Table 4.1. Incremental probabilities of machines A and B being available in the first 3 years

	Year 1	Year 2	Year 3[a]
Model A	0.1	0.2	0.3
Model B	0.02	0.05	0.13

[a] No capital expenditure will be permitted after year 3

Table 4.2. The values at the end of year 4

	After 1 year's use	After 2 years' use	After 3 years' use
Machine A	£ 0.45 million	£ 0.3 million	£ 0.15 million
Machine B	£ 0.4 million	£ 0.3 million	£ 0.2 million

Table 4.3. Decision tree for "buy now" option

Option no.	Year 1 alt		Δ_B	Δ_C	Σ_B	Σ_C	Year 2 alt		Δ_B	Δ_C	Σ_B	Σ_C	Year 3 alt		Δ_B	Δ_C	Σ_B	Σ_C	Year 4 alt		Δ_B	Δ_C	Σ_B	Σ_C	Option no.
1	red	(0.01)			0	1																			1
2	run		1	0.5	1	1.5	red	(0.03)			1	1.5													2
3							run		1	0.6	2	2.1	red	(0.09)			2	2.1							3
4													run		1	0.8	3	2.9	red	(0.27)			3	2.9	4
5																			run		1	1	4	3.9	5
6													upg	(0.05)	1	1.2	3	3.3	red	(0.27)			3	3.6	6
7																			run		1	0.7	4	4.0	7
8													A	(0.3)	1	1.6	3	3.7	red	(0.27)			3	3.7	8
9																			run		1	0.4	4	3.65	9
10													B	(0.13)	1	1.3	3	3.4	red	(0.27)			3	3.4	10
11																			run		1	0.25 (−0.4)	4	3.25	11
12							upg	(0.5)	1	1	2	2.5	red	(0.09)			2	2.5							12
13													run		1	0.64	3	3.14	red	(0.27)			3	3.14	13
14																			run		1	0.8	4	3.94	14
15													A	(0.3)	1	1.44	3	3.94	red	(0.27)			3	3.94	15
16																			run		1	0.4 (−0.45)	4	3.89	16
17													B	(0.13)	1	1.14	3	3.64	red	(0.27)			3	3.64	17
18																			run		1	0.25 (−0.4)	4	3.49	18
19							A	(0.2)	1	1.4	2	2.9	red	(0.09)			2	2.9							19
20													run		1	0.4	3	3.3	red	(0.27)			3	3.3	20
21																			run		1	0.48 (−0.3)	4	3.48	21
22													B	(0.13)	1	0.9	3	3.8	red	(0.27)			3	3.8	22
23																			run		1	0.25 (−0.4)	4	3.65	23
24							B	(0.05)	1	1.1	2	2.6	red	(0.09)			2	2.6							24
25													run		1	0.25	3	2.85	red	(0.27)			3	2.85	25
26																			run		1	0.3 (−0.3)	4	2.85	26
27	upg	(0.5)	1	0.9	1	1.9	red	(0.03)			1	1.9													27
28							run		1	0.54	2	2.44	red	(0.09)			2	2.44							28
29													run		1	0.72	3	3.16	red	(0.27)			3	3.16	29
30																			run		1	0.9	4	4.06	30

31													A	(0.3)	1	1.52	3	3.96	red	(0.27)			3	3.96	31
32																			run		1	0.4	4	3.91	32
33													B	(0.13)	1	1.22	3	3.66	red	(0.27)			3	3.66	33
34																			run		1	0.25	4	3.51	34
																						(−0.4)			
35							A	(0.2)	1	1.34	2	3.24	red	(0.09)			2	3.24							35
36													run		1	0.4	3	3.64	red	(0.27)			3	3.64	36
37																			run		1	0.48	4	3.82	37
																						(−0.03)			
38													B	(0.13)	1	0.9	3	4.14	red	(0.27)			3	4.14	38
39																			run		1	0.25	4	3.99	39
																						(−0.4)			
40							B	(0.05)	1	1.04	2	2.94	red	(0.09)			2	2.94							40
41													run		1	0.25	3	3.19	red	(0.27)			3	3.19	41
42																			run		1	0.3	4	3.19	42
																						(−0.3)			
43	A	(0.1)	1	1.3	1	2.3	red	(0.03)			1	2.3													43
44							run		1	0.4	2	2.7	red	(0.09)			2	2.7							44
45													run		1	0.48	3	3.18	red	(0.27)			3	3.18	45
46																			run		1	0.64	4	3.67	46
47													B	(0.13)	1	0.98	3	3.68	red	(0.27)			3	3.68	47
48																			run		1	0.25	4	3.53	48
49							B	(0.05)	1	0.9	2	3.2	red	(0.09)			2	3.2							49
50													run		1	0.25	3	3.45	red	(0.27)			3	3.45	50
51																			run		1	0.3	4	3.45	51
																						(−0.3)			
52	B	(0.02)	1	1	1	2	red	(0.03)			1	2													52
53							run		1	0.25	2	2.25	red	(0.09)			2	2.25							53
54													run		1	0.3	3	2.55	red	(0.27)			3	2.55	54
55																			run		1	0.4	4	2.75	55
																						(−0.2)			

purchased later it incorporates any upgradings available to date (but no subsequent upgrading is then possible). These machines incorporating upgrading still cost £ 1.0 million.

5) Neither upgrading nor replacement of machines interferes with the running of existing machines, which come on stream in the year *after* the one in which they are purchased. All costs are in year 0 present values at the relevant discount rate, and machines cannot be sold even if replaced. However, at the end of year 4 (the planning horizon) the values in Table 4.2 are to be credited.

6) Your organization has firmly decided not to put a money value on a QALY, its policy being to go for that course of action that minimizes the cost per QALY gained. It also takes the view that once it starts providing a service like this, it must keep going, even if it turns out to be more costly than expected.

7) You are asked to advise whether to buy the machine on offer now, or whether to wait until next year in the hope that things become cheaper.

Structuring the Problem

We can set this up as a simple binary choice – "buy now" *or* "wait". We can then systematically explore all the possible subsequent courses of action associated with each of these primary choices, work out the payoffs associated with each, and the way chance impinges on them. Where we have scope for subsequent choices, we must think our way into that situation and decide what we would do *if the situation then is what we expect it to be now.* This is a conditional (and hypothetical) choice and is not a firm commitment. What we will actually do when the time comes will depend on what information (and objectives) we then have.

Table 4.3 sets out the structure of the "buy now" branch of the decision tree. It contains 55 possible endpoints, and is constructed as follows. The first column labels the alternatives 1 to 55, with the time path of decisions, year by year, coded as follows: "red" = redundant (because of changed medical practice); "run" = run the (last) previously purchased machine (and do nothing else); "upg" = upgrade the previously purchased machine; "A" = purchase the rival machine A (whilst running the previously purchased machine); "B" = purchase the rival machine B (whilst running the previously purchased machine). In brackets, after each "decision" (except "run") is the probability of that "decision" being available. The machine becoming redundant is, of course, an overriding "decision", which, if it happens, takes the matter out of "our" hands. The decision "run" is always available, so will actually take on the residual probability if some other decision is preferred at that point or where "red" intervenes. (This will become clearer when we look at Table 4.5). Against each alternative the benefits and costs associated with it are shown, first in incremental terms ("ΔB" and "ΔC") and then in cumulative terms thus far ("ΣB" and "ΣC"). The benefits are measured in thousands of QALYs, the costs in millions of pounds, but to save space the units are suppressed in both cases. In the cost build-up, under "upg", "A" and "B" the setting-up costs are added to the costs of running the previous machine in the year in which that decision is made, and only one inclusive cost figure is shown. By contrast, in year 4 the end-period values (if any) of existing machines are shown separately in the "ΔC" column for the sake of clarity since the overall effect is sometimes to make "ΔC" negative in that year.

Table 4.4 does the same thing for the "Wait" alternative, which generates no less than 90 more alternatives (numbered 56–145 inclusive). The only new pieces of terminology here are pretty self-explanatory, namely: "Wait" = do nothing; "Buy Orig" = buy the original machine; "Buy Upg" = buy the original machine with the latest upgrading built in (if available). Option 145 is the waiting game throughout, yielding no costs and no benefits whatever happens! In all other respects, Table 4.4 follows the pattern of Table 4.3.

Doing the Arithmetic: The Expected Value Calculations

Tables 4.5 and 4.6 set out the calculations concerning the options whose payoffs were calculated in Tables 4.3 and 4.4 respectively. The general principle underlying the technique is to start at the end (year 4) and work back to the beginning (year 1) so as to decide which "lottery ticket" ("buy now" versus "wait") has the highest "expected value" (i.e. the value of each payoff multiplied by the probability of obtaining it). Each payoff has two "values", the benefits (in QALYs) and the costs (in pounds), and each pair of numbers is processed as if incommensurable, but in Tables 4.5 and 4.6 they are kept bracketed together, with benefits first, then a minus sign, followed by the cost figure. Thus the initial information given for each option in Tables 4.5 and 4.6 is merely the payoff data picked up from the final ("ΣB" and "ΣC") columns of Tables 4.3 and 4.4.

The method then proceeds as follows (using options 1–11 initially as an illustrative example). Options 4, 6, 8, and 10 represent what will happen if the machine becomes redundant in year 4, and there is a 0.27 probability of this being the case, so the "expected value" of this outcome is shown after the "=" sign. For instance, in option 4, the expected value of (3–2.9) 0.27 is (0.81–0.783), obtained by multiplying each term in the first set of brackets by 0.27. This leaves us with the residual probability of running the existing machine at 0.73, so against options 5, 7, 9, and 11 are shown the payoffs, probability, and expected values of that eventuality. Since options 4 and 5 *jointly* constitute one option at an *earlier* stage in the decision-making process, we need to add together their expected values to see what their joint value is, and it turns out to be (3.73–3.63). If we do the same for the joint options 6 and 7, 8 and 9, and 10 and 11, we obtain their joint values as (3.73–3.892), (3.73–3.664), and (3.73–3.291). If we look at all four of these joint options, since they all generate the same expected benefit (3.73), we can choose between them purely in terms of their costs. The least cost option is the last one (10 and 11) at 3.291, but we have only a 0.13 chance of having that one available to us, so there is a 0.87 chance that we may have to finish up with something else. The next most favourable option is (4 and 5) and this will certainly be available if we have reached that section of the decision tree, so it attracts the residual 0.87 probability. The other two joint options, (6 and 7) and (8 and 9), are therefore discarded and play no further role in the calculations, hence the double vertical lines blocking them off at this stage. What does continue to the phase of decision is 0.13 of (3.73–3.291), which comes to (0.485–0.428), and 0.87 of (3.73–3.63), which comes to (3.245–3.158), the sum of these amounting to (3.73–3.586). This represents the expected value of options 4–11 inclusive. Similar

Table 4.4. Payoff tree: "wait"

Option no.	Year 1 alt		Δ_B	Δ_C	Σ_B	Σ_C	Year 2 alt		Δ_B	Δ_C	Σ_B	Σ_C	Year 3 alt		Δ_B	Δ_C	Σ_B	Σ_C	Year 4 alt		Δ_B	Δ_C	Σ_B	Σ_C	Option no.
56	red	(0.01)	0	0	0	0																			56
57	buy	orig	0	1	0	1	red	(0.03)			0	1													57
58							run		1	0.5	1	1.5	red	(0.09)			1	1.5							58
59													run		1	0.6	2	2.1	red	(0.27)			2	2.1	59
60																			run		1	0.8	3	2.9	60
61													upg	(0.5)	1	1	2	2.5	red	(0.27)			2	2.5	61
62																			run		1	0.56	3	3.06	62
63													A	(0.3)	1	1.4	2	2.9	red	(0.27)			2	2.9	63
64																			run		1	0.4 (−0.45)	3	2.85	64
65													B	(0.13)	1	1.1	2	2.6	red	(0.27)			2	2.6	65
66																			run		1	0.25 (−0.4)	3	2.45	66
67							upg	(0.5)	1	0.9	1	1.9	red	(0.09)			1	1.9							67
68													run		1	0.48	2	2.38	red	(0.27)			2	2.38	68
69																			run		1	0.64	3	3.02	69
70													A	(0.3)	1	1.28	2	3.18	red	(0.27)			2	3.18	70
71																			run		1	0.4 (−0.45)	3	3.13	71
72													B	(0.13)	1	0.98	2	2.88	red	(0.27)			2	2.88	72
73																			run		1	0.25 (−0.4)	3	2.73	73
74							A	(0.2)	1	1.3	1	2.3	red	(0.09)			1	2.3							74
75													run		1	0.4	2	2.7	red	(0.27)			2	2.7	75
76																			run		1	0.48 (−0.3)	3	2.88	76
77													B	(0.13)	1	0.9	2	3.2	red	(0.27)			2	3.2	77
78																			run		1	0.25 (−0.4)	3	3.05	78
79							B	(0.05)	1	1	1	2	red	(0.09)			1	2							79
80													run		1	0.25	2	2.25	red	(0.27)			2	2.25	80
81																			run		1	0.3 (−0.3)	3	2.25	81

82	buy upg	(0.5)	0	1	0	1	red	(0.03)			0	1												82
83							run		1	0.45	1	1.45	red	(0.09)			1	1.45						83
84													run		1	0.54	2	1.99	red	(0.27)			2	1.99	84
85																			run		1	0.72	3	2.71	85
86													A	(0.3)	1	1.34	2	2.79	red	(0.27)			2	2.79	86
87																			run		1	0.4 (−0.45)	3	2.74	87
88													B	(0.13)	1	1.04	2	2.49	red	(0.27)			2	2.49	88
89																			run		1	0.25 (−0.4)	3	2.34	89
90							A	(0.2)	1	1.25	1	2.25	red	(0.09)			1	2.25							90
91													run		1	0.4	2	2.65	red	(0.27)			2	2.65	91
92																			run		1	0.48 (−0.3)	3	2.83	92
93													B	(0.13)	1	0.9	2	3.15	red	(0.27)			2	3.15	93
94																			run		1	0.25 (−0.4)	3	3	94
95							B	(0.05)	1	0.95	1	1.95	red	(0.09)			1	1.95							95
96													run		1	0.25	2	2.20	red	(0.27)			2	2.2	96
97																			run		1	0.3 (−0.3)	3	2.2	97
98	A	(0.1)	0	0.8	0	0.8	red	(0.03)			0	0.8													98
99							run		1	0.4	1	1.2	red	(0.09)			1	1.2							99
100													run		1	0.48	2	1.68	red	(0.27)			2	1.68	100
101																			run		1	0.64 (−0.15)	3	2.17	101
102													B		1	0.98	2	2.18	red	(0.27)			2	2.18	102
103																			run		1	0.25 (−0.4)	3	2.03	103
104							B	(0.05)	1	0.9	1	1.7	red	(0.09)			1	1.7							104
105													run		1	0.25	2	1.95	red	(0.27)			2	1.95	105
106																			run		1	0.3 (−0.3)	3	1.95	106

Table 4.4. Payoff tree: "wait" (continued)

Option no.	Year 1						Year 2						Year 3						Year 4						Option no.
	alt		Δ_B	Δ_C	Σ_B	Σ_C	alt		Δ_B	Δ_C	Σ_B	Σ_C	alt		Δ_B	Δ_C	Σ_B	Σ_C	alt		Δ_B	Δ_C	Σ_B	Σ_C	
107	B	(0.02)	0	0.5	0	0.5	red	(0.03)			0	0.5													107
108							run		1	0.25	1	0.75	red	(0.09)			1	0.75							108
109													run		1	0.3	2	1.05	red	(0.27)			2	1.05	109
110																			run		1	0.4 (−0.2)	3	1.25	110
111	wait		0	0	0	0	red	(0.03)			0	0													111
112							buy	orig	0	1	0	1	red	(0.09)			0	1							112
113													run		1	0.5	1	1.5	red	(0.27)			1	1.5	113
114																			run		1	0.6	2	2.1	114
115													upg	(0.5)	1	0.9	1	1.9	red	(0.27)			1	1.9	115
116																			run		1	0.42	2	2.32	116
117													A	(0.3)	1	1.3	1	2.3	red	(0.27)			1	2.3	117
118																			run		1	0.4 (−0.45)	2	2.25	118
119													B	(0.13)	1	1	1	2	red	(0.27)			1	2	119
120																			run		1	0.25 (−0.4)	2	1.85	120
121							buy upg	(0.5)	0	1	0	1	red	(0.09)			0	1							121
122													run		1	0.4	1	1.4	red	(0.27)			1	1.4	122
123																			run		1	0.48	2	1.88	123
124													A	(0.3)	1	1.2	1	2.2	red	(0.27)			1	2.2	124
125																			run		1	0.4 (−0.45)	2	2.15	125
126													B	(0.13)	1	0.9	1	1.9	red	(0.27)			1	1.9	126
127																			run		1	0.25 (−0.4)	2	1.75	127

128	A	(0.2)	0	0.8	0	0.8	red	(0.09)			0	0.8							128
129							run		1	0.4	1	1.2	red	(0.27)			1	1.2	129
130													run		1	0.48 (−0.3)	2	1.38	130
131							B	(0.13)	1	0.9	1	1.7	red	(0.27)			1	1.7	131
132													run		1	0.25 (−0.4)	1	1.55	132
133	B	(0.05)	0	0.5	0	0.5	red	(0.09)			0	0.5							133
134							run		1	0.25	1	0.75	red	(0.27)			1	0.75	134
135													run		1	0.3 (−0.3)	2	0.75	135
136	wait		0	0	0	0	red	(0.09)			0	0							136
137							buy	orig	0	1	0	1	red	(0.27)			0	1	137
138													run		1	0.5	1	1.5	138
139							buy upg	(0.5)	0	1	0	1	red	(0.27)			0	1	139
140													run		1	0.35	1	1.35	140
141							A	(0.3)	0	0.8	0	0.8	red	(0.27)			0	0.8	141
142													run		1	0.4 (−0.45)	1	0.75	142
143							B	(0.13)	0	0.5	0	0.5	red	(0.27)			0	0.5	143
144													run		1	0.25 (−0.4)	1	0.35	144
145							wait		0	0	0	0			0	0	0	0	145

Table 4.5. Buy now: expected value calculations

Option no.	Year 4			Year 3
1				
2				
3				(2–2.1) 0.09 = (0.18–0.189)
4	(3–2.9) 0.27 = (0.81–0.783)	(3.73–3.63) 1.0 [0.87]	= (3.245–3.158)	
5	(4–3.9) 0.73 = (2.92–2.847)	(2nd preference)		
6	(3–3.6) 0.27 = (0.81–0.972)	(3.73–3.892) 0.5	‖	
7	(4–4) 0.73 = (2.92–2.92)			(3.73–3.586) 0.91 = (3.394–3.26)
8	(3–3.7) 0.27 = (0.81–0.999)	(3.73–3.664) 0.3	‖	
9	(4–3.65) 0.73 = (2.92–2.665)			
10	(3–3.4) 0.27 = (0.81–0.918)	(3.73–3.291) 0.13	= (0.485–0.428)	
11	(4–3.25) 0.73 = (2.92–2.373)	(1st preference)		
12				(2–2.5) 0.09 = (0.18–0.225)
13	(3–3.14) 0.27 = (0.81–0.848)	(3.73–3.724) 1.0 [0.87]	= (3.245–3.24)	
14	(4–3.94) 0.73 = (2.92–2.876)	(2nd preference)		
15	(3–3.94) 0.27 = (0.81–1.064)	(3.73–3.904) 0.3	‖	(3.73–3.699) 0.91 = (3.394–3.366)
16	(4–3.89) 0.73 = (2.92–2.840)			
17	(3–3.64) 0.27 = (0.81–0.983)	(3.73–3.531) 0.13	= (0.485–0.459)	
18	(4–3.49) 0.73 = (2.92–2.548)	(1st preference)		
19				(2–2.9) 0.09 = (0.18–0.261)
20	(3–3.3) 0.27 = (0.81–0.891)	(3.73–3.431) 1.0		
21	(4–3.48) 0.73 = (2.92–2.54)	(1st preference)		(3.73–3.431) 0.91 = (3.394–3.122)
22	(3–3.8) 0.27 = (0.81–1.026)	(3.73–3.691) 0.13	‖	
23	(4–3.65) 0.73 = (2.92–2.665)			
24				(2–2.6) 0.09 = (0.18–0.234)
25	(3–2.85) 0.27 = (0.81–0.77)	(3.73–2.85) 1.0	=	(3.73–2.85) 0.91 = (3.394–2.594)
26	(4–2.85) 0.73 = (2.92–2.08)			
27				
28				(2–2.44) 0.09 = (0.18–0.220)
29	(3–3.16) 0.27 = (0.81–0.853)	(3.73–3.817) 1.0 [0.87]	= (3.245–3.321)	
30	(4–4.06) 0.73 = (2.92–2.964)	(2nd preference)		
31	(3–3.96) 0.27 = (0.81–1.069)	(3.73–3.923) 0.3	‖	(3.73–3.783) 0.91 = (3.394–3.443)
32	(4–3.91) 0.73 = (2.92–2.854)			
33	(3.–3.66) 0.27 = (0.81–0.988)	(3.73–3.55) 0.13	= (0.485–0.462)	
34	(4–3.51) 0.73 = (2.92–2.562)	(1st preference)		
35				(2–3.24) 0.09 = (0.18–0.282)
36	(3–3.64) 0.27 = (0.81–0.983)	(3.73–3.772) 1.0	= (3.73–3.772)	
37	(4–3.82) 0.73 = (2.92–2.789)	(1st preference)		(3.73–3.772) 0.91 = (3.394–3.433)
38	(3–4.14) 0.27 = (0.81–1.118)	(3.73–4.031) 0.13	‖	
39	(4–3.99) 0.73 = (2.92–2.913)			
40				(2–2.94) 0.09 = (0.18–2.65)
41	(3–3.19) 0.27 = (0.81–0.861)	(3.73–3.19) 1.0	=	(3.73–3.19) 0.91 = (3.394–2.903)
42	(4–3.19) 0.73 = (2.92–2.329)			
43				
44				(2–2.07) 0.09 = (0.18–0.243)
45	(3–3.18) 0.27 = (0.81–0.859)	(3.73–3.538) 1.0	= (3.73–3.538)	
46	(4–3.67) 0.73 = (2.92–2.679)			
47	(3–3.68) 0.27 = (0.81–0.994)	(3.73–3.571) 0.13	‖	(3.73–3.538) 0.91 = (3.394–3.220)
48	(4–3.53) 0.73 = (2.92–2.577)			
49				(2–3.2) 0.09 = (0.18–0.288)
50	(3–3.45) 0.27 = (0.81–0.932)	(3.73–3.278) 1.0	=	(3.73–3.538) 0.91 = (3.394–2.983)
51	(3–3.45) 0.73 = (2.92–2.346)			
52				
53				(2–2.25) 0.09 = (0.18–0.203)
54	(3–2.55) 0.27 = (0.81–0.689)	(3.73–2.697) 1.0	=	(3.73–2.697) 0.91 = (3.394–2.454)
55	(4–2.75) 0.73 = (2.92–2.008)			

Year 2		Year 1		
		(0–1) 0.01 = (0–0.01)		
(1–1.5) 0.03 (0.03–0.045)				
(3.574–3.452) 1.0 [X0.95X0.8] = (2.716–2.624) (3rd preference)				
(3.574–3.591) 0.5	(3.574 –3.409) X0.97 = (3.467 –3.307)	(3.497–3.352) 1.0 [X0.98] = (3.427–3.285) (2nd preference)		
(3.574–3.383) 0.2 [X0.95] = (0.679–0.643) (2nd preference)				
(3.574–2.828) 0.05 = (0.179–0.142) (1st preference)				
(1–2.9) 0.03 = (0.03–0.057)				
(3.574–3.663) 1.0 [X0.95] = (3.395–3.480) (2nd preference)			(3.497–3.338)	(3.497 –3.348)
(3.574–3.725) 0.2	(3.574–3.638) 0.97 = (3.467 –3.529)	(3.497–3.586) 0.5		
(3.574–3.168) 0.05 = (0.179–0.158) (1st preference)				
(1–2.3) 0.03 = (0.03–0.069)				
(3.574–3.463) 1.0 [X0.95] = (3.395–3.290) (2nd preference)	(3.574–3.454) 0.97 = (3.467 -3.350	(3.497–3.419) 0.1		
(3.574–3.271) 0.05 = (0.179–0.164) (1st preference)				
(1–2) 0.03 = (0.03–0.06)				
(3.574–2.657 0.97 = (3.467–2.577)		(3.497–2.637) 0.02 = (0.07–0.053)		

Table 4.6. Wait: expected value calculation

Option no.	Year 4		Year 3	
56				
57				
58				(1–1.5) 0.09 = (0.09–0.135)
59	(2–2.1) 0.27 = (0.54–0.567)	(2.73–2.684) 1.0 x 0.87	= (2.375–2.335)	
60	(3–2.9) 0.73 = (2.19–2.117)	(2nd preference)		
61	(2–2.5) 0.27 = (0.54–0.675)	(2.73–2.909) 0.5	||	
62	(3–3.06) 0.73 = (2.19–2.234)			
63	(2–2.9) 0.27 = (0.54–783)	(2.73–2.864) 0.3	||	(2.73–2.658) 0.91 = (2.484–2.419)
64	(3–2.85) 0.73 = (2.19–2.081)			
65	(2–2.6) 0.27 = (0.54–0.702)	(2.73–2.491) 0.13	= (0.355–0.323)	
66	(3–2.45) 0.73 = (2.19–1.789)	(1st preference)		
67				(1–1.9) 0.09 = (0.09–0.171)
68	(2–2.38) 0.27 = (0.54–0.43)	(2.73–2.848) 1.0 0.87	= (2.375–2.478)	
69	(3–3.02) 0.73 = (2.19–2.205)	(2nd preference)		
70	(2–3.18) 0.27 = (0.54–0.859)	(2.73–3.144) 0.3	||	(2.73–2.838) 0.91 = (2.484–2.583)
71	(3–3.13) 0.73 = (2.19–2.285)			
72	(2–2.88) 0.27 = (0.54–0.778)	(2.73–2.771) 0.13	= (0.355–0.360)	
73	(3–2.73) 0.73 = (2.19–1.993)	(1st preference)		
74				(1–2.3) 0.09 = (0.09–0.207)
75	(2–2.7) 0.27 = (0.54–0.729)	(2.73–2.831) 1.0	= (2.73–2.831)	
76	(3–2.88) 0.73 = (2.19–2.102)	(1st preference)		(2.73–2.831) 0.91 = (2.484–2.576)
77	(2–3.2) 0.27 = (0.54–0.864)	(2.73–3.091) 0.13	||	
78	(3–3.05) 0.73 = (2.19–2.227)			
79				(1–2.0) 0.09 = (0.09–0.18)
80	(2–2.25) 0.27 = (0.54–0.608)	(2.73–2.251) 1.0	= (2.73–2.251)	= (2.73–2.251) 0.91 = (2.484–2.048)
81	(3–2.25) 0.73 = (2.19–1.643)			
82				
83				(1–1.45) 0.09 = (0.09–0.131)
84	(2–1.99) 0.27 = (0.54–0.537)	(2.73–2.515) 1.0 0.87	= (2.375–2.188)	
85	(3–2.71) 0.73 = (2.19–1.978)	(2nd preference)		
86	(2–2.79) 0.27 (0.54–0.753)	(2.73–2.753) 0.3	||	(2.73–2.497) 0.91 = (2.484–2.772)
87	(3–2.74) 0.73 = (2.19–2.000)			
88	(2–2.49) 0.27 = (0.54–0.672)	(2.73–2.300) 0.13	= (0.355–0.309)	
89	(3–2.34) 0.73 = (2.19–1.708)	(1st preference)		
90				(1–2.25) 0.09 = (0.09–0.203)
91	(2–2.65) 0.27 = (0.54–0.716)	(2.73–2.782) 1.0	= (2.73–2.782)	
92	(3–2.83) 0.73 = (2.19–2.066)	(1st preference)		(2.73–2.782) 0.91 = (2.484–2.532)
93	(2–3.15) 0.27 (0.54–0.851)	(2.73–3.041) 0.13	||	
94	(3–3) 0.73 = (2.19–2.19)			
95				(1–1.95) 0.09 = (0.09–0.176)
96	(2–2.2) 0.27 = (0.54–0.594)	(2.73–2.2) 1.0	= (2.73–2.2)	= (2.73–2.2) 0.91 = (2.484–2.002)
97	(3–2.2) 0.73 = (2.19–1.606)			
98				
99				(1–1.2) 0.09 = (0.09–0.108)
100	(2–1.68) 0.27 = (0.54–0.454)	(2.73–2.038) 1.0	= (2.73–2.038)	
101	(3–2.17) 0.73 = (2.19–1.584)	(1st preference)		(2.73–2.038) 0.91 = (2.484–1.855)
102	(2–2.18) 0.27 = (0.54–0.589)	(2.73–2.064) 0.13	||	
103	(3–2.02) 0.73 = (2.19–1.475)			
104				(1–1.7) 0.09 = (0.09–0.153)
105	(2–1.95) 0.27 = (0.54–0.527)	(2.73–1.95) 1.0	= (2.73–2.038)	= (2.73–2.038) 0.91 = (2.484–1.089)
106	(3–1.95) 0.73 = (2.19–1.424)			

Year 2		Year 1		
	(0–1) 0.03 = (0–0.03)		(0–0) 0.01 = (0–0)	
(2.574–2.554) 1.0 [0.95] = (2.445–2.426 (2nd preference)				
	(2.574–2.537) 0.97 = (2.497–2.461)	(2.497–2.491) 1.0		
(2.574–2.754) 0.5				
(2.574–2.783) 0.2				
(2.574–2.228) 0.05 = (0.128–0.111) (1st preference)				
	(0–1) 0.03 = (0–0.03)			
(2.574–2.403) 1.0 [0.95] = (2.445–2.283) (2nd preference)				
		(2.497–2.350) 0.5		
(2.574–2.735) 0.2	(2.574–2.392) 0.97 = (2.497–2.320)			
(2.574–2.178) 0.05 = (0.128–0.109) (1st preference)				
	(0–0.8) 0.03 (0–0.024)			(0.20) 0.102
(2.574–1.963) 1.0 [0.95] = (2.445–1.865) (2nd preference)	(2.574–1.961) 0.97 = (2.457–1.902)	(2.497–1.926) 0.1	(0.206–0.103) x0.99 = (0.204–0.102)	
(2.574–1.247) 0.05 = (0.128–0.096) (1st preference)				

(extends to option no. 149 on p. 65) (extends to option no. 149 on p. 65)

Table 4.6. Wait: expected value calculation (continued)

Option no.	Year 4		Year 3	
107				
108				(1–1.75) 0.09 = (0.09–0.158)
109	(2–1.05) 0.27 = (0.54–0.284)	(2.73–1.197) 1.0	= (2.73–1.197)	= (2.73–1.197) 0.91 = (2.484–1.089)
110	(3–1.25) 0.73 = (2.19–0.913)			
111				
112				(0–1) 0.09 = (0–0.09)
113	(1–1.5) 0.27 = (0.27–0.405)	(1.73–1.938) 1.0 0.87	= (1.505–1.686)	
114	(2–2.1) 0.73 = (1.46–1.533)	(2nd preference)		
115	(1–1.9) 0.27 = (0.27–0.513)	(1.73–2.207) 0.5	‖	
116	(2–2.32) 0.73 = (1.46–1.694)			(1.73–1.932) 0.91 = (1.574–1.758)
117	(1–2.3) 0.27 = (0.27–0.621)	(1.73–2.264) 0.3	‖	
118	(2–2.25) 0.73 = (1.46–1.643)			
119	(1–2) 0.27 = (0.27–0.54)	(1.73–1.891) 0.13	= (0.225–0.246)	
120	(2–1.85) 0.73 = (1.46–1.351)	(1st preference)		
121				(0–1) 0.09 = (0–0.09)
122	(1–1.4) 0.27 = (0.27–0.378)	(1.73–1.75) 1.0	= (1.73–1.75)	
123	(2–1.88) 0.73 = (1.46–1.372)	(1st preference)		
124	(1–2,2) 0.27 = (0.27–0.594)	(1.73–2.164) 0.3	‖	(1.73–1.75) 0.91 = (1.574–1.593
125	(2–2.15) 0.73 = (1.46–1.570)			
126	(1–1.9) 0.27 = (0.27–0.513)	(1.73–1.791) 0.13	‖	
127	(2–1.75) 0.73 = (1.46–1.278)			
128				(0–0.8) 0.09 = (0–0.072)
129	(1–1.2) 0.27 = (0.27–0.324)	(1.73–1.331) 1.0	= (1.73–1.331)	
130	(2–1.38) 0.73 = (1.46–1.007)	(1st preference)		(1.73–1.331) 0.91 = (1.574–1.211)
131	(1–1.7) 0.27 = (0.27–0.459)	(1.73–1.591) 0.13	‖	
132	(2–1.55) 0.73 (1.46–1.132)			
133				(0–0.5) 0.09 = (0–0.045)
134	(1–0.75) 0.27 = (0.27–0.203)	(1.73–0.75) 1.0	= (1.73–0.75)	= (1.73–0.75) 0.91 = (1.574–0.683)
135	(2–0.75) 0.73 = (1.46–0.548)			
136				(0–0) 0.09 = (0–0)
137	(0–1) 0.27 = (0–0.27)	(0.73–1.365) 1.0	‖	
138	(1–1.5) 0.73 (0.73–1.095)			
139	(0–1) 0.27 = (0–0.27)	(0.73–1.256) 0.5	‖	
140	(1–1.35) 0.73 = (0.73–0.986)			
141	(0–0.8) 0.27 = (0–0.216)	(0.73–0.764) 0.3	‖	
142	(1–0.75) 0.73 = (0.73–0.548)			(0.095–0.051) 0.91 = (0.086–0.046)
143	(0–0.5) 0.27 = (0–0.135)	(0.73–0.391) 0.13	= (0.095–0.051)	
144	(1–0.35) 0.73 = (0.73–0.256)	(1st preference)		
145	(0–0)	= (0–0) 1.0 (2nd preference)	= (0–0)	

calculations are made for options 13–18, 21–23, and 25–26, which constitute the other basic choices at the beginning of year 4, within the earlier (hypothetical) decision (spanning all the options from 2 to 26 inclusive) of buying the machine in year 0 and running it in year 1.

The next phase of the calculation incorporates the possibility that whatever we have done up to then, there is a 0.09 possibility that it will be found to be redundant

Year 2		Year 1
(2.574–1.247) 1.0 = (2.574–1.247) 0.97	(0–0.5) 0.03 = (0.–0.015) = (2.497–1.210)	= (2.497–1.225) 0.02 = (0.050–0.025) (1st preference)
	(0–0) 0.03 = (0–0)	
(1.574–1.848) 1.0		
(1.574–1.688) 0.5		
	(0.161–0.08) 0.97 = (0.156–0.078)	(0.156–0.078) 1.0 [0.98] (2nd preference) = (0.153–0.076)
(1.574–1.283) 0.2		
(1.574–0.728) 0.05 = (0.079–0.036) (1st preference)		
(0.086–0.046) 1.0 [0.95] = (0.082–0.044) (2nd preference)		

at the beginning of year 3. This is what options 3, 12, 19, and 24 represent, so each of these has to be weighed against their respective complementary 0.91 probabilities that we shall be able to proceed along the options analysed above. Thus each of the earlier expected values for the joint options (4–11), (13–18), (21–23), and (25–26) has to be multiplied by 0.91 and their value, when added to the value of the redundancy risk, gives us (3.574–3.452), (3.574–3.591), (3.574–3.383), and (3.574–2.828).

We can now choose between them on a least-cost basis as before, from which it is obvious that the last one would be our first preference. But there is only a 0.05 chance of this being available (expected value (0.179–0.142), so we now turn to our second preference, which is the penultimate one. But this is only "available" with a 0.2 probability, so with a 0.95 chance that we may turn to it, its expected value is (0.679–0.643). The fall-back position, if neither of these is available, is 0.8 of 0.95 of (3.574–3.452), the first combined option, which generates an expected value of (2.716–2.624). Adding together these new expected values gives us (3.574–3.409) as the expected value of all the options from 3 to 26 inclusive, (although the options 12–18 have now dropped out of the picture).

At this stage the possibility of redundancy at the beginning of year 2 has to be brought in, and in this part of the decision tree this is represented by option 2, which has a probability of 0.03. When the expected value of this is added to 0.97 of our previously calculated expected value of (3.574–3.409), we obtain an expected value of (3.497–3.352) for options 2–26 inclusive. Similar calculations yield corresponding expected values of (3.497–3.616) for options 27–42, (3.497–3.409) for options 43–51, and (3.497–2.637) for options 52–55, each of which represents a set of choices to be made in year 1. Again our first preference is the least cost-combined option, and that is 52–55, but this has only a 0.02 probability of being available, generating an expected value of (0.07–0.053). Our second preference will be options 2–26, which, with the residual probability of 0.98, yields an expected value of (3.427–3.285). Adding these two together gives us (3.497–3.338), which then has a weight of 0.99 against option 1, which is the outcome (probability 0.01) that redundancy will occur at the start of year 1. Thus the expected value of options 1–55 is (3.497–3.348), and this is the key summary statistic for the "buy now" decision, if we go for it.

Table 4.6 does the same thing for all the options under the "wait" alternative. It proceeds in like manner, and the only complication is that the options numbered 111 onwards generate less benefits than the earlier ones, and option 136 et seq especially so. This means that we are forced to choose between blocks of options on grounds other than least cost. Here the rule we are given is to choose the least-cost-per-unit-of-benefit, i. e. choose those courses of action with the highest value of $\frac{\Sigma B}{\Sigma C}$.

On this basis we prefer options 133–135 $\left(\frac{1.574}{0.728}=2.162\right)$ to options 136–145 $\left(\frac{0.086}{0.046}=1.870\right)$, which in turn is better than 128–132, 121–127, or 112–120. Similarly in year 1, preference is given to options 107–110 (benefit: cost ratio 2.497 : 1.225 = 2.038) over options 111–145 (ratio 0.161 : 0.08 = 2.013), but both of these are markedly better than the ratios exhibited by any of the other options. At the end of the day, the "wait" strategy yields an expected value of (0.204–0.102). If this is compared with the "buy now" value of (3.497–3.348) it will be obvious that it yields a much better benefit: cost ratio, so the best strategy is to "wait".

Commentary

This example contained a moderate degree of complexity, but there is, of course, far more in the real world. However, if this extra complexity consists merely of further eventualities to be considered, it does not raise different issues of principle. I will therefore confine myself to some key issues that the example takes for granted.

The time horizon is arbitrary in the sense that problems seldom have natural and unique terminal points, and it is therefore a matter of judgement where, for analytical purposes, one chooses to truncate the planning horizons. This judgement will need to take note of the timing of any key *related* decisions (e.g. the commissioning of new premises), of financial planning or forecasting horizons (e.g. the assumption used here that no further purchases would be possible after year 3), the nature of the decisionmaking or review process, and so on.

The degree of risk is assumed to be reducible to probabilities associated with "states of the world", and these in turn are supposed to be independent of decisions that "we" make. It is not supposed that these probabilities are anything other than subjective estimates, though they may be the collective wisdom of "experts". The decision-makers are assumed to think in actuarial terms about "fair gambles", and not to be risk-averse (in the sense that a 0.5 chance of 1000 *plus* a 0.5 chance of 0 is valued the same as the certainty of 500. This is only likely to be true of organizations taking a large number of such decisions, no one of which is sizable in relation to its total operations. This is likely to be true of the British National Health Service in relation (say) to a particular scanner, but perhaps not to a small hospital faced with the same decision. In this latter case we would need to resolve these "expected values" into "certainty-equivalent values", which is a much more complicated form of evaluation.

We have assumed that benefits are reducible to a single unit of value (a QALY) and that these are known (or rather, explicitly estimated) for each alternative. This is often a source of uncertainty in itself, and the figure of 1000 used here may well be an "expected value" derived from a probability distribution over many possible benefit levels, depending on the reactions of clinicians, the local incidence of the relevant conditions or problems, the reactions of patients, etc. Moreover with multi-attribute benefit measures, assessment of gains becomes much more difficult unless dominance relationships emerge amongst the options.

It was assumed in this problem that benefits were not to be evaluated in money terms, though it would have made life much easier if they had. But it might also have changed the decision criterion, because we need then no longer work with benefit: cost *ratios*, but could have turned instead to the theoretically sounder criterion of the *difference* between benefits of costs. For instance, suppose that a QALY is worth £ 1000, then the benefit figures in the example can be interpreted as in millions of pounds, the same as the cost figures. It will immediately be observed that the "wait" alternative will now be valued at £ 0.204 million less £ 0.102 million (i.e. at £ 0.102 million) whilst the "buy now" alternative is worth £ 0.149 million (3.497 *less* 3.348), so the latter is now preferred to the former. This is actually too hasty a conclusion, however, because each choice that was made *within* each strategy needs to be reappraised according to this changed criterion, and the consequences reworked. It so happens that in this example the "buy now" alternative is unaffected, but in the "wait" alternative different choices would be made across options 112–145 in year 2 and across all options in year 1. The net effect of these changed preferences is to change the expected value of the "wait" strategy from (0.204–0.102) to (2.472–1.893), i.e. the new excess of benefits over costs is £ 0.579 million, which is still greater than the net benefits of the "buy now" strategy (still £ 0.149 million). The reason for the dramatic change in the "wait" strategy is that options 98–106 replace options 111–145 as the second preference in year 1 because although the latter has a higher *ratio* of benefits to costs it has a much smaller *difference*.

Thus the outcome can be quite sensitive to the decision rule used, though in this case the "wait" strategy remains the optimal one.

5 Discussion of Paper by Williams

J. F. Lacronique

Ministry of Health and Social Sciences, Paris

Let me start the discussion of Williams' paper by going back to the quotation from Banta's lecture on foetal monitoring. In his remarks Banta says "Questions that should have been asked 10 years earlier were asked for the first time". I think that here lies the central issue of the problem of evaluation – its timing. In Banta's account of the foetal monitoring story, I wonder if the question "Would it have been possible to ask the relevant questions about the new technology at an early stage?" would be no more possible than the question he actually asked. In fact, this is exactly why we are here – to answer this question. If the question were easy we would not be here.

To this question, many physicians would certainly give a negative answer – that it is futile, or simply impossible, to perform a good evaluation in the early stage of the development of a technology. In that case, we have just to deal with the "natural life cycle" of the technology and wait for the period of acceptance before discovering whether the application of the technology is (was) appropriate. The problem is then utilization review rather than technology appraisal. On the other hand, if we take the opposite standpoint – that evaluation is to be undertaken at the earliest possible stage – we have to deal with research into and the philosophy of technical progress. Practically, I cannot see any real example of such analysis, except the temporary moratorium for recombinant DNA experimentation and research on the building of a totally implantable artificial heart. In both of these examples, the result was only a delay in the funding by government grants and no more.

I would like now to turn to the issue of using the information derived from evaluation studies. The principal target for information is the medical profession, because it is physicians who decide whether to employ a new technology or to drop one that is obsolete or unsafe. Special attention should be paid to those technologies that are used mostly because they are money-makers. Take a special example – thermography, about which there seems to be a medical consensus as to its lack of therapeutic value although the debate on this has at times been bitter. I personally tried to persuade the Social Security administration to withdraw this procedure from the list of reimbursable procedures. But I did not succeed for the authorities do not want to raise further controversy on this subject. Thus, a critical issue in any discussion of evaluation has to be an examination of the various possible ways by which relevant and reliable information can be brought to the principal decision-maker – the user. Since the user is invariably a physician it is clear that we still have a long way to go in making them receptive to economic information. Thus, I agree strongly with the clinical decision-making approach, as illustrated by the works of McNeil and Fineberg, because it speaks a language that physicians understand.

This is not to say that physicians should stay only among their own kind. I do believe in teamwork. But I would like to see the economists paying more attention to the language they use, and I make the plea that they increase the relevance of their work so as to render assistance to the daily clinical practice of medicine. Such studies (McNeil, Fineberg etc.) precede the inclusion of a new method into the routine arsenal of health care. They include, of course, randomized trials. In my opinion there is a need for an intermediate position between the anecdotal first kind of study and the randomized or otherwise controlled studies. This intermediate type of study would owe to the first its applied nature and to the second its scientific methodology. A basic difference between this and the anecdotal ad hoc approach is that the middle way would routinely subject to scrutiny all relevant factors and not merely specific incidents.

This new approach should, moreover, focus on the quality of the routinely accepted technology as it is commonly used. At this level, the concern is not so much with the effectiveness, but is to do with meeting set standards. For example, in the case of renal dialysis, the issue is not so much on the efficacy of the machines, or their cost-benefit aspects, but simply on the way the machines are utilized – what kind of patients are treated? Accompanied by what kinds of other treatments? What kinds of diet should be prescribed to limit its costs? My own experience has convinced me that the questions that are actually asked about the technology of kidney replacement are more of the type "Can we instal machines near vacation resorts so as to let the patients have a normal holiday life?" or "How can we make renal transplant more attractive to surgeons or the nephrologist?", rather than "Is an artificial kidney worth its costs?"

I do not underestimate the value of cost-effectiveness analysis (CEA) but I think that the criteria for choice are in practice quite different for new medical equipment from what they are for capital projects in general. Therefore, I disagree with Williams when he classes effects on local or national employment, the balance of payments, and so on, as being of secondary importance. In my experience, these are the most important variables that actually influence decision-making, because we are dealing not with the merely technical but with highly political matters.

The second point is this: evaluations should never be considered to be definitive. However, since our objective is not merely cognitive, but aimed at helping decision-makers, there is the possibility that the conclusions of an evaluation may dramatically change the fate of a given technology, especially when the issue is to finance a project or let it die.

Williams devotes the major part of his paper to a plea for CEAs. I certainly do not have anything against CEA but I wonder if this is the crucial issue. Why do we need to evaluate technology today more than we did 10 or 20 years ago? There have been at least two classic approaches to evaluation, they have both been around a long time, and today there is more a need for a new spirit rather than a new methodology. One classic approach is the critical study of faults in the provision of services that physicians have observed. Such ad hoc evaluations can employ sound scientific methods, but their objectives are always of a limited pragmatic nature – to find out why something untoward has happened and to try to prevent it from happening again. This is the most primitive approach to evaluation since it implies that the damage has been done and the only benefit is the prevention of similar occurrences in the future. This kind of action – or rather reaction – is however still all too prevalent, which is why we need a more forward-looking method of proceeding.

The second classic approach is the method that epidemiologists started to use some 20 years ago to assess the differential effects of drugs in patients. Let me stress this point, for I have been exposed for 2 years to the difficulty of dealing with demands for implementation of various medical technology (e.g. positron imaging, neutron therapy, endocochlear-multielectrode audio-prosthesis, computerized medical records of numerous kinds, nuclear magnetic resonance). The consistent experience that I recall is one of discomfort and frustration simply because I played the role of the villain: I have been accused of being opposed to the advancement of science and to the well-being of mankind, of weakening the development of French industry, as well as some things I dare not tell you. Very few people are willing to accept a role that exposes one so brutally, especially when one shares the same fascination as everyone else for modern sophisticated technology. This is a very important point: is anyone strong enough to use evaluation data in such a fashion as to have a real impact on the use of a technology?

I will not discuss the pages that Williams devotes to definitions of key concepts. Let me just say that the mere need for these definitions proves that we are dealing with a subject that is subtle and potentially misleading, and even sometimes not far from rhetoric. I would nonetheless like to stress one point in Williams' definition of very costly technology. We in France had a law passed in 1970 according to which a particular technology was to be considered costly if it had the potential for permitting excessive use as well as having a high initial purchase cost. This applies, for example, to renal dialysis or to echo tomography. It also applies to laboratory equipment. I would also like to express my total agreement with the two definitions excerpted from Suchman's book, and will add one remark: evaluations should be repeatable, and in terms of international cooperation this means that an evaluation performed in one country may not apply to another.

6 Renal Replacement Therapy, Computerized Axial Tomography, and Cimetidine in Peptic Ulcer Disease

D. Taylor

Office of Health Economics, London

Introduction

In the 30 years from 1950 to 1980 the health care systems of Western Europe and North America passed through a remarkable process of expansion. In 1950 the average outlay on health care represented around 3% of the gross national product. Today the equivalent figure is of the order of 8%. This represents more than a sixfold increase in health spending in real terms. Those countries that have enjoyed the greatest economic growth in the last 3 decades have tended to divert the largest amounts of "new money", in both absolute and relative terms, into their health sectors.

Until the start of the 1970s the public and most of the leaders of the Western industrialized nations welcomed this trend. Many commentators automatically equated more health spending with better health. This, they hoped, would make the population more productive in economic terms. Whilst even those cynical about the direct consequence of extra health spending often believed that large sums spent on items like new hospitals at least purchased political good will and enhanced social stability. The very optimistic thought that health outlays would naturally stabilize at a "reasonable" level.

This last view implies that health care demand relates to finite, clearly definable needs, the satisfaction of which would halt the rise of, or in some circumstances actually start a decline in, medical expenditures. But this has not proved to be the practical experience of the developed countries. Population aging, rising consumer expectations, "cost-drift" associated with changes in sizes, structures, and rewards of the various medical manpower groups, and the introduction of new diagnostic and therapeutic technologies – all are examples of factors that have acted continuously to drive up health service expenditures.

Faced with the fall off in economic growth following the mid-1970s' oil crisis and suggestions that investment in health may have reached a period of declining marginal returns, governments and consumers have recently turned their attention to stopping the escalation of health costs. Strategies for attempting to ensure value for money include: imposing fixed overall budgets on health spending (as in the UK); influencing capital investment through, for instance, certificates of need regulations (the United States) or other capital spending controls (West Germany); introducing safety and efficiency regulations governing the market introduction of medicines and medical devices; and placing greater emphasis on the evaluation of, and dissemination of information about, technological innovations. In this last context there are a number of recent examples of increased national and internatioal activity. These include, for instance, in the United States the work of the albeit shortlived National Center for Health Care Technology (1978–1981) and the Office of Technology Assessment, founded by Congress in 1972 (see for illustration, office of Technology Assessment 1978 a, b, 1980 a, b). In Europe in 1980 a joint Nordic countries/WHO consultation examined British, Swedish, and American technology assessment programmes (World Health Organization 1980). The European Community's Directorate V is currently funding a major study on technology evaluation and management in the medical sector.

The objective of this volume is to present a comprehensive analysis of the methodological issues and problems involved in the analysis of technologies relevant to health care, via a detailed look at three areas. First, renal dialysis and transplantation, which became generally available in the 1960s. Second, computerized (axial) tomograhic (CAT or CT) scanning, a diagnostic technology introduced in the early 1970s. (This field is examined particularly in the context of brain scanning.) And, third, the use of the pharmaceutical product cimetidine to treat peptic ulcer disease, an innovation made available in much of the Western world during the late 1970s. The goals of this chapter are, first, to present background material about the historical development and basic nature of the technologies used in these three areas. Second, to outline the patterns of their diffusion and current supply in the industrialized Western nations. Third, to indicate some general economic points that may be drawn from the first two sections and to conclude by relating these to the problems underlying the processes of technology and health planning, particularly in the economic context.

Development Histories and Technical Aspects

Renal Replacement Therapy

Chronic or end-stage renal failure is a relatively uncommon condition in the industrialized nations, where the control of infectious diseases has cut its incidence very considerably in the last century or so (McKeown 1976). The annual incidence in subjects under 60 years of age is in the order of 40 individuals per million of the total population. If older individuals are included, then the projected incidence rises to between 60 and 150 per million per annum, depending on the assumptions made (Office of Health Economics 1978; Fineberg and Pearlman 1981 a). The higher figure of this range would include individuals dying of other causes who enter irreversible kidney failure.

In much of the Third World, where age-specific occurrence rates are probably an order of magnitude greater, resource constraints negate the possibility of any form of renal replacement therapy. Kidney failure victims meet a lingering, wasting death. But in Europe and North America the last half century or so has seen the emergence of a number of technologies that can offer long term survival to sufferers. The therapeutic choices available are indicated in Fig. 6.1.

Animals were experimentally dialysed before the First World War. That is, creatures such as dogs that had had their kidneys removed were kept alive by means of a machine which took from their blood wastes the kidneys normally dispose of. It was

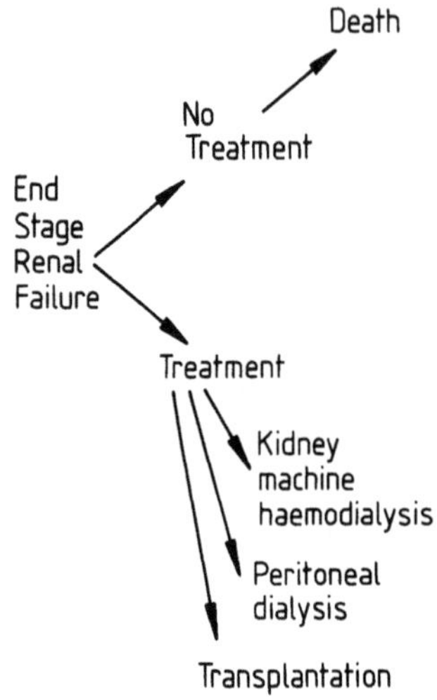

Fig. 6.1. Therapeutic choices in the management of end-stage renal failure

passed over a membrane permeable enough to let molecules of substances like urea diffuse out into a cleansing, dialysate fluid on the other side, but impermeable enough to prevent larger bodies like the blood cells passing through. Some early twentieth century experiments also involved the peritoneal dialysis of animals, a method referred to later in the text. However, the technique was not suitable for use in man. The semi-permeable membranes then available were unsatisfactory, a problem not solved until the development of synthetic cellulose acetate as a potential membrane material in the 1930s. Also improved anti-coagulents were needed to stop the blood clotting outside the body. Purified heparin, the first suitable agent, again only became commercially available in the 1930s.

After these two key developments had taken place, the way was open for trials of human haemodialysis. Kolff, working in Holland in 1943, constructed a rotating drum artificial kidney as a treatment for acute renal failure. Therapy based on his technique has subsequently saved the lives of many people who were temporarily without normal kidney function. But health workers in the 1950s were not able to supply the long-term therapy needed by those who had entered end-stage renal failure resulting from, say, the various forms of nephritis (for example "glomerulonephritis"), cystic renal disease, and factors like phenacitin abuse or kidney-damaging hypertensive illness. This was because the patients' blood vessels were damaged by the access method then employed. Repeated dialysis destroyed all the sites available for exchanging the blood. But in 1960 a novel type of junction, known as the Quinton-Scribner shunt, was developed in America. Using the then new materials teflon and silastic this acted as a durable artificial blood vessel via which the patient and his or her kidney machine could be linked. Yet it had to be replaced from time to time, was subject to occasional failures leading to blood loss, and also suffered the disadvantage of being external to the patient's body. This if nothing else sometimes proved psychologically distressing.

In 1967 an alternative American technique, commonly known as the Cimino-Brescia internal fistula, was introduced. This involves joining a peripheral artery to a nearby vein, which subsequently thickens. It then becomes possible to access the circulatory system by venepuncture using a wide-bore needle. Although this can be painful it has a number of advantages, including reduced clotting risk. Over 80% of patients on haemodialysis today use the Cimino-Brescia fistula, together with dialysis machines incorporating semi-permeable membranes.

Dialysis typically involves treatment every 2 days, lasting for periods of 3–8 h depending on the needs of the patient. The quality of life that results is variable. Some patients, especially those using home-based machines at night, can have a fairly satisfactory existence. But for others there are both physical and psychological problems and side effects. Psycho-social factors are particularly influential in determining survival (Wai et al. 1981).

A more satisfactory form of treatment may thus be kidney transplantation. Once again, this was first done on animals at the turn of the century. But the problem of immune rejection of grafts meant that the procedure was not attempted in man until the 1950s. The first long-surviving graft, involving a transplant between identical twins who in normal circumstances do not reject each other's tissue, was achieved in 1956. In 1960 the first immunosuppressive drug was introduced, and it was that which opened the way to large scale transplantation programmes. Since then further work on the nature of the human immune system and the use of immunosuppressive medicines has increased the viability of this form of renal replacement therapy. But even so the average 5-year cadaver graft survival probability is still only about 35%. And many renal failure sufferers are either not suitable for or cannot obtain a suitable organ replacement. Research may in the future generate new forms of immunosuppression, which will lift some of the restrictions on transplantation. But for the present there are still a number of patients who cannot benefit from either the latter or conventional haemodialysis. For them the only alternatives are haemofiltration or some form of peritoneal dialysis.

Haemofiltration involves the extraction of toxic substances such as urea from a patient's blood by filtration under pressure against a cellulose screen. The plasma and toxic wastes pass through and are disposed of, whilst the remaining blood constituents are made up with a suitable replacement fluid and passed back into the patient. For individuals suffering from some forms of blood pressure or from "dialysis dementia" (side effect of dialysis believed to be related to the build up of toxic levels of aluminium), this may be a worthwhile form of therapy. But it is expensive.

In recent years rather more attention has been paid to forms of peritoneal dialysis. In this the peritoneum, the lining of the abdomen cavity, is filled with dialysate fluid, into which toxic materials pass from the blood vessels on the other side of the peritoneum. The technique is simple and effective in clearing even relatively large molecules. Initial work on the treatment of patients with acute renal failure with intermittent (that is occasional, intensive) peritoneal dialysis was done by Ganter in Germany and Heusser and Werder in Switzerland in the 1920s. Yet access to the peritoneum was difficult, and the complications caused by treatment were often fatal. However, in the 1960s Tenckhoff in the United States reduced this barrier by developing a special peritoneal dialysis catheter designed to give a permanent point of entry to the body cavity. And in 1976 a Russian/American, Popovich, introduced the basis of a technique now known as continuous ambulatory peritoneal dialysis (CAPD) (Popovich et al. 1978). This involves a constant process of gradual exchange, with dialysate fluid permantly in the body cavity. It was pioneered in practive by Oreopolous in Canada in 1977 (Oreopolous et al. 1980).

Some renal specialists hope that because CAPD is less complex than conventional techniques involving a kidney machine, more people, especially older subjects, will be able to use it in their own homes. Economic savings may be significant. Yet for the moment it too is not without problems. Peritonitis is still a fairly frequent complication, despite some attempts to control it with prophylactic antibiotic therapy.

For such reasons research into improved ways of treating endstage renal failure is thus continuing. One possibility is that ways will be found of regenerating dialysate fluid in situ in the peritoneum. Another is that orally administered substances could promote gastro-intestinal excretion of blood-transported wastes. This last could well act as a valuable supplement to techniques like CAPD, so contributing to the gradual, largely unplanned evolution of therapies capable of prolonging the survival of, and hopefully granting an acceptable life-style to, people unfortunate enough to enter end-stage renal failure.

Computerized Axial Tomography

In November 1885 Wilhelm Roentgen, working in the University of Würzburg in Bavaria, discovered "X" rays (the "X" stood for an unknown quantity). Over the course of the following century, Roentgen's work has proved to have many applications in health care, the most widely appreciated of which relate to medical imaging. CT scanning is one of the most important developments in the history of this last area. Its significance is that whereas in conventional X-ray pictures internal structures are superimposed one on top of another, in CT scans a cross-section of the body being examined is provided. Masking effects, most troublesome in the case of the brain and spinal neural structures that are completely encased in bone, are eliminated. Also in conventional X-ray images it can be very difficult to distinguish between adjacent soft tissues of similar densities. Scanner images are usually easier to interpret.

A scanner involves mounting an X-ray source on a gantry, on the opposite side of which are sensitive X-ray detectors (Fig. 6.2). The patient lies inside this structure, which surrounds him or her like a hoop. It turns a series of small, rapid steps and the intensity of the X-rays transmitted through the body is recorded at each point. The resulting mass of data is converted by computer into a cross-sectional image of the body, which in the case of the best modern machines relates to a slice only a millimetre or so thick.

The concept of tomography (from the Greek "tomo" cutting, and "graphy", to write) is several decades old. Conventional tomographs (made by moving an X-ray source in a curvilinear manner in one direction above a subject and an X-ray film in the opposite direction under the subject) were to some extent able to "blur out" unwanted structures. And by the early 1960s researchers such as Oldendorf, Cormack, and Kuhl in the United States had constructed elementary scanners which used relatively simple image reconstruction techniques.

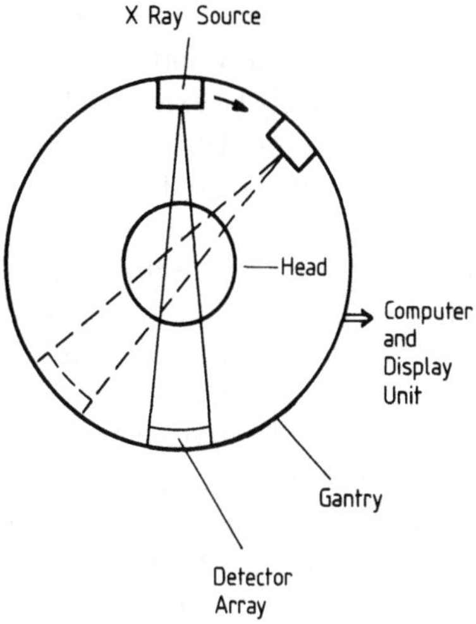

Fig. 6.2. Schematic diagram of CT scanner

In 1967 Hounsfield was able to utilize a mathematically accurate method of image reconstruction to produce cross-sectional pictures of inanimate objects. The British company he worked for (EMI) requested assistance from the Department of Health and Social Security to develop a prototype brain scanner. This was installed in the Atkinson Morley Hospital in 1971 and was followed by four other experimental, partially state funded, machines (Stocking and Morrison 1978). Hounsfield's belief in the new technology's value to radiology was swiftly confirmed. The alternative methods of investigating the brain then commonly used included cerebral angiography (involving the injection of radio-opaque material into the carotid artery); pneumoencephalography (which requires replacement of the cerebrospinal fluid bathing the nervous system with air or other gas); and isotope scanning (injection of radioactive material into the blood and photography with gamma-cameras). They are more prone to side effects and are less effective.

The first commercial brain scanner was sold to the Mayo clinic in 1973. The first whole-body scanner, developed by Ledley, was installed in the Georgetown University Center in 1974. The reasons why the early machines were brain rather than whole-body scanners (that is, had gantries with a diameter capable of accepting only the patient's head) were basically twofold. First, those with a smaller distance between the X-ray source and the detectors opposite were perhaps easier to construct. Second, the early technology required a total scan time of some 300 s. Body movement would have made the image impossible to reconstruct clearly.

The first commercial body scanner, marketed by Pfizer, cut scanning time to 150 s. This was swiftly followed by a British (EMI) machine with a scan time of 18–20 s–an easy breath-holding period for most people. Today the best machines available have a scan time of under 2 s. Commercial competition has led to a very high rate of product improvement in the scanner market, so much so that purchasers may well be advised to ensure that machines are designed so that they can be updated to incorporate new software/hardware as it becomes available.

Developments like these, combined with the greater resolving power of modern installations, mean that the distinction between body scanners and brain scanners has largely become outmoded. Most machines now purchased have whole-body scanning capability, although this does not necessarily mean to say that their use should routinely be extended beyond the head and the spinal structures. This decision depends on the benefits to be expected from the various ways in which CT scanners might be used.

It would be beyond the scope of this paper to investigate the latter area in detail. However, it is of note that Fineberg et al. (1977) have argued that in this context there are five questions to be asked of scanner technology: (1) technical capability – does the device perform reliably and deliver accurate information? (2) diagnostic accuracy – does use of the device permit accurate diagnoses? (3) diagnostic impact – does use of the device replace other diagnostic procedures, including surgical exploration and biopsy? (4) therapeutic impact – do results obtained from the device affect planning and delivery of therapy? (5) patient outcome – does use of the device contribute to improved health of the patient? Currently available machines are so sophisticated that for many conditions, perhaps the most important of which is cancer, the answers to the first two or three of these questions will at present often be positive, although in a variety of instances scanning complements rather than replaces other technologies. It is usually with regard to the last two questions that the answers are either uncertain or negative. That is, in areas other than brain scanning the future of the technology will hinge on the evolution of therapeutic interventions. For example, if effective systemic anti-cancer drugs are developed, whole-body scanning may become generally more useful but not essential or particularly cost-effective. If, alternatively, effective cancer therapy based on, say, the highly accurate delivery of some type of radiation is introduced whole-body scanning could well be an integral part of care planning and delivery. In such a context it might be regarded as highly cost-effective and cost-beneficial.

However, there is a final point to add here. It is that although CT scanning was the most exciting medical imaging advance of the 1970s, rivals are now emerging. Ultrasound imaging was another important British advance generated in the 1960s and 1970s. Today CT ultrasound machines are becoming available. Although these will not be of value in brain investigations they may be very useful in other contexts. Also, perhaps more significantly, the viability of imaging involving nuclear magnetic resonance effects is now actively being investigated. In Britain there are several projects already in progress, and American, European, and Japanese companies are also investigating the field.

In some areas it may thus be that CT X-ray scanning will become outmoded. One advantage that new alternatives may offer is freedom from the albeit small risks associated with even minimal X-ray dosages. In other instances it seems likely that the new imaging techniques will serve a complementary role, so adding further dimensions to the already complex problems surrounding resource allocation in this field (Wagner 1981; Stocking 1982).

The Treatment of Peptic Ulcer Disease

Peptic ulcers are lesions of the mucous membrane lining the stomach and the small intestine or duodenum. They commonly cause epigastric pain and may also result in events such as sudden, heavy blood loss and perforation. The latter permits entry of the contents of the upper digestive tract into the body cavity. Thus they are frequently incapacitating and sometimes life-threatening. Peptic ulcer disease is, when untreated, of chronic duration, although after a period ranging from 7 to 15 years typical subjects tend to recover, at least partially. A variety of factors, the mechanisms of which are not fully understood, may initiate the formation of gastric or duodenal ulcers. What is clear is that relatively high concentrations of stomach acid contribute to the disease(s) processes. The latter are referred to in the plural because although peptic ulcer is a convenient general term epidemiological observations suggest that gastric and duodenal ulcers are to an extent discrete states.

Most studies indicate that the incidence rate of duodenal ulcers is about four times that of those situated in the stomach – say about 1–1.5/1000 adults compared with 0.3/1000, respectively. Gastric ulcers are evenly distributed between sexes, whilst those of the duodenum are roughly twice as frequent in men. From mid-life onwards the onset rate stays fairly stable. It is conventionally "guesstimated" that about one man in ten will suffer a duodenal ulcer before retirement age. But the incidence of the disease has been falling in the West in recent years, so this figure may be a little high. Even so peptic ulcer disease remains a significant cause of long-term morbidity within the working population (Fineberg and Pearlman 1981b).

Treatment has developed along two lines, medication and surgery. In both a key goal is to reduce stomach acidity and so to promote healing and prevent recurrence. Surgery also often has reconstructive goals. The pattern of treatment choices is illustrated in Fig. 6.3.

The historical background to the development of cimetidine by the American company Smith, Kline and French has been described by Dollery (1978). The basic understanding that acid was involved in the digestive process began to emerge in France and Italy in the eighteenth century, when scientists lowered perforated capsules into the stomachs of experimental animals and extracted samples of the gastric juice. But it was not until the first half of the nineteenth century that it was found to contain hydrochloric acid. It was the Russian, Pavlov, working in the opening years of the twentieth century, who showed that the gastric tissue's excretion of acid was mediated by the vagus nerve. This discovery opened the way to the important surgical innovation of vagotomy, described briefly later in this paper.

Regarding chemotherapy the use of atropine and other anticholinergic drugs in attempts to control stomach acidity stemmed from their inhibitory effects on the vagus nerve. But this, like special diets recommended by many nineteenth- (and twentieth-) century physicians, was of little real value. However, the avoidance of mucosal irritants is obviously desirable, as may be the use of antacids – alkaline substances that offset the effects of excessive stomach acid. One of the earliest (and simplest) of the latter to be employed in medical practice was sodium bicarbonate. It is effective, but can cause systemic alkalosis.

Carbenoxolone, a drug derived from liquorice, has been available in some countries from about the mid-1960s. It improves the resistance of the stomach and duodenal lining to damage from acid. Certain bismuth preparations have a direct protective effect. But what is arguably the major therapeutic breakthrough came from initially academic theorizing on the role of histamine in controlling gastric acid secretion. First synthesized by German chemists in 1907, histamine had for many years been

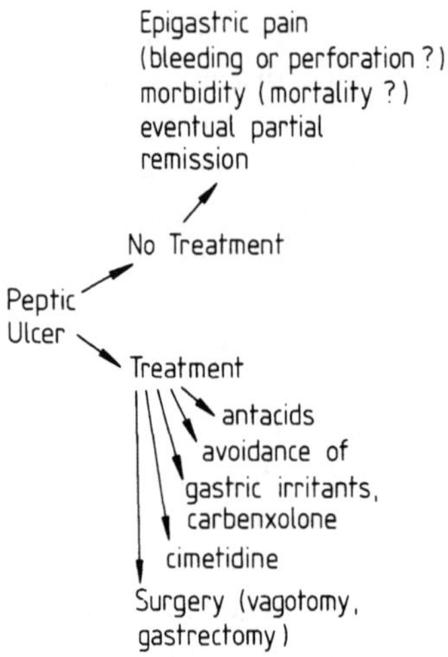

Fig. 6.3. Pattern of treatment choices in peptic ulcer

suspected of involvement in this area. Yet conventional anti-histamines have no effect in ulcer disease.

In 1966 Ash and Schild suggested that there might be two types of histamine receptor, those being termed H_2 being involved in the control of stomach acid levels. Black, working in the SKF laboratories in England, decided to seek out a drug that would block the (then theoretically existent) H_2 receptors in the stomach. He and his colleagues produced over 700 variants of the histamine molecule before announcing an initial success in 1972. Burimamide showed that the H_2 theory was realistic but was not itself clinically useful. The next drug tested, metiamide, was effective but in human trials in 1974 was shown to have undesired side-effects on the blood's white cells. Cimetidine finally was approved for the market in Britain in 1976.

The significance of the drug is that it acts to block the initial release of stomach acid, an effect hitherto achieved only by surgery. The side effects of surgical intervention are, however, relatively high. In the short term there are the immediate operative and post-operative risks. In the longer term reduced stomach size can lead to discomfort associated with the "dumping syndrome". Food is rapidly emptied from the stomach into the intestines, leading to symptoms like flushing and diarrhoea. And there is also a low risk of cancer of the digestive tract after peptic ulcer surgery.

Regarding the history of the alternatives to medical interventions it would be beyond the scope of this short introductory paper to go into the details of areas like X-ray therapy for this condition or the background of gastric freezing treatment. This first was of limited value and relatively dangerous; the second was adopted rapidly in the United States but was in British trials also shown to be ineffective and, in some instances, harmful.

As to surgery the two key types of techniques are partial gastrectomy and vagotomy (Ellis 1979). The former was introduced after anaesthesia had led to a wave of surgical innovation at the start of the twentieth century. It peaked in popularity in the 1920s and 1930s. In simple terms gastrectomy involves cutting away areas of the stomach wall (the parietal cell mass), and reforming the stomach to form a much smaller organ. Ulcerated parts of the doudenum just below the stomach may be bypassed and then a new link made with the rest of the intestine. Vagotomy was introduced by Dragstedt. He initially cut the vagus nerve relatively high up (truncal vagotomy), which led to reduced stomach acid secretion but also to unwanted side effects. Although these can in part be overcome by interventions aimed at facilitating adequate stomach drainage, surgeons now prefer some form of selective vagotomy. At its most refined this cuts off nervous stimulation to the parietal cells alone. However, because of improvements in medicines the need for surgery has been reduced. Its indications are becoming increasingly seen as being confined to reconstruction work (when the passage of food is blocked or restricted) or emergency treatment, as in cases of ulcer perforation and uncontrollable bleeding. And even in the latter case conventional surgery may become obsolete.

In the late 1950s fibre-optic endoscopy was introduced. This allows physicians visually to inspect the digestive tract. The head of the endoscope, which contains a light source and an optical system, is passed down the patient's throat. The light travels back along flexible fibres to the observer. Diagnostic accuracy in relation to peptic ulcers has been greatly improved by this invention. Now the technique may be complemented by lasers, employed as surgical tools. The combination of the use of such devices to stop ulcer bleeding with sophisticated pharmacological aids to healing may soon relegate operations like gastrectomy to the history books.

The Diffusion of Technology and the Supply of Care

Renal Dialysis and Transplantation

Of the three areas considered in this paper the most adequately monitored across Europe is renal replacement therapy. This is due to the work of the European Dialysis and Transplant Association (EDTA), an independent body established by renal specialists in 1964. Tables 6.1–6.3 present EDTA data relating to the expansion of services in Europe during the last decade. The figures shown raise three sets of points worth special emphasis in the context of this paper. The first is that as with other technologies the supply of renal replacement therapies is a function of two broad factors – the structure of the health services of any given country and the overall wealth of that country. In the earlier years of the 1960s nations like Britain and Denmark, with strong central planning capabilities in the health sector, were the first to initiate comprehensive care programmes. But as the technology of dialysis and transplantation became better established, richer nations increased rapidly the number of patients being accepted for care. It is of note that America had a new patient acceptance rate of around 60 patients million of the population in 1980, or more than twice the EDTA register average.

Following on from this, the second point is that Britain in particular has adopted rather different policies from the rest of Europe. For instance, two thirds of dialysis patients in the UK use home machines. This is unique. In most countries well under one-fifth of the total receive home dialysis. Against this Britain has only one hospital dialysis centre and ten hospital dialysis stations per million people, compared with around 4 and 40 respectively, for France, Germany, Spain, and Italy col-

Table 6.1. End-stage renal failure patients alive on treatment – 1970, 1975, and 1980 (UK Transplant 1981)

1970			1975			1980		
Country	PMP		Country	PMP		Country	PMP	
	Total	Grafted		Total	Grafted		Total	Grafted
Denmark	58.5	34.1	Denmark	129.6	74.4	Switzerland	259.7	88.6
Switzerland	45.7	13.4	Switzerland	119.8	41.9	Israel	238.1	35.9
Sweden	36.5	14.9	Israel	119.7	14.8	Belgium	233.1	64.9
Netherlands	31.3	5.0	Belgium	102.4	31.2	France	228.6	29.8
Belgium	28.8	9.8	France	94.7	11.1	Fed. Rep. Germany	208.0	17.6
United Kingdom	24.7	5.6	Luxembourg	90.0	0	Denmark	202.0	94.1
France	23.6	2.8	Netherlands	84.8	21.3	Italy	197.0	14.1
Finland	20.6	7.6	Sweden	83.9	39.1	Netherlands	185.5	55.9
Ireland	19.0	3.1	Italy	74.0	4.77	Sweden	178.1	83.9
[a]			Fed. Rep. Germany	71.9	3.6	Luxembourg	177.5	5.0
			Norway	70.5	51.8	Spain	144.5	11.8
			Finland	67.4	40.8	Cyprus	143.3	26.7
			United Kingdom	65.4	24.3	Finland	134.6	87.7
			Austria	54.5	18.2	Austria	133.9	25.9
						Norway	133.7	88.8
						United Kingdom	127.6	56.3
						Greece	118.6	14.8
Total registry	15.2	2.1	Total registry	47.8	9.2	Total registry	117.6	21.6

Abbreviation: PMP, patients per million population

[a] Only nations with above EDTA average rates are shown

Table 6.2. New end-stage renal failure patients – 1970, 1975, and 1980 (UK Transplant 1981)

1970			1975			1980		
Country	PMP		Country	PMP		Country	PMP	
	Total	Grafted		Total	Grafted		Total	Grafted
Denmark	35.5	11.4	Luxembourg	50.0	1.1	Israel	61.6	27.6
Switzerland	22.5	4.3	Isreal	36.2	10.3	Cyprus	56.7	11.7
Sweden	15.8	9.0	Switzerland	31.7	12.7	Sweden	48.4	20.1
Belgium	14.1	5.2	France	28.6	8.3	Switzerland	48.3	24.1
Netherlands	12.1	3.1	Sweden	27.8	17.4	Luxembourg	47.5	35.0
France	11.9	2.4	Belgium	27.5	11.6	Fed. Rep. Germany	44.5	18.9
Israel	10.8	1.2	Norway	27.4	14.3	France	42.6	16.7
Luxembourg	10.0	0	Austria	26.3	13.7	Belgium	41.5	23.1
Norway	9.2	2.1	Finland	26.3	13.6	Norway	38.3	20.7
United Kingdom	9.2	3.8	Denmark	26.1	17.6	Finland	38.1	18.5
Austria	8.7	5.8	Fed. Rep. Germany	25.4	10.6	Spain	37.0	9.5
Fed. Rep. Germany	8.3	3.6	Italy	23.2	8.0	Italy	34.2	14.1
Finland	7.7	3.2	Netherlands	19.4	6.7	Austria	33.7	19.3
[a]			United Kingdom	16.1	7.1	Netherlands	32.4	12.9
						Denmark	28.8	22.4
						United Kingdom	24.6	9.1
Total registry	7.6	2.6	Total registry	15.3	6.2	Total registry	24.6	7.7

Abbreviation: PMP, patients per million population

[a] Only nations with above EDTA average rates are shown

Table 6.3. Number of transplants – 1970, 1975, and 1980

1970			1975			1980		
Country	PMP		Country	PMP		Country	PMP	
	Total grafts	cadaver grafts		Total grafts	cadaver grafts		Total grafts	cadaver grafts
Denmark	27.4	24.3	Norway	24.7	16.7	Finland	29.0	20.4
Sweden	12.4	11.9	Denmark	22.3	21.5	Switzerland	23.0	21.3
Switzerland	8.7	8.4	Sweden	19.3	16.5	Sweden	22.7	14.0
Belgium	6.7	5.7	Finland	15.7	14.2	Denmark	20.4	14.7
Norway	5.5	3.4	Switzerland	13.9	13.9	Israel	20.0	17.0
Iceland	5.0	0	United Kingdom	11.9	10.4	Norway	19.5	11.2
United Kingdom	4.5	3.9	Austria	11.3	10.9	United Kingdom	16.9	14.4
Netherlands	2.9	2.8	Belgium	8.6	8.0	Belgium	14.7	11.2
Austria	2.7	2.7	Netherlands	8.1	8.0	Iceland	12.2	9.4
Israel	2.3	1.2	Israel	6.5	5.6	Netherlands	10.4	8.7
Finland	2.1	0.6	Ireland	5.4	4.8	France	9.4	7.8
Ireland	2.1	2.1	France	4.8	4.4	Austria	7.5	6.9
[a]						Dem. Rep. Germany	6.9	6.8
						Fed. Rep. Germany	6.7	5.2
Total registry	2.1	1.8	Total registry	4.1	3.6	Total registry	6.6	5.3

Abbreviation: PMP, patients per million population

[a] Only nations with above EDTA average rates are shown

lectively. Britain in 1980 had nearly 6% of all its dialysis patients on CAPD, compared with an EDTA average of just over 2% (UK Transplant 1981).

Just under a half of all living British kidney patients have a graft; and in 1980 the number of kidney transplants done was equal to two-thirds of the total number of new UK kidney failure patients accepted. For the EDTA nations as a whole the equivalent proportions are around one-fifth and one-quarter. The basic explanation for such discrepancies is indicated in Table 6.4. British provision developed at a time when it was thought that only relatively fit, young patients would be suitable for treatment, and that their quality of life would be best maintained by a transplant or by home dialysis. Neither of these treatment modes are desirable for a large proportion of older subjects. But not surprisingly, perhaps, many older people (and their families) want to obtain renal replacement therapy.

Other European and North American countries have developed hospital facilities for caring for their elderly and otherwise less independent end-stage renal failure victims. Britain has not, although CAPD may be suitable for some such subjects. (In some British clinics today up to half of new patients are started on this form of haemodialysis). It is a matter of debate whether this is due to an informed analysis of all the social and monetary costs and benefits involved or to crude "economic" considerations (Office of Health Economics 1980). There is a case to be made both for and against the British strategy. But what is certain is that few other countries would have the planning and allied machinery for enforcing such successful control over the expansion of high-technology medical care.

The third point to be made is that current renal patient survival figures indicate that on a new patient acceptance ("flow") rate of 40–60/million population/year, an equilibrium level of patients living either on dialysis or with a graft will probably approach 500/million population. This is nearly twice even Switzerland's current "stock" figure. The full cost of renal replacement therapy will not be expressed in most health care systems until the twenty-first century. Such flow and stock (or incidence and prevalence) calculations affect many areas of health care.

Table 6.4. Acceptance of new end-stage renal failure patients by age and country for 1978 (Office of Health Economics 1980)

Age-group (years)	Rate per million population			
	West Germany	France	Italy	United Kingdom
15	2.3	3.9	3.5	4.0
15–24	13.1	13.9	12.5	17.7
25–34	22.8	27.6	22.0	26.9
35–44	41.7	34.2	37.2	33.1
45–54	58.8	59.8	55.7	43.5
55–64	71.3	69.5	69.5	22.7
65–74	49.9	56.6	52.2	3.5
75+	8.6	17.6	7.3	0
Total	30.9	39.4	29.0	19.2

Computed Tomographic Scanning

As has already been described brain scanners first became commercially available in 1973 and whole-body scanners in 1974. Subsequently the United States and Japan have adopted this technology most enthusiastically. As Table 6.5 shows by 1979 the former had installed over 1200 machines, with at least one available in four out of five hospitals. Japan had at that time the second highest provision. But there the ratio of brain to body scanners was notably different according to the Office of Technology Assessment (1981 a). Although the material shown in Table 6.5 is now a little outdated (Britain now has installed about 80 machines, half of which have whole-body capability, whereas Japan's stock of scanners has risen dramatically) it is quite clear that European uptake has been much more controlled.

The basic question is "why should the US and Japan together in 1979/80 have had some seven scanners million population whilst Sweden had only two and France and Britain nearer one?". The answer in France's case may have been partly to do with national economic policy and the desire to develop domestic industry. But in Britain's case such restraints could hardly have been relevant. In reality the explanation lies more in the market structure for health care and the extent of government control over the evaluation and purchase of capital equipment like scanners. (They typically cost around £400000 each.) Despite the US's experiments in areas like "certificate of need" legislation, that country basically has a fee for items of service system in health. Physicians act as entrepreneurs. If demand for items like scans exists or can be created amongst consumers, then US physicians will supply, provided it can be done economically, that is at a profit. By contrast in Britain health authorities control capital spending tightly. The most salient factor is that the National Health Service (NHS) operates within a strictly limited overall budget. A

Table 6.5. Distribution of installed CT scanners by country for 1978 and 1979 (Office of Technology Assessment 1980[b])

	March 1978				1979			
Country[a]	Number of Scanners			Scanners per million population	Number of Scanners			Scanners per million population
	Head	Body	Total		Head	Body	Total	
United States	337	668	1005	4.6	400	854	1254	5.7 (Feb)
Japan	180	112	292	2.6	304	212	516	4.6 (Apr)
West Germany	51	42	93	1.5	U	U	160	2.6 (July)
Australia	U	U	U	U	7	21	28	1.9 (Jan)
Canada	U	U	U	U	9	29	38	1.7 (May)
Sweden	8	5	13	1.6	8	6	14	1.7 (Feb)
Netherlands[b]	U	U	U	U	U	U	20	1.4 (Jan)
United Kingdom	36	16	52	0.9	39	18	57	1.0 (Jan)
France[c]	10	2	12	0.2	20	10	30	0.6 (Jan)
Iceland	0	0	0	0.0	0	0	0	0.0 (Jan)

Abbreviation: U, unknown

[a] Ranked by scanners per million population in 1979

[b] The Netherlands planned to install 30 head scanners and body scanners at the time this data was collected

[c] In France an additional 21 scanners were authorized in July 1979

strong case has to be made for the extension of any expensive technology, diagnostic or curative. Whether the stringency the UK authorities have shown has been in the public interest is, however, once again a matter of debate. But it may be observed that in the case of CT scanning the social security and/or insurance-based health systems of Europe appear to have acted more like the British than the American model.

A final point to add in this context is that in Britain a substantial number (over half) of the scanners recently deployed in NHS units have actually been purchased with money donated by the public and then given to the health authorities. This bypasses controls imposed by government, although in some localities the NHS is now refusing such "gifts" unless they are accompanied by pledges to meet running costs as well.

Cimetidine

At the start of the 1970s surgical interventions aimed at treating peptic ulcer disease were running in the UK, US, and Holland at a level that was around twice the figure for 1980. In part this fall was related to an apparent underlying reduction in the prevalence of the disease. But in the latter half of the 1970s, coinciding with the introduction of cimetidine, the drop in surgery rates accelerated notably. The new drug and its promotion by the innovating company had a swift and significant effect on both the provision of health care and, according to new British data, on the level of incapacitating peptic ulcer disease morbidity experienced by the population.

Fineberg and Pearlman (1981b) have described the initial diffusion of cimetidine. They noted that after its introduction in the UK in November 1976 the FDA[1] in the United States recognized its clinical promise and expedited the process of its approval for marketing. This was finally granted in America in August 1977. The indications accepted were duodenal ulcer disease – at first for only 8 weeks' treatment – and hypersecretary conditions like the Zollinger-Ellison syndrome and hormone-secreting tumours. Yet there was a very rapid spread of the medicine's use in US clinical practice. Fineberg stressed that a substantial proportion of cimetidine prescribed in America, perhaps as much as a half, is for patients with problems like acid reflux and gastritis. In Britain too interest has been shown in non-ulcer H_2 antagonist applications, such as pancreatitis. The result of cimetidine's swift diffusion was that in 1979 it was consumed by some 10 million individuals worldwide. Since that time, as Table 6.6 indicates, the volume consumption of the medicine has continued to expand. One factor in this process has been its extended employment for prophylactic purposes.

Perhaps the most important point to make regarding the available data is that there appears to be significantly less variation in overall cimetidine use between countries like Britain and America than in CT scanning and renal replacement therapy. The 1980 crude per capita volume consumption ratio between the US and the UK was around 1.8:1. In, say, the case of new patient acceptance rates for dialysis or transplantation the equivalent figure was about 2.4:1. The deployment of CT

1 Food and Drug Administration, USA

Table 6.6. Index of volume (kg per capita) consumption of cimetidine, US and UK, in the first 4 of years medical use. (use × quarter, year 1 = 100). Not adjusted for age/sex population variations

	Year				Quarter[a]
	1	2	3	4	
US	46	200	347	461	1
	100	240	384	506	2
	145	292	414	526	3
	187	318	438	559	4
(Mean – year 1/year 4 = 4.2)					
UK	77	141	218	259	1
	92	157	222	255	2
	108	178	214	276	3
	124	207	243	310	4
(Mean – year 1/year 4 = 2.75)					

[a] Quarter 1 year 1 in the UK began January 1977, in the US it began August 1977
Source: Smith, Kline and French (personal communication)

scanners per unit population was over 5:1. The factors underlying this observation include the possibility that there is relatively more professional certainty and confidence about the role and value of the pharmaceutical product than in the two other instances; that different financial pressures are at work; and that promotional and other distributional influences have been important.

Conclusions

The data in this paper suggest a number of points regarding the evaluation of medical technologies and the factors influencing their diffusion. The key one is that as far as the latter area is concerned budgetary controls on either overall or capital spending, coupled with regulations affecting medical fee structures, appear to be the main determining factors. The process of evaluation seems in many instances to occur independently, after a particular technology has already achieved widespread usage. What limits there are to the diffusion process thus tend to be set by relatively arbitrary forces.

This is a disturbing conclusion. It can be convincingly argued that it would be desirable to associate more closely the processes of technology evaluation and diffusion. This would enable rational planning and resource allocation decisions to be made and the systems of incentive and control within health sectors to be adjusted accordingly.

At a time when, as the introduction to this paper noted, pressure to restrict health care funding is relatively high, it is important to stress that spending limits per se cannot ensure "value for money". If the well-being of a population is to be raised to the highest possible levels purposeful efforts have to be made to ensure that the greatest marginal benefit is obtained for each extra unit of cost. Unfortunaltely, however, there are substantial barriers to the achievement of such a goal. As the three development histories that have been outlined indicate "revolutionary" medical technologies are normally the end result of prolonged, gradual, and largely unpredictable processes of evolution. They usually cannot be anticipated, and their final emergence and uptake can be relatively swift and (not least for political reasons) difficult to control. It would thus seem that health care agencies are going to have to develop capabilities in technology evaluation geared to providing early, in-service analysis if provision is to be made in an efficient manner.

Such activity requires coordinated inputs from medical, economic, and other social-science-oriented professionals. It also demands considerable administrative skills to ensure that the intentions formulated by interdisciplinary planning teams are actually translated into operational realities. With prospects like effective but costly cancer treatments, viable mass liver transplantation programmes, and implantable or portable artificial hearts and lungs on the not too distant horizon it is a fairly urgent priority for health care providers to gain improved expertise in technology evaluation and diffusion direction.

It may be argued that at present it is health care systems like the British NHS that have advanced furthest towards achieving patterns of care that optimize the balance of costs against benefits (Office of Technology Assessment 1980b). Yet not all commentators would see such a model as an attractive one on which to base calls for improved medical technology evaluation. With examples like the British record in renal replacement therapy in mind even those who do not reject "socialized medicine" on ideological grounds may fear that consumers' interests might in practice be neglected in systems like the NHS. And a few observers, some based within medicine itself, argue in particular that economics and health care do not mix; they feel that the "dismal science" is also an inhumane one and that to introduce it into the health sphere is wrong. "What about", they ask, "factors not normally measured in cash terms, like suffering and lost life?".

It is with some broad introductory remarks on the potential contribution of economics to medical technology evaluation that this paper ends. The answer to the above question is, of course, that comprehensive economic analyses do take into account such matters. Sophisticated cost-benefit studies attempt to gauge *all* a population's preferences and implicit evaluations, including those in areas where money transactions are not normally involved. Money values are simply used as a generic, common expressor of value to allow broad comparisons and choices between alternative programmes to be made.

Provided that people's values in a given context can be clearly established, and that the interrelationships within and consequences of any given set of human transactions can be understood accurately, the skills of economists can be employed to identify the most efficient allocation of resources possible. And in the case of cost-effectiveness analysis, the purpose of which is to identify the most economical ways of achieving a given, accepted goal rather than to help to choose between different objectives, the methodological and associated problems are in any case less complex.

However, there are some balancing or cautionary points to be noted when the role of economics in the "real world" is considered. For instance, in some cases values are not sufficiently homogenous to allow meaningful aggregation. In others even the measurement of monetary costs can be misleading. It is often precisely because vital information is not available and rational choice difficult that "experts" like economists are called in to assist policy formation.

By making explicit the implicit evaluations underlying policies economists serve to question established assumptions and, hopefully, can help promote workable concensus. But in the final analysis they cannot replace political process and compromise as the final arbiter of questions like "who should be given life-saving but costly care?". As the eighteenth century Scottish philosopher David Hume pointed out, there is a sense in which what "ought" to be done must in the end be decided by the heart rather than the head.

Part II

Dialysis

7 A Review of the Clinical Evaluation of Dialysis

A. Colombi

Kantonsspital Lucerne

Kidney Function, Kidney Failure

In comparing the effectiveness and cost of different types of kidney replacement therapies, one must bear in mind the complexity of human kidney function. It consists not only of elimination and regulation of water, salts (electrolytes), acids, and metabolic end products, but also of hormone production and metabolism of many substances, hormones, and vitamins. Any form of dialysis can replace only the elimination function and even this in a very restricted manner. The main kidney functions are as follows:

Regulation of water balance
Regulation of electrolyte balance
Regulation of acid-base balance
Elimination of waste products
Production of hormones
Activation of vitamin D_3
Metabolism of hormones and other substances

The elimination capacity of human kidneys, even in endstage renal failure, had been underestimated during the initial 15 years of long-term dialysis treatment. The kidney elimination capacity is an important factor in considering dialysis treatment as in many instances it may equal or exceed the dialysis capacity. Many patients in the 1960s had their kidneys removed as a result of the overestimation of the potential of the dialysis procedure and the underestimation of the remaining kidney function. By the elimination of metabolic waste products through dialysis uremia is avoided. Uremia is a metabolic intoxication imparing all organ systems in differing degrees. Its manifestations are as follows:

Encephalopathy
Polyneuropathy
Pericarditis
Cardiomyopathy
Gastrointestinal Disorders
Fluid retention in the lungs
Hypertension
Osteodystrophy
Microangiopathy
Hyperparathyroidism
Anaemia
Amenorrhoea/impotence
Hypophyso-gonadal dysfunction

There is an enormous amount of medical literature on the subject of uremic toxins. This field of discussion will not be gone into in detail here other than to point out some difficulties encountered by the nephrologist in using laboratory data as measurable parameters of uremia. The data resemble the visible top of an iceberg, with an invisible bulk of really toxic substances such as guanidine succinic acid, methylguanidine, phenols, etc., and last but not least the so-called middle-molecules (MM), polypeptides of a molecular weight range of 350–2000 daltons. Determination of these toxins can be performed only in highly specialized research laboratories. It is not available for the physician following the patient on dialysis. If dialysis is sufficient, long-term clinical manifestations of uremia (pericarditis, hypertension, neuropathy, osteodystrophy, severe anaemia), should not develop or should even disappear if they were previously present.

Kidney Replacement Systems

The main structure of a kidney replacement system is the semipermeable membrane, which filters the blood by means of one or more of the four following transport mechanisms: diffusion of solutes due to a concentration gradient, convective solute transport during ultrafiltration, osmotic water shift due to an osmotic gradient, and ultrafiltration due to hydrostatic pressure gradient. Different dialysis systems utilize different transport mechanisms. Haemofiltration consitsts exclusively of ultrafiltration and convective solute transport. Haemodialysis, when drum-kidneys were used, mainly utilized osmotic water transport. Today, haemodialysis employs hydrostatic rather than osmotic water movement. With peritoneal dialysis hydrostatic ultrafiltration is not feasible because the pressure gradient cannot be controlled within the peritoneum. Absorption, a further way of eliminating solutes from the blood, has been used to regenerate the dialysis solution by means of membrane-coated active charcoal. The Redy System is to date the only absorption-based procedure in use to any extent.

We have only recently been furnished with a wide variety of kidney replacement therapies for patients with end-stage renal disease. Haemofiltration has been added to haemodialysis and continuous ambulatory peritoneal dialysis (CAPD) has also become a viable alternative to intermittent peritoneal dialysis (IPD) and haemodialysis. Not more than 4 years old, it is already competing with a newer mode of treatment, the continuous cycling peritoneal dialysis (CCPD).

In the early days of long-term dialysis treatment it was claimed that the treatment should be started as soon as the glomerular filtration rate (GFR) decreased to less than 5 ml/min. More recently, Funk-Brentano and Man (1981) specified that with a GFR of less than 3 ml/min the patient risks getting impaired nervous function (uremic neuropathy) (Table 7.1).

Table 7.1 summarizes the weekly clearances of two small molecular and two MM substances in the healthy human kidney and the above-mentioned dialysis sys-

Table 7.1. Weekly clearance rates (in litres)

	Molecular weight (daltons)	Kidney (168 h)	Haemodialysis (15 h)	Haemofiltration (9 h)	CAPD (168 h)
Urea	60	1008	125	54	56
Creatinine	113	1200	99	58	50
Vitamin B_{12}	1355		15	30	45
Inulin	5200	1200	4	63	28

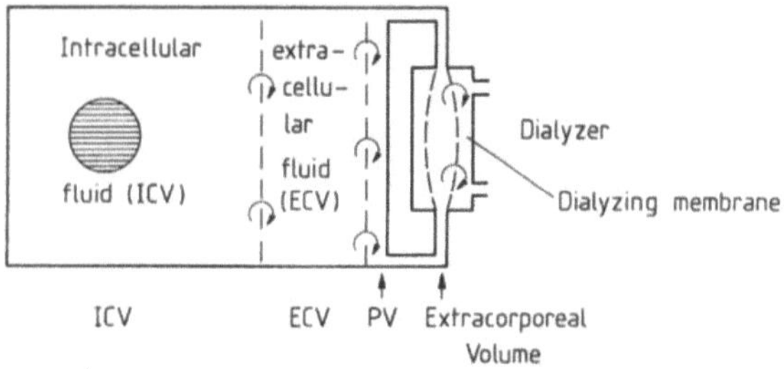

Fig. 7.1. "Cleaning" of body fluid with extracorporeal dialysis. *ICV*, intracellular fluid volume; *ECV*, extracellular fluid volume; *PV*, plasma volume (is part of the extracellular volume)

tems. If 5 ml/min or 50 l/week of creatinine clearance is a minimum clearance, one can see that none of the replacement systems go much beyond this limit. As an MM model for clinical purposes vitamin B_{12} has been introduced because of its molecular weight of 1355 daltons and because it can be measured rather easily by the clinical laboratory. Inulin slightly exceeds the upper limit of MM substances. Table 7.1 shows that for the human kidney, the molecular weights up to this range do not influence the clearance values. This is in contrast to all dialysis systems with mainly diffusive solute transport.

The ultrafiltration capacity is another important feature in any haemodialysis system. It is optimally about 3 ml/h/mm Hg, which corresponds to a volume loss of 2.3 l during a 5-h dialysis with a mean transmembranous pressure gradient of 150 mm Hg. Furthermore the ultrafiltration rate should be constant. With haemofiltration, however, ultrafiltration should exceed 100 ml/min.

Because of the long contact time with the patient's blood dialysis material must be biologically compatible. Problems have arisen from PVC blood lines, causing skin lesions (necrotizing dermatitis) in some patients. Cuprophane, a widely used membrane material, contains significant amounts of copper. Other materials promote blood coagulation and aggregation of white blood cells.

Any kind of kidney replacement therapy consists of a series of cleaning procedures working consecutively (see Fig. 7.1). Thus the patient's blood cleared in the dialysis filter re-enters the vascular system to clear the extracellular fluid space. This in turn builds up a concentration gradient, which eliminates waste products from the intracellular fluid space by diffusion. This process accounts for the long duration of any dialysis procedure.

Preparing the Patient

Dialysis is certainly among one of the more expensive therapeutic procedures. Because of this a high success rate is expected. This is possible only with the patient's cooperation, i.e. with the patient's motivation and determination. An evaluation of the patient's attitude is easy when he seeks help early in the course, but may be almost impossible when he sees the nephrologist only in terminal renal failure. The reason for this delay is mainly the oligosymptomatic character of most chronic renal diseases.

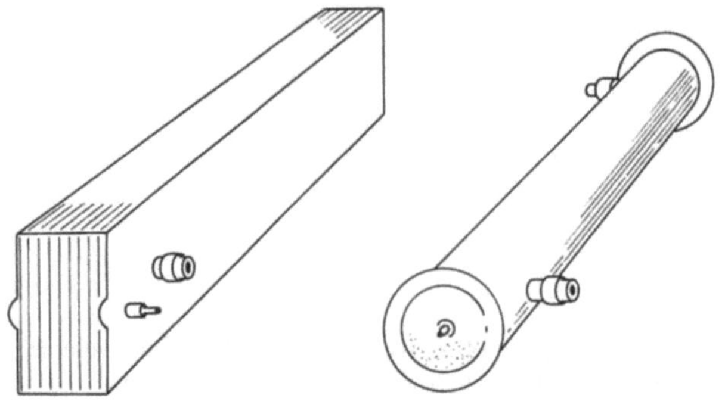

Fig. 7.2. Two different types of dialyser

Preparation of the patient for long-term dialysis includes the construction of a vascular access in one arm when the progression of the disease towards end-stage renal failure becomes evident. Preferably a few months prior to haemodialysis, an arteriovenous fistula (Cimino-fistula) is made in the patient's forearm. If the patient's original veins are not suitable the saphenous vein from the patient's leg may be transplanted. Other materials to be used in performing a vascular access are bovine grafts, umbilical cord grafts, and the more preferred polytretrafluorethylene (PTFE) grafts. Bovine grafts tend to produce aneurysms and the major problem with the PTFE graft is perivascular infection.

To choose the ideal starting point for dialysis is difficult. The aim of a well-timed beginning is to avoid uremic complications on one side and not to expose the patient to unnecessary risks from the treatment on the other. Usually a remaining kidney function with a GFR of 5 ml/min – in other words approximately 5% of normal – is a useful starting limit except for diabetics who need dialysis earlier to avoid severe ocular complications. The GFR can easily be derived from serum creatinine level using a nomogram (age and sex of the patient are taken into account). Clinical symptoms, however, such as increasing blood pressure, decreasing lean body mass, itching, epistaxis, nausea, and vomiting are important indicators for the necessity of renal replacement therapy.

Haemodialysis

Today proportioning systems are used almost exclusively in haemodialysis. These machines mix soft water with the concentrate to form the desired dialysis solution, which is warmed to body temperature. A negative-pressure valve connected to a dialysate pressure monitor allows increased transmembranous pressure by adding negative dialysate pressure to positive pressure in the blood compartment. A blood leak is detected by a photoelectric-cell system on the dialysate back-flow site. The new generation of kidney machines disposes of a regulatory system. This guarantees controlled ultrafiltration, a considerable improvement in dialysis procedure.

The blood side of the dialysis system includes blood lines, blood pump, air detector, and above all the dialyser itself, where the solute transport takes place across the semipermeable membrane. The efficiency of the filter is dependent on the quality and thickness of the menbrane as well as on the design of the dialyser. Membranes used in dialysers have a thickness of 8–30 μm.

In the Kiil kidney or parallel plate dialyser dialysis occurs through a number of planar membranes. In the capillary kidney the membrane consists of capillaries (Fig. 7.2). Capillary kidneys have two advantages – a maximum surface area and a turbulant dialysate flow by the capillary structure itself. These two conditions for an optimal effect are achieved in Kiil-type dialysers by sophisticated surface reliefs of the supporting structures. The counter-current flow of blood and dialysate within the dialyser ensures a constant concentration gradient over the whole filter.

Special attention should be given to ultrafiltration during haemodialysis. Increase in body weight between two dialysis sessions and the deviation from the "ideal" weight can be controlled by the volume loss to be reached during dialysis. To ensure the correct volume loss, corresponding values for the transmembranous pressure (TMP) may be taken from a nomogram. While the patient undergoing dialysis may be put on a scale, the necessary pressure gradient may be deduced empirically or a dialysis machine with controlled ultrafiltration may be used as mentioned earlier.

Dialysis fluid composition conforms to the abnormalities of the uremic patient's blood. A low potassium concentration sufficiently eliminates K^+, while sodium is primarily eliminated by convective transport, i. e. by ultrafiltration. Therefore, dialysate concentration is only slightly inferior to serum concentration. The Ca^{2+} concentration in the dialysis fluid is such as to guarantee a constant calcium influx to the patient. This Ca^{2+} substitution should represent a supplement to the oral Ca^{2+} intake, and by increasing the Ca^{2+} concentration in the serum it should stop parathyroid hormone secretion. However, the duration of this mechanism is too short to be effective in preventing the patient from developing secondary hyperparathyroidism. As a consequence of the increased serum Mg^{2+}, the dialysate concentration of Mg^{2+} is usually low. If glucose is added, the glucose concentration in the dialysis solution is approximately 200 mg%, thus increasing the total dialysate osmolarity to about 300 mosmol/l.

Small molecular clearances do not differ significantly among the various dialysers in use, whereas the MM clearances depend very much on the material and thickness of the membrane used. The following measures increase MM clearances: increase of membrane surface area, increase of dialysis time, use of highly permeable membrane material, increased use of convective solute transport. An increased surface area is usually connected with a higher priming volume of the dialyser and thus with an increase in the extracorporeal volume. An increase of dialysis time is often tolerated by the patient unless it is not related to bed-rest. Membranes with a significantly higher MM clearance usually have higher ultrafiltration rates and thus require the combination of a proportioning machine and controlled ultrafiltration. This is especially true of the RP dialyser from Rhône-Poulenc. Such dialysers are more expensive as well. The good results of haemofiltration, indeed, are due to convective solute transport.

With dialysers of about 1-m^2 surface area the patients are usually dialysed

3–5 h/week. Since a reduction of dialysis time after many months will increase uremic organ manifestations in the patient, such a reduction must be carefully considered. The patients request a reduction in dialysis time usually when ultrafiltration is not under control. As we pointed out earlier solute transport among the different body compartments is a time-consuming procedure.

During haemodialysis complications may originate from both machine and patient. From the patient's side the most frequent problem is low blood pressure (hypotension) arising from excessive or precipitated volume withdrawal. Hypotension as a consequence of bleeding due to anti-coagulants is an exception. Cardiac arrhythmias and anaphylactic or septic shock are equally rare reasons for a low blood pressure during dialysis.

An increase in blood pressure during dialysis accompanied by a headache is usually a sign of the disequilibrium syndrome. If extracellular solute removal exceeds that of the intracellular space considerably, an osmotic intracellular water shift will lead to cerebral oedema resulting in the disequilibrium syndrome. This complication is often the consequence of a high predialytic solute accumulation and low dialysate osmolarity. The disequilibrium state, furthermore, is responsible for the postdialysis syndrome – fatigue, inability to concentrate, muscular weakness, headache, and exhaustion. As a consequence of these troubles many patients are unable to work after dialysis for several hours. The main advantage of an evening dialysis lies in the re-equilibration during sleep. With continuous dialysis procedures, such as CAPD and CCPD, desquilibrium syndrome and postdialysis syndrome are nonexistent.

Other complications are due to the vascular access. Infections after cannulation may occur as well as thrombosis and bleeding. Aneurysmatic enlargement of the Cimino-fistula may give rise to cardiac failure, thromboembolism, or simply to local pain. Complications with the equipment may be due to insufficient water softening (hard-water syndrome), defective dialysate compostion (haemolysis), blood leak, air leak (air embolism), and coagulation within the extracorporeal circuit. Water softening is tested by the soaptest and coagulation, usually by the antithrombin time measurement. Dialysate conductivity and blood and air leaks are monitored by the dialysis machine.

Haemofiltration

Haemofiltration has gained much interest during recent years. Not only the shortening of dialysis time but also a greater elimination of MM with fewer side effects than dialysis may be the reasons for this. The membrane material for haemofilters is either polysulphone, polyamide, or polyacrylonitrile. During each treatment 20–30 l of ultrafiltrate are gained and an equal amount of substitution fluid is infused either before (predilution) or after (postdilution) the filter. This sterile electrolyte solution increases costs considerably. In order to guarantee a constant replacement of the ultrafiltrate with a sufficient amount of warmed substitution fluid a haemofiltration machine is required. Today, it seems that the patients who tend to be hypertensive while on haemodialysis would profit from haemofiltration. Since the serum osmolarity does not change significantly during haemofiltration, volume depletion is better tolerated than with haemodialysis.

Besides the considerably higher costs and the lower elimination rate of small molecules, an increased loss of hormones must be considered a disadvantage of haemofiltration. However, the loss of parathyroid hormone (PTH) again is advantageous in preventing hyperparathyroidism. The decreased loss of small-molecular substances is compensated for by the combination with dialysis (haemodiafiltration).

Continuous Ambulatory Peritoneal Dialysis

The year 1978 will certainly enter dialysis history as a milestone when Popovich et al. published their clinical results on CAPD. Although it was known since the mid-1960s that patients with chronic peritoneal dialysis treatment did well, long-term peritoneal dialysis succeeded only in the form of CAPD mainly for logistical reasons. With a dialysate flow of 2–4 l/h, small-molecular clearances were much lower compared to with haemodialysis. Since within the system blood circulation / dialysate flow / peritoneal surface, dialysate flow was the only variable factor, attempts were made for over 2 decades to increase this flow. The result was the Di Paolos semi-continuous peritoneal dialysis reaching a flow of 10 l/h. Popovich et al. abruptly stopped this trend by accepting even very low clearances and increasing dialysis time to a maximum. Their dialysis system in fact brought many advantages. It is the tragedy that the CAPD looks so simple that many physicians are led to perform it in a careless way with the inevitable consequence of bad results, which are even worsened by poor patient selection.

The procedure in CAPD consists of filling the peritoneal cavity three to five times a day with 2 l dialysate. The time allowed for the fluid to remain in the peritoneum lasts 4–8 h during which the empty bag stays attached to the peritoneal catheter in order to avoid infection from disconnection. The 8-h rhythm during the night allows the patient an ordinary sleep. The four dialysate changes at 0700, 1200, 1700, and 2200 hours need 30 min each but fortunately fall at convenient times of the day.

From the metabolic viewpoint CAPD is very effective. By the continuous character of this treatment solutes are stabilized at a level determined by their generation rate and the daily dialysate volume. In this form of dialysis a high MM clearance combines with an ideal small-molecule elimination rate. Phosphate excretion is higher than with haemodialysis so that in most patients oral phosphate binders are unnecessary. Parenteral Ca^{2+} substitution takes place constantly provided dialysate Ca^{2+} concentration is high enough and ultrafiltrate Ca^{2+} does not exceed Ca^{2+} reabsorption from the peritoneal cavity. With these conditions the considerable increase in haematocrit found in CAPD patients is not astonishing. In five patients transferred to CAPD after 3–8 years on haemodialysis treatment we observed an increase in haematocrit from 23% to 39%!

Volume withdrawal by means of the hyperosmolar dialysis fluid is very easy. However, experience has taught us to be restrictive with dialysate of high osmolarity because the large amount of glucose absorbed leads to hypertriglyceridemia and obesity. Adequate elimination of volume and substances with pressor activity rends more patients on CAPD normotonic than with usual haemodialysis.

Frequent complications of CAPD are hernias, hyper- and hypovolemia, hypokalemia, and obesity; but the most serious problem is peritonitis. Peritoneal infection is defined as a cloudy dialysate outflow with 50 or more leucocytes per mm^3. Abdominal symptoms such as pain, nausea, vomitus, diarrhoea, and fever are frequent but not necessarily present. *Staphylococcus epidermidis* and *Staph. aureus* are responsible for 67% of peritonitis as indicating the source of infection. Yet in a considerable number of cases isolation of the germs is difficult. The treatment of peritonitis consists of short lavages, addition of antibiotics to the dialysate, and other measures. It has been proven that peritonitis can be prevented by a series of precautions, namely:

1) Correct implantation and positioning of the catheter
2) Sterile dialysis fluid and safe connectors
3) Safe dialysate exchange procedure
4) Use of sterile gloves and masks
5) Specialized CAPD staff and units
6) Dialysate warming system that is "safe" from the bacteriological viewpoint
7) Immediate antibiotic prophylaxis follwing incidents with possible infection
8) Serious training for the patient
9) No additives to the dialysate except insulin and antibiotics
10) Careful examination after every infection episode

In a well-guided CAPD programme, the peritonitis rate is lower than one episode per patient-year. Such a programme can be offered to the patient as a viable alternative to haemodialysis or haemofiltration. We recommended it moreover to all patients showing a great interest in fast and good social rehabilitation because the short training of 1–2 weeks, the rapidly increasing haematocrit and well-being, and the short time spent for the treatment itself favour rehabilitation.

Rehabilitation

Good medical rehabilitation is the *conditio sine qua non* for social rehabilitation; but whoever treats dialysis patients knows as well that only the outlook for social rehabilitation makes medical rehabilitation possible. Reintegration is easier the fewer the complications and complaints the patient has, including troubles arising from the treatment as well as the renal disease. Thus a careful treatment will also facilitate rehabilitation.

The loss of hours from work has been diminished by dialysis procedures, such as self-care dialysis, limited-care dialysis, and especially home-dialysis treatment. However, the time factor is not the main advantage of these forms of active self-care. The main advantage of these procedures is of a psychological nature. The dependence on dialysis staff, machines, on a fixed dialysis schedule, on diets, on the help of other family members often leads to depression. Further reasons for the depressive tendency are partly due to exchanges within the family life and sexual problems, whereas self-treatment gives the patient more independence, confidence, and self-esteem. If on the other hand dependence increases, depression will turn into regression or even aggressive behaviour. This aggression may even be demonstrated against those who do their best to help the patient.

To judge the working capability of dialysis patients is difficult. This depends on age and profession, on the mode of dialysis procedure, on medical and psychosocial fitness and attitude, and finally on the patient's family background. Patients just before retirement age will willingly accept their pension, saying that they have done their job and are going to enjoy the few years left. Furthermore, those who do strenuous physical labour will be handicapped in advance by uremic myopathy, polyneuropathy, myatrophy due to the negative N-balance, and lack of physical training. Anemia is another factor that decreases physical capacity, and with elderly patients cardiovascular and cerebrovascular diseases lead to a further decrease in the ability to work. In addition to these handicaps neuropsychological troubles render reintegration rather difficult, there is namely a decreased ability to concentrate, early fatigue, weakness of memory, and insomnia.

Although statistical reports on rehabilitation should be considered with caution some of the data given by the European Dialysis and Transplant Association (EDTA) will be discussed in the following section. In the international report (1980) col-

Table 7.2. Degree of rehabilitation (1–6) in 21 European countries

Country	Percentage of patients in each rehabilitation category in 1979					
	1[a]	2	3	4	5	6
Austria	37.9	11.0	13.8	14.8	18.6	3.8
Belgium	22.1	30.4	10.9	18.4	16.8	1.3
Bulgaria	13.0	17.0	19.0	36.0	15.0	0
Czechoslovakia	20.6	36.0	5.1	28.5	9.8	0
Denmark	34.9	18.1	7.2	7.2	28.9	3.6
Fed. Rep. Germany	27.7	18.7	15.7	13.6	20.7	3.6
Finland	10.2	37.3	1.7	15.3	30.5	5.1
France	38.6	22.4	12.4	14.1	10.7	1.8
German Dem. Rep.	15.2	51.6	8.2	3.2	19.1	2.6
Greece	28.1	25.0	20.3	11.7	13.3	1.6
Hungary	17.8	26.0	15.1	30.1	11.0	0
Israel	44.6	24.3	12.6	9.9	8.1	0.5
Italy	62.9	17.5	7.1	6.7	5.1	0.6
Netherlands	18.2	28.3	17.0	9.1	25.9	1.4
Poland	19.3	35.1	7.9	24.6	12.3	0.9
Portugal	47.4	34.2	5.3	0	10.5	2.6
Spain	40.7	25.4	12.4	10.6	9.9	1.0
Sweden	12.1	27.1	7.1	16.4	30.0	7.1
Switzerland	19.9	47.4	8.7	7.7	14.8	1.5
United Kingdom	33.2	16.3	19.1	14.1	14.9	2.5
Yugoslavia	13.6	19.1	7.4	37.0	22.5	0.3
Total Registry	36.6	22.8	11.9	12.9	13.9	1.9

[a] 1, able to work full-time
2, able to work part-time
3, able to work but no work available
4, able to work but pension is higher
5, unable to work
6, unable to care for self

lected from 30 European and Middle East countries, 54550 patients on dialysis treatment or with renal transplants were recorded (*Table* 7.2).

From the data in Table 7.2 one can see that overall 59.4% of the patients work full- or part-time and another 24.8% would be able to do so but do not either because an adequate job is lacking or because the job would bring in less than social security. While only 56% of hospital-dialysed males and 69% of females work, the numbers for home-dialysed patients are 75% and 89%, respectively. It is obvious that countries with a so-called high social standard such as Sweden, the Federal Republic of Germany, and Finland have a low rate of working dialysis patients (39%, 46.4%, 47.5%, respectively) in contrast to 61% in France and 67.3% in Switzerland. After transplantation the rate of patients unable to work is less than 7%, and 67% of all patients work full-time.

Results of Dialysis Treatment

On 31 December 1980, 48408 patients were alive in Europe on haemodialysis, 2749 patients were on peritoneal dialysis, and 12394 patients were alive with a functioning kidney graft. Within that year a total of 14084 new patients had entered a dialysis programme. Divided by the population of 573 million this means 117.6 treated patients/million population. However, the national numbers vary greatly between Turkey (3.9/million) and Switzerland (259.7/million).

The percentage of home-dialysed patients shows enormous variations among different countries (Table 7.3). While home treatment is nonexistent in the German Democratic Republic, in Austria 9.5% of the patients are treated with this form of dialysis. The numbers of France and the Federal Republic of Germany are slightly above the European average of 16%. The percentage of home-treated patients has increased in Switzerland slowly but steadily during the last decade, while the United Kingdom has always led with home-dialysis. The reasons for these differences are well known. In the USA and the Federal Republic of Germany the costs of dialysis are covered by social security and the establishement of private dialysis centres has lead to a secondary decrease in home-dialysis.

Cumulative survival on dialysis and transplantation can be derived from Fig. 7.3. The mean 5-year survival for hospital dialysis is 54% and the 10-year surviv-

Table 7.3. The porportion of home-dialysis versus the total number of patients on dialysis in six different European countries

	Total patients	Home patients	Percentage
German Dem. Rep.	622	0	0
Austria	725	69	9.5
Fed. Rep. Germany	10837	2058	19.0
France	9926	2162	21.8
Switzerland	1031	286	28.0
United Kingdom	3839	2458	64.0
Europe	59347	9677	16.0

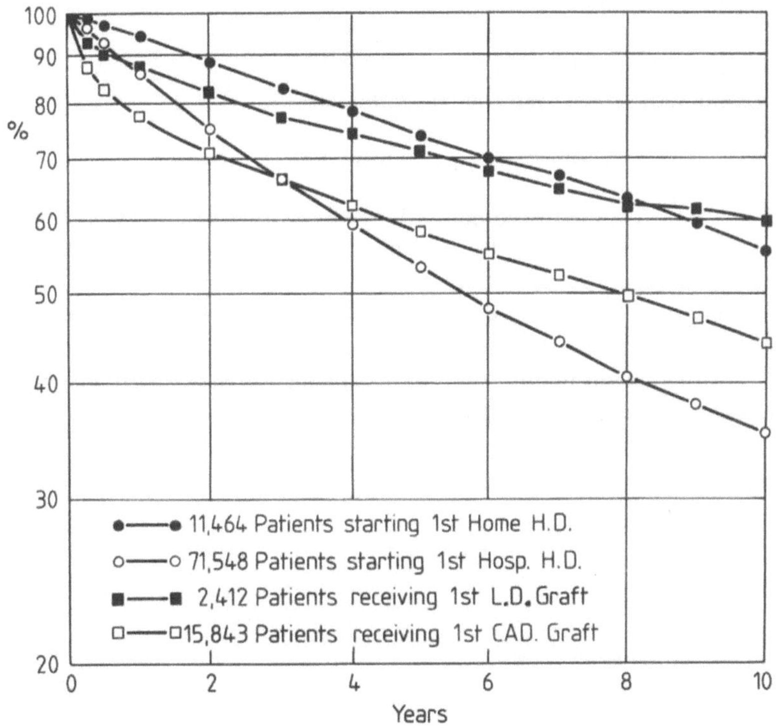

Fig. 7.3. Cumulative survival on dialysis and transplantation

al rate is 36%. For patients with cadaveric donor grafts the figures are slightly better (54% and 48%). In contrast, home-dialysis patients have a much better prognosis with survival rates of 75% and 56%, respectively. Both the 5- and the 10-year survival rates decrease considerably with age. The three main causes of death in dialysis patients (hospital) are cardiovascular (5.17%), infections (1.46%), and cerebrovascular accidents (11.59%) per 100 patients at risk. Suicide accounts for 0.09%.

Economic Aspects

For anyone working in the field of kidney replacement therapy, economic aspects should not be taboo. To consider these aspects of treatment does no harm to the patient per se. In Switzerland the cost for the treatment of 1200 dialysis patients exceeded the 40 million Swiss francs limit in 1981. In 1970 the corresponding expenses were 2 million Swiss francs, 14 million Swiss francs in 1975, and 28 million Swiss francs in 1978. Although a ceiling of 2000 patients has been predicted, the 100-million Swiss franc cost-ceiling will be reached within this decade.

Possibilities for reducing dialysis cost include:

A clear plan for treatment (avoidance of complications)

Rational drug therapy

Comparison of cost and quality of dialysis material
Provision for dialysis material through pool systems
Reutilization of disposable material
Promotion of self-dialysis (home haemodialysis, CAPD)
Promotion of renal transplantation
Avoidance of the development of private dialysis centres

All these factors lowering cost for dialysis treatment have been widely considered in Switzerland since the beginning of long-term dialysis treatment. Unfortunately, the relatively large number of small dialysis centres in this country (5.1 centres/million population) is in opposition to a further increase in self-dialysis because the training requires corresponding teams and facilities. Perhaps the CAPD will help us in the future to make further progress in this respect. It is not just by chance that the United Kingdom and Switzerland have the highest rates of CAPD patients in Europe.

8 Discussion of Paper by Colombi

J. D. Pole

Department of Health and Social Security, London

I begin with an attempt to summarize Colombi's excellent paper but very much from an ignorant economist's point of view. If I may say so I thought that Colombi's approach to his task was very nicely judged in the sense that the paper is informative about the clinical aspects without being too far above the heads of the nonmedical participants.

Kidneys are complex organs and Colombi begins by drawing attention to the important fact that dialysis cannot compensate for all the complex renal functions but only for those that involve the elimination of toxic waste products produced by the metabolic processes. Even in this respect dialysis is only partially successful and in order to be effective to a tolerable degree in eliminating toxins, it requires either a large membrane area, which implies a relatively large artificial kidney, or a long period of dialysis. And as an economist, to start off with I thought I spotted an interesting trade-off here, which may well be solved differently for people of different ages and so on.

The author concludes by tactfully affirming the relevance of economic considerations by offering a number of suggestions for the cost-effective development of services. These include various specific measures to promote technical and operational efficiency. The development of self-dialysis is the preferred cost-effective mode, drawing on experience in Switzerland, avoiding the establishment of small private treatment centres.

One constraint on my discussion of the clinical aspects of dialysis is its perfectly obvious effectiveness, in general terms. Dialysed, one is probably alive and moderately comfortable – or perhaps moderately uncomfortable. Undialysed, one is almost certainly dead, and in this sense the medical evaluation of dialysis lacks the excitement of the close-run thing, which it tends to have in the case of many other advanced medical technologies. Should one then go to the opposite extreme and assert that only economic criteria are important in evaluating dialysis? If so – regression analyses demonstrate it to a certain extent – then the rate of dialysis depends on the national income level (to pre-empt any comment on the subject I might point out that the UK actually lies on the regression line). In fact, the clinical effectiveness of treatment is very variable. It varies with a large range of factors including the characteristics of the patient and almost equally the characteristics of his or her spouse, age, intelligence, education, smoking, obesity, and psychological attributes of various kinds. Another aspect that one must consider in this context is the quality of life. Colombi draws attention very fairly to the substantial social and psychological handicaps involved for patients in dialysis and hence the need to balance these contraindications against the progressive physiological deterioration of the patient in determining when to begin dialysis. Perhaps someone has already formalized this decision situation in an interesting way and it would be interesting to hear from them.

I was very interested by Colombi's discussion of the various modes of dialysis, broadly defined. It appeared that none of them dominates the others and again the process of allocating patients to treatment modes is bound to be full of interest to economists. Colombi's paper also covers rather briefly the question of outcome. Unfortunately, neither in Colombi's paper nor elsewhere have I seen an attempt at standardization of outcomes in relation to patient characteristics so that little that is scientific can be concluded from this analysis about the relative merits of different modes of treatment. Nevertheless, the value of dialysis to the patient is clearly established in general terms and the advantages of home-dialysis also appeared to emerge fairly clearly. Also very important are the aetiology of renal failure and any complications, such as diabetes or hypertension, which used in the past to be critical contraindications but may now be less so. So far as intervention is concerned, the mode of treatment is clearly important, though its importance in terms of apparent outcome may be somewhat exaggerated by the evident patient selection bias that occurs.

Not only the mode but also the provider of treatment may be important. In the case of transplantation, it seems that the most important factor in the outcome is where you have it done. Now this is not at all an uncommon situation in surgical procedures. What is perhaps uncommon in the UK is that, according to the published statistics, London is not the best place to have it done. Variation in outcome for transplantation seems to be absolutely critical in relation to the cost-effectiveness of transplantation as a mode of treatment for chronic renal failure and in the centres with the highest graft survival transplantation is clearly way ahead. In those that have the poorest graft survival it seems that it is very doubtful whether transplantation is cost-effective.

Variation in outcome by centre is probably less for dialysis but larger centres are almost certainly better, among other things, at the important task of training patients for self-dialysis. Against this background, perhaps I could invite our medical colleagues to address the questions of how far the determinants of treatment are clinical, economic, or even sociological. It is not unknown, especially in Switzerland, for economists to take an interest in sociology (usually in their old age), and it seems that from the point of view of the sociology of professions and organizations the treatment of chronic renal failure may throw interesting light on the decision-making process in hospitals and the role of clinicians in resource allocation.

I mentioned earlier the strong relation internationally between national income per head and the rate of maintenance dialysis. It has been noted in various places that not only the total amount of finance provided but also the manner in which it is provided can have important effects on the extent and mode of treatment for chronic renal failure. But the attitudes of referring physicians and of the accident surgeons who supply the grafts may also be very important in the choice of mode. Other important factors are the availability of physical resources, allocated beds, and number of transplant surgeons, trained nurses (this seems to be a particular constraint), and other trained ancillary personnel. So it is not entirely a matter of finance and the question I am interested in focusing on is how far it is a question of finance and how far other factors of a more clinical kind are relevant not only to the choice of mode but to the total extent of maintenance care.

There is a great diversity among countries in the extent to which they utilize different modes of treatment. To some extent this clearly reflects the economic and organizational factors already referred to, but to what extent does it reflect the absence of consensus on the relative clinical effectiveness of different modes? Is the choice of mode a matter of comparative indifference to clinicians? If not it would seem appropriate to try to resolve the matter of outcome in a systematic way and this would involve the use of measures of outcome as well as of cost. What would be the appropriate measures? Survival rates, obviously, but also physical and psychological morbidity and rehabilitation status in terms of capacity to fulfil normal tasks such as work appropriate to a patient of a certain age. These are obvious possibilities. Would controlled trials of mode be feasible?

Now, I have said nothing about prevention and of course when a patient presents with chronic renal failure, there is no alternative to treatment unless it is non-treatment. But in the longer term prevention may have a role. After all, the incidence of chronic renal failure has fallen a great deal in developed countries since the nineteenth century to its present low level.

I conclude with five questions:

1) How far are the limits to dialysis effectively set by clinical considerations and how far do they depend on economic or sociological factors? Or in other words, how relevant is the question of clinical evaluation to extend to dialysis?
2) How far does the divergence in choice of mode between countries reflect clinical considerations and how far does this choice of mode also reflect economic, sociological, organizational, or historical factors? That is to say, how far is the question of clinical evaluation relevant to the choice of mode?
3) To the extent that clinical evaluation is relevant in these respects, how far is it being systematically carried out and what are the prospects for future work?
4) What is the potential role of prevention?
5) And finally, I just throw this one in in case everything else fails, what does the future hold in relation to the development to other life-saving but costly medical technology?

Summary of Workshop Discussion

Following Pole's discussion the advantages and disadvantages of the different techniques used in the support of impaired kidney function were as follows. The limits to dialysis are set by technical, sociological, and economic factors.

Haemodialysis needs a machine and filters, which are expensive. The patient has to be connected to the machine by a vascular shunt, which constitutes the main technical problem in performing haemodialysis. Potential complications originate from machine failure. Dialysing time (3 × 5 h/week) creates opportunity costs. Even the costs of operation are high, e.g. in Switzerland 63000 Swiss francs/patient/year.

Haemofiltration poses the same problems as haemodialysis. Treatment time per patient might be shorter than with haemodialysis (12 instead of 15 h/week), but the operating costs of the machine are higher. Today haemofiltration is used in 5%–8% of all cases, the rest receive ordinary haemodialysis.

Continuous ambulatory peritoneal dialysis (CAPD) has the advantage that most patients can be treated at home. The main problem is again a technical one: a tube inserted into the patient's abdomen must allow free exchange of the dialysate solution to and from the peritoneal cavity. Infection (peritonitis) is a risk; the rate of infection is about one infection episode per patient every 2 years. In such a case the patient needs to be hospitalized for approximately 2 weeks. The costs of CAPD in Switzerland are in the order of 16000 Swiss francs: about one-quarter of those of haemodialysis.

Kidney transplant needs either a living or cadaver kidney donor. If successful, the transplant organ will function like a normal kidney, but failure and rejection of the transplanted organ is a risk. The yearly costs for patient follow-up and control is between 1500 and 3000 US dollars. If enough donors could be made available transplantation would be a good solution to the problem of terminal kidney failure. But even then the transplant procedure is limited by age (patients over 55 or 60 years not being suitable) and the presence of diseases (patients with cardiovascular diseases or severe diabetes are not suitable). The choice of alternatives of conservative methods (dialysis, haemofiltration, and CAPD) reflects the problem of clinical evaluation: there are patients in whom you cannot insert a shunt – these patients will not be on dialysis; patients with diabetes do better on CAPD than on dialysis; both methods are suitable for patients being prepared for transplantation and for patients with rejection of transplanted kidneys.

The main question is not *what* to do but *when* to start special diets, *when* to start dialysis, *when* to consider transplantation. To the extent that clinical evaluation is relevant in these respects, further systematic research is needed.

As far as prevention of end-stage renal disease is concerned, high blood pressure (hypertension) should be treated, but the main reason for terminal renal failure is glomerulonephritis, a condition which at the present state of knowledge is very difficult to cure except in a limited number of cases.

9 Economic Evaluation of Dialysis

K.-M. Pedersen

Odense University

Introduction

More than 100000 patients receive chronic haemodialysis throughout the world. In Europe alone well above 40000 patients received haemodialysis at home or in hospital in 1979. The stock of patients on various treatment modalities for chronic renal failure (CRF) has been increasing by roughly 15% a year during the last part of the 1970s as shown in Table 9.1. The costs of treating patients suffering from CRF have

Table 9.1. Stock and flow figures, 1979, for 31 member countries of the European Dialysis and Transplantation Association (EDTA), including several Mediterranean contries(European Dialysis and Transplantation Association 1980)

	1976	1977	1978	1979
Patients on file (dead or living)	51154	60371	70892	91866
Patients alive	34215	39735	44914	52515
Treatment modality for patients alive				
Haemodialysis	27343	31297	35001	40645
Peritoneal dialysis[a]	436	545	839	1583
With functioning graft	6307	7402	9074	10287
New patients	9440	10116	10523	12258
Transplant operations performed	2654	3086	3538	3295
Total deaths	3269	3480	3705	5123

[a] The dramatic increase from 1978–1979 was mainly due to continous ambulatory peritoneal dialysis (CAPD), see glossary at end of book for a short description of the treatment modalities

Table 9.2. Actual and projected Medicare costs for end-stage renal disease, 1974–1976 (actual), and 1981–1983 (projected) in United States (Rettig 1977)

Fiscal year	Costs of Medicare ($ million)	Total national costs ($ million)	Patient population
1974	242.5	286.2	18848
1975	404.6	479.5	25654
1976	573.3	684.2	31631
–	–	–	–
1981	1667.7	1992.7	53077
1982	1941.7	2321.6	55911
1983	2235.1	2674.3	58391

of course increased at least proportionately with the stock. To give an indication of the size of the costs, consider Table 9.2.

The US costs are only the financial costs to Medicare and thus exclude copayment by patients on home dialysis, approximately 20%. Some European figures can be added. In West Germany it is estimated that in 1982 the costs will amount to roughly DM 1.2 billion for a patient population of about 16000 (Clade 1980). For the United Kingdom the approximate running costs of dialysis and transplantation in 1976 were £22.1 million (Office of Health Economics 1978). If capital costs are added, the corresponding figure is £25 million. The patient population was approximately 4500. Japanese figures (Office of Technology Assessment 1980) indicate that in 1976/1977 20000 patients were under treatment, 160 per million population, at a cost of $624 million.

When looking at these figures it has to be remembered that the costs – incomplete, minimum figures – do not refer to ultimate costs, i.e. treatment costs when the patient pool has reached equilibrium (inflow of patients equals outflow). Consider, for example, the treatment rates in Table 9.3. It is clear that the main generator of costs is the number of people on treatment at a given time. From Table 9.3 it is seen that the number on treatment has increased by 80%–100% over a 5-year period. In most countries the equilibrium level has not been reached yet. Thus, one estimate is that the UK treatment rate per million will ultimately rise to about 340 per million – based on the assumption that new cases per year will increase to 40 per million, compare with Table 9.3. With unchanged proportions in the various treatment modes, the cost of treating these people would rise to about £120 million in terms of 1976/1977 prices. (Office of Health Economics 1978).

In economic terms dialysis and transplantation programmes in many countries are considerable, often between 1%–2% of the health budget. As an example of medical technology[1] dialysis is interesting partly because of the size of the programme, partly because it was introduced relatively early, namely early in the

Table 9.3. Treatment rates per million population – stock and flow figures (European Dialysis and Transplant Association)

	Stock			New flow		
	1972	1975	1979	1972	1975	1979
Australia	24.1	55.1	119.6	12.4	25.3	37.5
Belgium	58.5	102.7	205.9	22.1	25.9	48.2
Denmark	88.4	132.4	181.2	32.0	28.7	25.7
East Germany	17.4	28.4	55.6	9.4	10.5	19.0
Israel	26.6	117.0	200.8	23.0	38.6	51.9
Sweden	65.5	85.4	149.5	20.1	28.7	37.4
Switzerland	78.1	136.1	220.8	25.4	34.2	39.7
United Kingdom	38.2	62.0	111.2	12.8	14.5	21.7
West Germany	37.8	87.7	160.9	17.3	29.6	37.0

1 "Medical technology" is taken to refer to the wide range of equipment, drugs, and procedures employed in the care of the patient.

1960s[2]. As a case study dialysis should provide ample evidence about the use and influence of economic evaluation along with evidence as to whether early promises and assessments have come true. In the next section some of the economic questions are summarized and discussed briefly. This is followed by a review of two examples of cost-benefit analysis (CBA). A discussion of a number of points pertaining to the usefulness of CBA is postponed to the third section where it will be discussed in connection with some examples of cost-effectiveness analysis. In the final section so-called cost analyses are discussed with a view to the usefulness of this kind of analysis.

Some Economic Questions in Technology Evaluation

In terms of a hierarchy of decisions with respect to a given technology, in case of dialysis, one might be interested in answers to the following questions:

a) Should the technology be introduced at all as a therapy? In particular if other technologies compete for resources. This is the "level of resources question"
b) If yes, should dialysis and/or transplantation be available for all people who may be expected to benefit, regardless of costs?
c) If yes, what are the expected ultimate costs of such a strategy?
d) If no to b), which patients should be selected?
e) For b, c, and d – what are the optimal treatment modality combinations? This is the question of "allocation of resources between treatments"
f) Should economic evaluation be a one-shot phenomenon or should it be a continuous monitoring?

The analytic approach needed to answer these questions differs, but roughly involves CBA for a, cost-effectiveness for e, cost-analysis for c and f, along with statistical models for projecting patient populations. For instance, one line of reasoning with respect to a could be the following:

> The difficulty of putting a value on human life, apart from livelihood, is well known. Of equal difficulty would be the measurement of benefit due to a reduction in orpanhood ... Finally, and perhaps most important ... in the absence of overwhelming costs (as reflected by an appreciable fraction of the GNP), treatment for end-stage renal disease should be made available to all persons qualified to receive it from a medical standpoint. The reasons for this decision are the irreversibility of the decision not to do so, as far as an individual is concerned; the existence for the first time of a technology capable of prolonging the lives of persons otherwise doomed to a early death; ... and the fact that the patients are known and identifiable, not members of a statistical distribution, enhances the community's interest in doing something in their behalf (Gottschalk 1967).

The above quotation is of particular interest because it nicely summarizes some of the much debated points surrounding the use of CBA and specifically the valuation of life. Furthermore, the above arguments along with reasons like the fact that some

2 See Glossary for a short description of the technology.

veterans were already receiving free care in Veterans Administration Hospitals and that some countries, each poorer than the US, were committed to delivering this service to the entire population etc. in 1968 led to the conclusion that the role of the US federal government should be expanded considerably in this area[3]. Once this recommendation had been made, the problem that remained for analysis was how best to discharge this responsibility. This basically entails an analysis attempting to answer one question: Under existing conditions of knowledge regarding the cost and end-results of treating patients with chronic renal disease, what is the best mix of centre/hospital-dialysis, home-dialysis, and kidney transplantation? Such a question is answered by means of cost-effectiveness analysis, CEA (point e above). CEA follows logically from the above line of reasoning (if any economic evaluation is wanted at all). With respect to the American experience Rettig (1976) notes that the Gottschalk committee was not asked to do a cost-benefit study of providing treatment but a cost-effectiveness study of how to provide such treatment. The commissioning entity, the Bureau of the Budget, saw the experts as having competence on the latter question, while the former question was to be reserved for senior policy makers. Based on the above line of reasoning one of the best known CEAs was carried out based on the committee's data, namely that of Klarman et al. (1968).

However, implicit in the arguments used above at least one assumption is hidden: CEA is a relatively simple exercise and less controversial than CBA. This is usually not the case, in particular not when two or more types of outcomes/effects, say life expectancy and "quality of life", are sought. If only one outcome such as life-years gained is preeminent, other outcomes may be neglected. Where all outcomes, such as reduced mortality, changed morbidity, less disability, are considered one must – like in CBA – arrive at common or weighted measures of outcome for alternative programme. These issues will be addressed in the Cost-Effectiveness Analyses section. We now turn to CBA.

Two Cost-Benefit Analyses

In the late 1960s several studies appeared in the US and established the significance and cost of kidney disease (Burton 1969; Gottschalk 1967; Hallan and Harris 1968; LeSourd et al. 1968). Only one of these studies was a CBA. The study by LeSourd et al. was done for the National Center for Chronic Disease Control (the Kidney Disease Control Programme). One of the aims of the study was to carry out a benefit-cost analysis of a limited number of select kidney disease programmes. The analysis was intended to supplement the programme analysis carried out that same year, 1967/1968, the Gottschalk Committee's analysis. Benefits in the analysis were supposed to be both economic and health-related. The study appears to be the first rigorous CBA of a kidney treatment programme. Treatments considered were home- and hospital-haemodialysis, and transplantation.

The cost-benefit approach adopted was that which subsequently has become known as human capital (HC)-based CBA as opposed to the "willingness to

3 Reference is made here to the Gottschalk (1967) report. In 1968 the first steps leading to a general coverage of treatment for CRF were taken in the US and in 1973 Medicare benefits were extended to virtually all patients with CRF.

pay"-based approach[4]. The *format* of the HC-based CBA is simple. Following Weisbrod's (1961) lead the monetary losses that accrue as a result of morbidity and mortality are:

1. Indirect costs
   a) The loss of economic production due to premature death (of a member of the labour force)
   b) Temporary and/or intermittent losses of economic production due to sickness
   c) Decreased production efficiency due to disease-induced debility
2. Direct costs
   a) The economic costs of detection, treatment, rehabilitation, and capital investment in medical facilities

In the case of CBA (as opposed to the cost-of-illness format above) of a contemplated treatment programme, the indirect costs become benefits, namely, "saved costs". More precisely, a fraction of the costs become benefits. The size of the fraction depends among other things on the efficacy of the treatment. Depending on the disease under consideration the direct costs may become benefits too, for instance in connection with a disease-eradication programme. The costs in the CBA are the costs of the new programme, say an eradication programme. In terms of the monetary measuring rod used, it is assumed that a person's wages are a reasonable measure of his productivity. To conduct a CBA some *epidemiological* information must be present: (1) incidence and/or prevalence of disease, (2) number of cases discovered and/or treated, (3) treatment or diagnostic techniques actually or potentially available, (4) cure rate and survival period for the various treatment modalities/ techniques, and ideally, (5) some indication of the "quality of life" (rehabilitation, social function) etc. after treatment.

In the LeSourd study all benefits and costs were obtained by *cohort analysis,* i.e. by relating costs and benefits to the present and future history of a cohort. Usually a cohort of 1000 people is studied for, say, 20–30 years. To translate the analysis into equivalent economic terms, the cohort must be characterized in terms of sex, age, potential earnings, and morbidity and mortality patterns. LeSourd et al. assumed: (1) the cohort was composed of 50% males and 50% females, (2) average age for both groups was 45 years in the 1st year of the programme, (3) cohort attrition for centre- and home-dialysis was based on two assumptions – (a) 15% of the original cohort dies during the 1st year of treatment, and (b) in each subsequent year 10% of the remaining individuals die[5]. Rehabilitation in terms of ability to work was as-

4 For further discussion of these two CBAs see the section "Two Cost-Benefit Analyses".

5 It is obvious that in any analysis assumptions like these are crucial and must reflect the best available medical evidence. They refer to the American experience in the mid-1960s. For easy reference and comparison the European 1979 figures are:

	Percent of patients surviving after	
	5 years	10 years
Hospital-haemodialysis	53.2	35.6
Home-haemodialysis	74.0	55.6
1st live-donor graft	71.2	60.0
1st cadaver graft	58.1	44.2

Source: EDTA (1980), Table 17

sumed to bo equal to 70%, i. e. it was assumed that 70% of the surviving members of the dialysis cohort were able to maintain each year 100% of the earnings of a healthy individual of the same age and sex. For the remaining 30% a 50% earnings potential was assumed[6].

The results for haemodialysis and transplantation may be summarized as in Table 9.4. The benefit-cost ratios are calculated by forming a fraction of discounted

Table 9.4. Benefit-cost ratios for USA 1968, 1000 patients cohort followed 30 years, 6% discount rate (LeSourd et al. 1968)

		High[e]	Low[e]	"Best estimate"[e]
Centre benefit-cost ratio		0.29	0.21	0.25
Home benefit-cost ratio		0.86	0.34	0.65
Transplantation[a]	0.85	–	–	–
Transplantation[b]	1.05	–	–	–
Transplantation[c]	0.97	–	–	–
Transplantation[d]	1.23	–	–	–

[a] 75% 2-year suvival rate, centre with 60 transplants, including research costs
[b] as [a] but without research costs
[c] as [a] but peritoneal dialysis prior to transplantation
[d] as [c] but without research costs
[e] data from various sources

Table 9.5. Results from England and Wales, 1972 cost-benefit ratios, 1000-patient cohort followed for 20 years, 10% discount rate

	A[a]	B[b]	C[c]	D[d]
Hospital-dialysis	6.4	7.0	3.2	12.7
Home-dialysis	3.2	3.5	1.6	6.3

[a] Assumptions: *survival* after 6 years – hospital 50%, home 63.4%, and extrapolations based on a negative exponential function for subsequent years, *rehabilitation:* hospital – years 1–3, 30%, 52%, and 60%, respectively, 60% in subsequent years; home – years 1–3, 45%, 65%, and 75%, respectively, and 75% in subsequent years. Wage rates used were annual average rates for males and females. Discount rate: 10%. Capital costs distributed over 20 years.
[b] as [a] but with a 14% discount factor,
[c] Low cost case – half of [a]
[d] Low average earnings, half of [a]

6 For comparison consider the following 1978 American figures

	Percent			
	Disabled		Not working	
	Before	After	Before	After
Centre-haemodialysis	3.1	49.5	10.9	20.9
Home-haemodialysis	2.7	37.4	8.2	14.3

Source: extracted from Table 16 in Bryan (1969) and Levans (1979). For European figures see EDTA (1980), Tables 19–21

benefits and costs. If the ratio is greater than 1, benefits exceed costs and investment is "profitable" provided that no other relevant possibilities with greater ratios exist. Put differently, given limited resources, it is possible to rank-order projects according to their benefit-cost ratios.

Buxton and West (1975) carried out a similiar HC-based cost-benefit analysis for long-term haemodialysis for England and Wales. Their results, in terms of *cost-benefit ratios* are presented in Table 9.5 under various assumptions. Despite differences in assumptions and time and place, the American and English data show the same result: In terms of benefits and costs of haemodialysis, costs clearly outweigh benefits. In an attempt to cope with uncertainty about a number of parameters sensitivity analyses were carried out in both studies. In no case did it change the general picture of costs markedly exceeding benefits. From case C in Table 9.5 it is also clear that the crucial factor appears to be the costs of treatment. The American figures seem to indicate that transplantation is "socially profitable" when research costs are excluded. However, it is clear that the benefits are too high due to the unrealistic assumptions about rehabilitation. If adjustments are made for this fact the ratios in all cases will be less than 1.

A more critical discussion of the results the methodology will follow the section on CEA.

Cost-Effectiveness Analyses

If for some reason one is not interested in doing a CBA, for instance because the decision-makers are not interested in an answer to the general question of whether or not resources should be allocated to a given project, economic evaluation may still be carried out by means of CEA whereby answers to a narrower set of questions are analysed. CEA and CBA are two related but still distinctly different approaches to evaluation of health practices. In a sense the key difference between CEA and CBA is the valuation of the benefits/outcomes of a health practice. Ideally, in CBA all outcomes/benefits are valued in money terms, including loss of life and limb along with quality of life and other intangibles. CEA serves to place priorities on alternative treatments (expenditure categories), as noted previously, but without requiring that the dollar-value of life and health be assessed[7].

Two typical CEA situations can be envisaged, both involving two or more treatments: (a) given or assuming that the alternatives under consideration have the same clinical effectiveness in terms of whatever outcome measures are thought appropriate – which procedure is the least costly? i. e. in this situation cost differences between two alternatives are important; (b) outcomes are not the same, either with respect to type of outcome or level of outcome. Assuming that outcomes vary with respect to level (e. g. life expectancy or "quality of life"), one might attempt to cost the units of outcome, for instance cost per life-year gained, and then compare the

7 For two short easy to read introductions to CEA see Weinstein and Stason (1977) and Shepard and Thompson (1979); and for an example with a reasonable methodological discussion see Culyer and Maynard (1981).

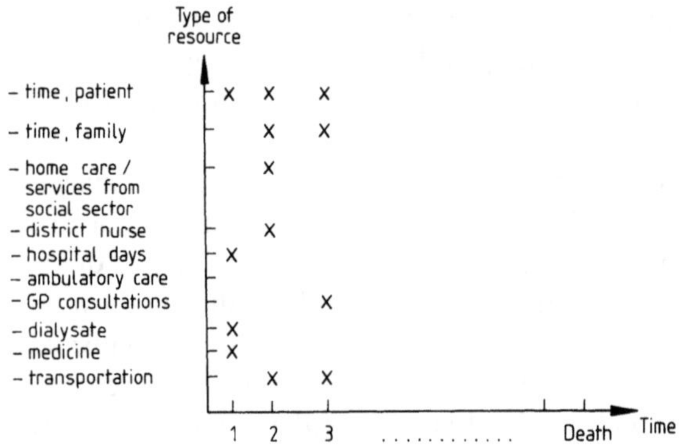

Fig. 9.1. "Treatment-resource profile"

alternatives this way. It is this latter version of CEA that has been used in studies of dialysis and transplantation (see Table 9.6).

The characteristic feature of CEA[8] is the simultaneous inclusion of *costs* and *end-results* of the treatment. The latter distinguishes CEA from cost analyses. CEA can be conducted from various perspectives, for instance from (a) a sectoral point of view, i.e. the health care sector or even narrower, for instance a hospital, and (b) a broad societal perspective. The perspective in particular influences the cost side. In connection with medical technology evaluation the societal perspective ought to be taken. Ideally, therefore, social costs are the costs sought. One way to picture this is to look at the "treatment-resource profile" (Fig. 9.1).

Looking at "costs" this way may help to dispel a number of common mistakes or poorly understood notions. First, we disregard from which sector resources are drawn or, put differently, resources drawn from different sectors are included on an equal footing. In relation to home-haemodialysis, resources from the social sector (e.g. home care) are undoubtedly important – and disregarded in many perhaps all studies encountered by the author. Similarly, there is no doubt that input of patient time is important in all forms of dialysis as is the input of time by family members, in particular in connection with home-haemodialysis. Second, we can separate the quantity, e.g. number of hours, litres of dialysate, from the price/value question, i.e. can the hourly wage be used as a reasonable price for an hour? Third, and more or less as a logical consequence of the previous point, we are *not* looking at expenditure flows. In the present context this means that we are not only disregarding who finances costs (patients, third party, or government), but the perspective on transfer payments, for instance disability pensions to disabled dialysis and transplantation patients or sick pay, is clear from the figure: they are excluded (whereas they would be included in a typical, sectoral expenditure analysis). The reason for exclusion is the societal perspective on the cost issue. From the viewpoint of society as a whole transfer payments merely imply that what one pays in taxation another receives, i.e. there is no net change in resource use, merely a reshuffling of purchasing power.

After this brief review we can now turn to five CEAs of dialysis and transplantation (Table 9.6). The general result emerging from the table is that for *dialysis*, home-

8 As has been demonstrated in the section "Some Economic Questions in Technology Evaluation" this also is true for CBA.

Table 9.6. Results and assumptions in five CEAs

Authors	Year	Country	Cost per life-year saved[a]						Model	Discount rate (%)	Time-span (years)
			1	2	3	4	5	6			
Klarman et al. (1968)	1968	USA, $	4200	11600	2600				Cohort	6	40
Stange and Summer (1978)	1978	USA, $	16986	26547		15007	12982		Cohort	7 costs life-years	10
Roberts et al. (1980)	1980	USA, $	≈14000	≈26000			16000	≈8000	Simulation of 10000 patients	5 cost 7 life-years	onset of uremia to death
Ludbrook (1981)	1981	UK, £	5150–5800	7100 11200	3250–4650				markov chain	7 cost	
Barnes (1977a)[c]	1977	USA, $	31000	170000			27000	22000	Cohort	5	5

[a] 1, Home-dialysis; 2, hospital/centre-dialysis; 3, transplantation and dialysis; 4, Facility dialysis to cadaveric transplantation; 5, Home dialysis to cadaveric transplantation; 6, Live-denor tranplant + dialysis [b] Cost figures read from a bar-diagram [c] per survivor in a single cohort, 5 years total

dialysis is systematically cheaper than hospital-dialysis. Comparing *dialysis* and *transplantation* it is seen that transplantation is the cheaper alternative. Note, however, that in the case of cadaveric transplantation the difference between home-dialysis and transplantation is neglible. In the latest American analysis only the live-related-donor transplant is better than dialysis[9].

The policy implication of these results – consistent over a 13-year period – seems to be that resources for treating CRF should be shifted towards increasing the transplantation rate, in particular, efforts should be directed at increasing live-donor transplantations. However, a bottleneck in this connection is the availability of kidneys. In the absence of a well-organized organ-exchange network or in the case of legal problems, this bottleneck may be the real constraint on expansion of the transplantation programme.

With regard to the question of allocation of resources between treatments there is not much doubt as to the favourable position of transplantation. This is basically due to very low costs, because survival, in particular during the 1st year, is lower than for the alternative. However, both from a medical and economic point of view one is interested in *patient selection,* or put differently, allocation of resourves between patients. In only two of the above studies was this issue addressed (Roberts et al. 1980; Ludbrook 1981).

Discussion of CEA Assumptions

Three elements enter any CEA – epidemiological parameters, e.g. survival rates, a model, e.g. a cohort model, and the cost data. A CEA is no better than the weakest link. These elements therefore will be investigated in turn.

The Epidemiological Parameters

It is almost a truism, but nevertheless often overlooked: Inadequate epidemilogical information makes for inadequate CEA and CBA. When judging the above results it is obvious that the results are only as valid as the underlying epidemiological parameters allows. The crucial assumptions have been presented already and will not be discussed further as they undoubtedly reflect the best present knowledge. There are two problems worth commenting on. When comparisons are made between centre-dialysis and home-dialysis it is assumed that we are more or less looking at

9 This is obviously due to the rather low survival probability for cadaveric transplants, see note 5. Survival *probabilities* used by Roberts et al. (1980) are:

	Transplantation		Home and hospital dialysis
	live	cadaveric	
Year 1	0.83–0.85	0.60–0.63	–
Year 2+	0.89–0.98	0.96–0.87	–
Year 1–3			0.80–0.90
Year 16+			0.51–0.88

The assumptions used by Stange und Summer (1978) were similar to those of Roberts et al. Ludbrook's (1981) assumptions were not stated explicitly, but references were made to EDTA figures. Thus the data in note 5 probably are indicative of the assumptions.

two substitute treatments, implying that centre-dialysis patients might just as well have been home-dialysis patients and vice versa. While this is undoubtedly true to some extent, it is also true that some kind of conscious selection of patients takes place – on average heavy and/or troublesome patients are left for centre-dialysis. This may create a bias in the comparisons, as does the fact that some of the centre mortality is undoubtedly "home-dialysis mortality", either because mortality occurs while training for home-dialysis or when home-dialysis patients are being centre-dialysed due to complications. The extent of the latter type of bias is difficult to assess.

The other problem is related to the fact that survival information is lacking for the long term. Some models use work with 20–30-year time horizons. Usually survival information is only available for 10–15 years, at least information of reasonable quality. Beyond that, survival figures are "guesstimates". Some of the, possibly erroneous, medium and long-term assumptions may be compounded by the particular "model" used. Model refers to the method used to combine the epidemiological assumptions (data input) and data requirements (data output from the model) for CEA and CBA.

Types of Model

Three models have been used in the CEAs reviewed here: the cohort model, Markov-chain models, and simulation models. In the *cohort model* the epidemiological inputs consist of survival data, either aggregated or sex- and age-specific, and the output is a time profile indicating how many of the cohort are on treatment at given points in time; it allows for relatively easy calculation of average or median life expectancy of an individual in a cohort. This output gives not only the time profile of outcomes but also the time profile of the costs incurred for treatment of the cohort. This is indispensable for the calculation of present values. However, the cohort model embodies an assumption about independence of treatments under consideration. It is easy to overlook that patients move among treatments. It is rather difficult to incorporate this in the cohort model, and in some instances it is crucial to be able to do this. Thus, home-dialysis presupposes for practical purposes that back-up centre facilities are available either for short- or long-term use by home-dialysis patients – and for their initial training. The cohort model thus simplifies the real treatment process considerably. The degree of simplification depends on whether only one or multiple cohorts are considered. The inclusion of multiple cohorts implies that a new cohort of patients is included annually[10]. It thus becomes possible to consider end-results and costs in a more realistic programme setting. This also ought to include the assumption that programmes are expanding, i.e. the selection criteria are relaxed over time[11].

---

10 For a rather general cohort model see Barnes (1977 a), in particular the appendix where the general formulaes are developed. Stange und Summer (1978) use a multipel-cohort model for some of their calculations – a total of ten cohorts are considered – the period is 10 years.

11 Thus EDTA figures indicate that in many European countries, e.g. France, West Germany, and Italy, but not the UK, acceptance rates for dialysis expressed in terms of number of patients per million of the population in different age-groups have increased markedly from 1974–1978 for the age-groups 55–64 years, 65–74 years, and 74+ years (Figure 1 a, b, EDTA 1980).

Use of a simple *Markov model* enables one to consider the transitions between treatment modalities in detail and allows for easy calculation of mean stay time in each state. Markov models were developed quite early for planning purposes (see Farrow et al. 1971; West et al. 1974; Pliskin et al. 1976 1976; Rimm et al. 1978). These models mainly differ with respect to the number of "states" included and thus the number of treatment combinations allowed. Ludbrook (1981) appears to have been the first to use this model in a CEA context; the author notes that it is a very compact method of analysis making it possible to consider the treatments in more detail than in cohort analysis, and the probabilities can be re-estimated as new data become available. However, some of the assumptions underlying the Markov models are not tested, in particular the stationarity assumption, i.e. that the transition probabilities are stable over the period considered. Two other assumptions not tested are the Markov property, i.e. the "no-memory" property of the transition probabilities, and the homogeneity assumptions, i.e. that everybody in a group has the same transition probability. Some of the results of a Markov-chain analysis may be rather sensitive to departures from the assumptions. The use of Markov-chain models thus has a price, but the gains undoubtedly outweigh the costs. It would be useful to move away from the simple Markov models to semi-Markov models allowing for variable duration in each state (these durations are treated as stochastic variables in a semi-Markov model).

The final model is the *computer simulation model,* which allows for great flexibility; there is no doubt that this approach is to be preferred to both the cohort and the Markov models, because many possibilities can be tested without much trouble by means of standard simulation programmes. The important point to oberserve is that it becomes relatively easy to include rather detailed epidemiological information.

Overall it must be concluded that only in the case of a single cohort model must one be cautious when interpreting CEA results, such as those of Klarman et al. (1968).

Cost Components and Assumptions

With regard to the models it was noted that it was rather important to be able to simulate a full-programme – and possibly expanding programmes. The cost figures ought to reflect this too[12]. However, the cost figures usually used at best reflect average costs for a limited number of facilities or even patients[13]. However, if the results of the analysis are used for a recommendation that certain programme components should be expanded or contracted, the expected (marginal) costs undoubtedly would be higher than the average cost figures on which the programme analysis was based (even with unchanged selection criteria). As an illustrative example consider Fig. 9.2.

---

12 In this connection it is of interest to note that in the study by LeSourd et al. (1968), the scale of operation was included for the transplantation alternative, namely 60, 75, and 90 transplants per year. For the smallest scale all benefit-cost ratios were less than 1.

13 Thus, Ludbrook's figures are (unpublished) figures from the Department of Health and Social Security. However, they appear to be the same figures as used by OHE (1978), where a fuller description is given: a) 36 patients admitted for transplantation in 1974–1975 were followed-up through to the end of 1976; counting the costs generated by them at 1976/1977 prices; b) for comparison, a sample of 20 patients destined for home-dialysis were also followed-up.

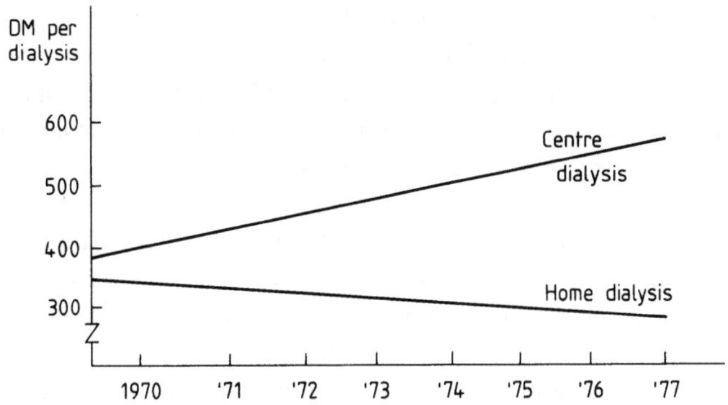

Fig. 9.2. Development in costs of home- and centre-dialysis in West Germany. Centre figures are national averages, whereas the home dialysis figures are from "Kuratorium für Heim Dialyse Neu Isenburg". (Modified from Clade 1980)

According to the source prices are current annual prices. It cannot be ruled out that inflation has developed differentially for the two modes, but it cannot explain away the trend. No doubt, the increase in the costs of centre-dialysis to some extent is due to increasing marginal costs of treatment associated with facility expansion along with relaxed selection criteria, which may have operated differentially[14]. The important observation heres is related to the possible erroneous policy use of CBAs and DEAs, which do not reflect reasonable assumptions as to marginal costs. However, for practical purposes it might be claimed that one in general would expect the pattern exhibited in Fig. 9.2 and this just reinforces the general conclusion from Table 9.6.

We turn now to the more detailed examination of the cost figures used. If Fig. 9.1 is used as a point of departure, it must be noted that in none of the studies were *time costs* included. This holds both for home- and centre-dialysis. In terms of working time centre-dialysis is undoubtedly the more costly because dialysis usually takes place during the normal working hours for hospital personnel as well as in the working hours of the patient. If this were included, centre-dialysis would become even more costly than home-dialysis[15]. On the other hand, the exclusion of the

14 The numerical development in the number of patients in West Germany has been as follows:

	No. in hospital	No. home	Transplants
1972	1596	509	148
1977	4981	1747	478

The average age of patients who started hospital-haemodialysis in West Germany in 1974 and 1979 was 44.4 and 50.0 years, respectively. For grafted patients the corresponding figures are 33.6 and 35.1 years.

15 See Crichton et al. (1981) for a description of a ten-bed haemodialysis unit operating 24 h a day – during the day as a fully assisted regular "centre"-haemodialysis unit, during the night as a self-care dialysis unit. The latter programme was offered to patients unable for social reasons to carry out home-haemodialysis who did not wish to waste time during the day. Not only was valuable patient time saved, but operating costs for the self-care unit were more than 50% lower than for the day-care unit.

input of family time for home-dialysis may seriously understate the costs of home-dialysis[16]. From a societal point of view the exclusion of time costs is deplorable, in part because the real costs then cannot be estimated, in part because it might distort the comparisons. However, on balance it probably would not change the rank-ordering of treatment modalities discussed earlier.

Transport costs are another relatively important cost component missing in all the studies. In relation to the treatments considered it makes centre-dialysis appear less costly than actually is the case. However, one must not overlook travel costs for home-dialysis patients to back-up centre facilities for routine examinations[17].

Morbidity costs are often neglected. Annual hospitalization[18] costs for each method of treatment can be substantial, in particular for transplantation[19]. If one recalls the negligible difference between cadaveric transplantation and home-dialysis, this component may be crucial[20].

The last cost component to be commented on here is related to home-dialysis. The training for home-dialysis usually takes place in a regular hospital dialysis unit or a special training unit. It is clear that these costs must be assigned to the home-dialysis cost figures[21]. Furthermore, home-dialysis to some extent takes place in the hospital, i.e. in event of complications and for control[22].

The general impression of the cost side of CEAs is that a rather narrow cost concept is employed. Time and transportation costs are never/rarely considered, and morbidity costs are only included in a few cases. As indicated in the discussion these omissions on balance probably do not change the rank-ordering of treatments. However, they become important if the CEAs are used either for calculation of total costs of treatment programmes, or if programmes are expanded or changed without reflection based on a CEA. As an example of the former, consider the results of the multiple-cohort model used by Stange and Summers (1978). Three options were investigated: shifting 1000 patients a year (a) from facility- to home-dialysis, (b) from facility-dialysis to transplantation, and (c) from home-dialysis to

---

16 Despite the fact that this argument has played an important role in the American discussion no study has apparently been undertaken of the issue.

17 In non-CEA/CBA contexts they have been estimated, see for instance Hoffstein et al. (1976) and Schippers and Kalff (1976). Hoffstein et al. (1976) found that travel costs ranged between 14% and 21% of the total average cost in dollars per dialysis. The Dutch figures were lower, 7% of annual treatment costs.

18 Over and above what is needed in connection with routine dialysis and routine post-transplant check-ups.

19 Some relevant hospitalization figures are provided in EDTA (1980), Figure 33 and Table 22. If one compares hospital-haemodialysis and first cadaveric transplant patients in the age-group 35–54 years, one finds that in both groups more than 9% of the patients were hospitalized for more than 3 months during the 1st year of treatment, falling to 2%–5% for subsequent years.

20 It appears to have been included in the cost figures used by Roberts et al. (1980) and Stange and Summer (1978).

21 In Hoffstein et al. (1976), four separate home training units were included and had the highest cost per dialysis – $190.09 vs. $158.58 and $43.13 for hospital- and home-dialysis, repsectively. Training costs were included by Roberts et al. (1980) and made up 17% of the 1st-year costs of home-dialysis.

22 Buxton and West (1975b) estimated that about 5% of the dialyses given to Cardiff home-dialysis patients were given in hospitals. Roughly the same percentages were noted by Roberts et al. (1980).

transplantation. The overall results were estimated to be: life expectancy unchanged and $241 million saved for a, life expectancy reduced by 7%–17% and $279–330 million saved for b, and life expectancy reduced by 10%–20% and $103–143 million saved for c. However, the cost figures used do not include time costs, which is important for option a, but with respect to b and c morbidity costs as measured by hospital costs were included. Furthermore, and this point relates to expansion or change along with the previous discussion of average versus marginal costs, available evidence seems to indicate that the assumed (average) cost relationships do not hold with nonmarginal changes[23]. It seems to be generally recognized (e.g. Diaz-Buxo and Chandler 1980) that unless new end-stage renal patients are introduced to home-training from the very beginning it is practically impossible to keep a high rate of home-dialysis.

In order to keep a state of readiness to provide competent and immediate dialysis home-training to new patients and adequate facilities must be available at any time. This will (may) result in an intermittent under-utilization of facilities, which in turn translates into higher costs to provide this specialized service. Diaz-Buxo and Chandler claim that we tend to apply the familar industrial rule that costs of production drop as volume increases. Unfortunately, this is not the case with home-training (Diaz-Buxo and Chandler 1980). For low levels of training for home-dialysis, i.e. 10% of the patients in a programme, the chances are that no particular provision will be made to accommodate these patients in special facilities. However, if home-training rates increased to 20%–25% or even to 50% – which is currently the aim in the US – special provisions must be made and costs per case most likely will increase.

The point of the above is not necessarily that a more careful costing exercise would change the direction of the recommendations. Rather, the size of possible savings may be exaggerated, and differences on the margin are not as great as they appear to be on average.

If one were to give a recommendation for future CEAs it would be that more attention ought to be paid to the cost side. As a minimum the cost categories indicated in Fig. 9.1 ought to be discussed along with the patient and/or centre base for cost calculations *and* this discussion should be included in the article. Otherwise it is difficult to accumulate comparable evidence[24]. *Ideally,* the resource use associated with a treatment should be investigated as an integrated part of clinical trials, i.e. ascertained prospectively and not retrospectively as is the case now. Often availability of accounts and book-keeping conventions rather than economic cost conventions are decisive for how "costs" are calculated. If collected prospectively and/or with the same vigour as clinical data are collected, the cost side of CEAs might improve considerably.

---

23 In the example, a shift of 1000 patients/year is equal to 10%–15% of the new patients in a given year.

24 There is no doubt that it is a rather dubious comparison that is made in Table 9.6. The cost concepts employed differ considerably.

The Broader Perspective

In this section the broader treatment perspective will be considered whereas the broader analytic questions, i.e. the omission of "quality of life" considerations from the CBAs and CEAs discussed so far along with other issues will be discussed below.

With all medical technologies there is a tendency towards being caught by the treatment/curative aspects – simply because most technologies are treatment technologies (definitely not curative technologies in the case of chronic renal failure). This usually means that the overall strategy (treatment/prevention and research priorities) is neglected in connection with the economic evaluation – and consequently neglected in the ensuing policy debate. There are several reasons for this bias. One has just been mentioned, but at a more fundamental level the necessary aetiological information is often lacking[25]. And this aetiological knowledge seems to be a prerequisite for analysis of prevention strategies. Reasonably good knowledge has ac-

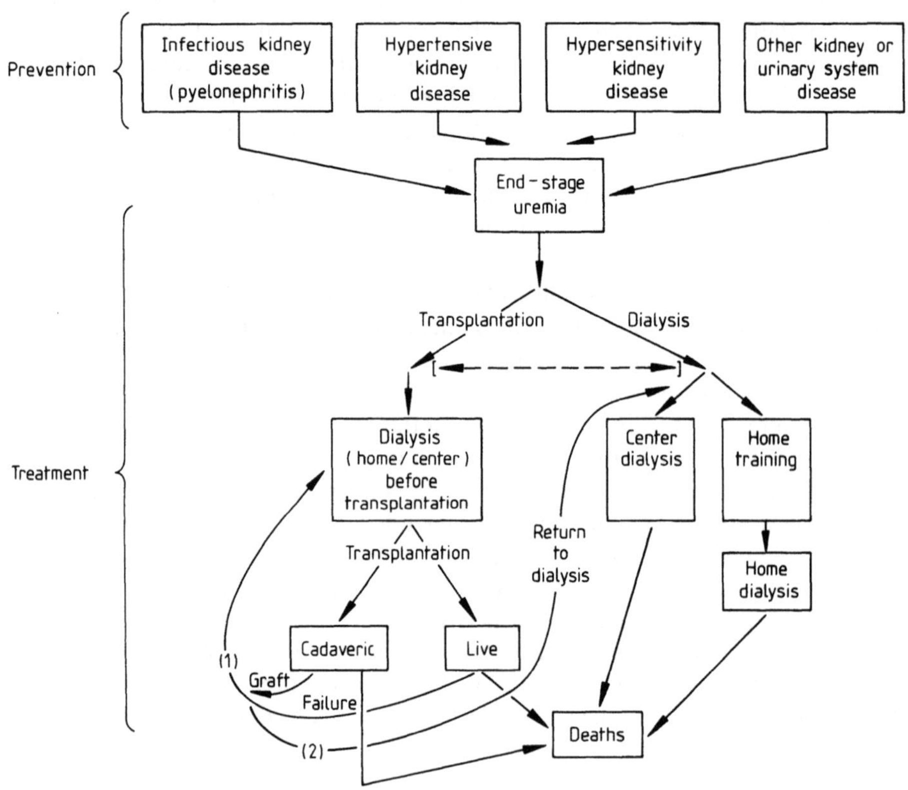

Fig. 9.3. The overall prevention and treatment strategy

25 We are here disregarding the fact that professional groups with vested interests in given medical technologies bloom quickly in and along the wake of a new technology and may cause and reinforce this bias. The same holds for patient associations. Some of these issues are considered in the literature on diffusion of technologies. For a formal model see Monheit (1978) or, at a more general level, Russell (1979).

cumulated concerning kidney diseases leading to end-stage uremia. In Fig. 9.3 a rough sketch is given of prevention and treatment strategies.

In the present context it is of interest to note that the only analysis where treatment and prevention strategies were considered simultaneously is that of LeSourd et al. (1968). They give a careful description of the then typical medical basis for programme design of preventive and treatment programmes. A CBA, based on the same principles as described earlier, was carried out for a *Streptococcus*-screening programme and a bacteriuria-screening programme. With respect to the former it was thought that it was highly probable that a screening programme designed to identify persons harbouring known nephrogenic organisms could significantly reduce the incidence of acute glomerulonephritis and thereby reduce the incidence of chronic glomerulonephritis, which can often be expected as a sequela – and this in turn can lead to end-stage uremia. Benefit-cost ratios of 46.9 and 130.0 were found for the *Streptococcus* programme[26]. The ratios in the bacteriuria-screening programme ranged between 7.5 for school children and 12.8 for industrial workers – all ratios were calculated for 100000 person-programmes.

A cost-benefit approach to overall research strategy has also been attempted – at least in a loose sense (see Statens Medicinska Forskningsrad 1976). The identified research areas, among these the aetiological and preventive activities had a prominent place, had been picked with a view to the economic aspects. However, no stringent CBA was carried out.

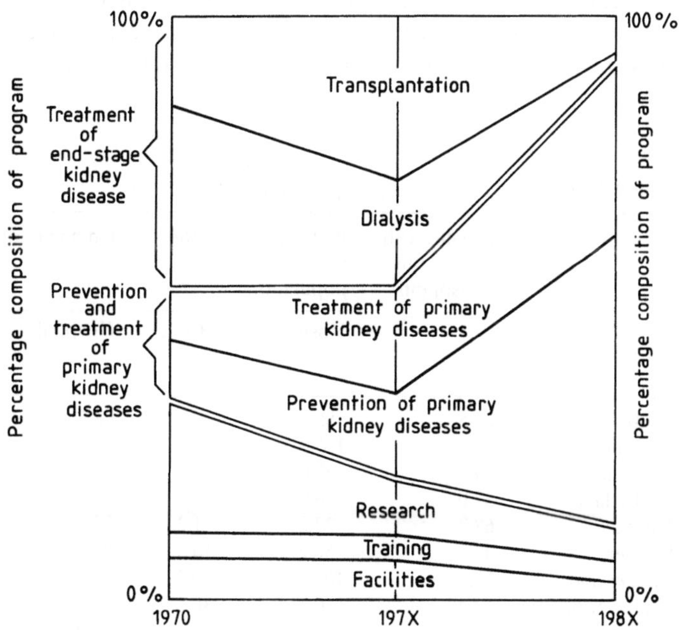

Fig. 9.4. Hypothetical effects of advancing state of the art on future programme composition

26 Screening 100000 adults. See Table 5.4 in LeSourd et al. (1968). For 100000 children the ratios were 14.6 and 39.2 – for programme costs of $200000 and $75000.

In view of the above considerations it may be of interest, if only historical, to consider Fig. 9.4 (based on Burton 1969 and Grosse 1970) where a hypothetical, anno 1970, future programme mix is pictured. The important thing to note is not the exact percentages, but the trends. It is almost superfluous to note that these trends have not materialized. In a speculative vein one may wonder whether there is a tendency towards "crowding out" by treatment-oriented medical technologies – this crowding out is perhaps helped in part by lack of aetiological knowledge (see Menz 1971, 1975).

The Present Treatment Pattern

From an economic – and also clinical point of view – home-dialysis has been advocated as the "best" form of treatment, or even optimal mode of dialysis therapy, for years. In view of this it is of interest to have a look at the present treatment pattern (Table 9.7). It is striking that in many countries the home-dialysis rate is very low – and lower than necessary. Medical opinion on the percentage of patients that can be on home-dialysis ranges from 10%–90% and in specific countries will depend on the age-composition of patients and other medical complications, e.g. diabetes. However, as long as medical opinion differs, it must be of interest to note that it can differ so much that the consequences (cumulative) become as great as the right-hand columm in Table 9.7 indicates. The economic consequences of these treatment patterns are considerable. Roughly the most expensive programmes are characterized by low home-dialysis rates and low percentages of patients with functioning grafts. It is interesting to note that in the UK where the budget constraint has been very real for years, home-dialysis is used in 65% of all cases. This has to be contrasted with Norway and Austria at the other extreme. It is seen that with the exception of Norway, countries with high home-dialysis rates also have relatively high per-

Table 9.7. Treatment patterns in Europe and the US for 1979

	Percent with functioning transplants[b]	Patients on haemodialysis per million population		On haemodialysis (%)		
		Hospital	Home	Hospital	Home	
					1979	1977
Austria	20.5	85.3	10.2	93.6	6.7	4.9
Belgium	29.0	123.9	10.0	92.5	7.5	7.3
Denmark	50.2	57.6	17.5	76.8	23.2	22.4
Netherlands	32.0	86.0	9.1	90.5	9.5	9.4
Norway	68.7	27.8	1.2	95.8	4.2	5.8
Sweden	47.7	50.2	14.5	77.0	22.3	22.4
Switzerland	33.1	101.9	30.5	77.0	23.0	24.0
United Kingdom	43.4	20.5	36.5	35.9	64.1	66.3
United States[c]				88.0	12.0	

[a] Calculated from Table II, European Dialysis and Transplant Association (1980)
[b] Percent of total number of CRF patients alive
[c] Bryan and Evans (1980a and b) give these figures; n = approx. 26000 patients but undoubtedly it is a minimum figure, compare with Table 9.2

centages of patients with functioning transplants, giving a rough indication of economically efficient dialysis-transplantation programmes.

It would need a separate study to try to explain how and why such divergent patterns emerge. It suffices to note that financing and reimbursement systems may dramatically influence choice of treatment. Thus the copayment clause for home-dialysis in the US has undoubtedly been very decisive in bringing about a decline in home-dialysis from 1973 onwards. This example points towards an area that ought to be an integral part of economic evaluation of medical technologies, namely, the effects of various incentive and reimbursement schemes.

It is surprising that home-dialysis is not used more extensively when there are good economic and clinical reasons for doing so. In general, considerable inertia seems to come to prevail with respect to treatment modalities and treatment procedures. One example where economic savings could be realized without changing outcome is the re-use of dialysers. In this case one can study the reluctance to change or try out a new procedure, re-use of dialysers, for economic reasons and unchanged outcomes. Consider the following: "Financial constraints have made it necessary for many physicians to decide to reuse 'disposable' dialysers. Ethical responsibility for this decision must remain with the clinician" (Wing et al. 1978). In Wing et al. (1978) it is also interesting to note that seven units thought that the practice was potentially very dangerous. However, in terms of mortality and morbidity it appears that re-use of dialysers is no worse than not re-using dialysers. In view of the fact that dialysers are expensive (7%–10% of the costs of a dialysis), and re-use might free resources for other beneficial uses in the dialysis area, the reluctance to do so is a bit surprising. Wing et al. (1978) estimated that were the present rate of re-use to be eliminated, for instance due to fears of litigation, the extra expenditure would at the present re-use rate be almost £1 million/year – for this money, 150 patient-years of home-dialysis could be financed[27]. With a given budget, trade-offs are made all the time, implicitly and explicitly! It is going to be interesting to see how fast (or slowly) CAPD is going to replace home- and centre-haemodialysis. It is roughly 20% cheaper[28] than home-dialysis and in terms of outcome CAPD on many counts appears to be superior to haemodialysis[29].

On the "Narrowness" of CEA and CBA

Both CBA and CEA are often accused of being "narrow, economic" analyses. The exact implications, however, are rarely made clear. The examples presented here are admittedly narrow in the sense that the only outcome considered is survival time

---

27 See also Ogden et al. (1981) and Siemsen et al. (1980) for further discussion and economics of re-use. A sample quotation from Ogden may illustrate the various interests: "Given the present technical, legal, medical, and economic concerns, the re-use of single-use dialyzers should be discontinued!"

28 von Fuchs (1979) and Robson et al. (1978) note that "an impressive advantage" of CAPD is a marked decrease in running costs, which are cut to almost one-third of those in intermittent peritoneal dialysis (IPD), i.e. $5000/year – and IPD is considerably cheaper than haemodialysis.

29 For further clinical and outcome aspects of CAPD, see among others Weinman et al. (1980), Oreopoulos et al. (1980), and Robson and Oreopoulos (1978).

(and rehabilitation). In some areas this would be less of a problem, but in dialysis and transplantation this is not the case. The quality of the survival time in terms of rehabilitation, social functioning etc. differs considerably between treatments and cannot be disregarded lightly. As an example consider the following lists of "psychosocial costs" compiled by Abt (1977): home-dialysis is characterized by discomfort; disrupted professional and work relations; loss of community contributions and participation; segregation, isolation, and discrimination; immobility; dependency; limitation of normal activities such as work, social life, sex, recreation; furthermore, loss of self-esteem, anxiety, and worry and depression can be expected. Hospital-dialysis may be described similarly with the following added – greater loneliness, limitations, and inconvenience as well as reduced opportunity to enjoy the home environment. Hospital-dialysis and transplantation involve some worry and the inconvenience of follow-up checks during the period after discharge from hospital. Other aspects can undoubtedly be added, for instance dialysis dementia in some patients, i.e. a clinical neurological syndrome consisting of speech disorder, apraxia, and progressive dementia. In 1977, 157 patients were registered for this European Dialysis and Transplant Association 1977). Bone pain is another problem for dialysis patients[30].

From the viewpoint of CEA and CBA the problem is how these important aspects are to be integrated. In the case of CBA some kind of method of translating data on the duration and severity of pain, inconvenience, and anxiety into costs commensurable with other more regular costs is needed. Otherwise the quality of life factors cannot rationally be weighed against the quantity of life, i.e. survival time. In this connection Abt (1977) notes that a major motivation for his own attempt in this direction is that by placing a monetary "price" on pain etc. it becomes tangible. Ceteris paribus, when weighing a tangible aspect like longevity against previously intangible benefits such as reduced pain "many human physicians, like most rational individuals, would tend to give more weight to the tangible side of the balance" Abt (1977). There is no doubt that by focusing on survival this aspect is implicitly considered to be more important than quality of life, i.e. in many cases a longer survival time is considered to be better than a shorter survival time but with better quality of life.

The particular approach taken by Abt was to use "shadow prices" for the various aspects of quality of life. Shadow prices of quality of life factors can be estimated in so far as we can determine what people are willing to pay to be rid of them. In most cases, however, such willingness to pay prices is not immediate. Considerable imagination must be exhibited when indentifying shadow prices – often too much imagination. For instance, the loss of home privacy and comfort in the hospital can be estimated from what is paid on average to achieve it beyond a similar level of purely physical convenience attainable in rented rooms.

> Assuming one can rent a standard room with shared use of a bathroom and kitchen for about $ 1000 a year and that the average private apartment or home rental is about $ 3000 a year, the annual loss of privacy and aesthetic choice is estimated conservatively at the difference of $ 2000 per year. (Abt 1977).

30 For other aspects see Levy and Wynbrandt (1975) and Levy Schribner (1974).

Another approach can be taken – and applicable in connection with CEA, where one needs a method of weighing quality of life against survival to arrive at a rank-ordering of treatments. One approach is to use decision analysis, which provides a systematic approach to such considerations, and the use of one of the approaches, the construction of multiattribute utility functions, forces one to be explicit about preferences and trade-offs. Recently methods have been developed to estimate utility functions for life-years and health status/quality of life[31]. It would be digressing to enter into a thorough discussion of these possibilities. One should just note the possibility and the feasibility of the idea.

Sackett and Torrance (1978) published a study where the general public's preferences were "quantified" by means of a utility function. A series of „scenarios" describing the physical, social, and emotional characteristics, limitations, and duration of different health states was applied to a random sample of the general public in order to determine their social utility. The scenario for hospital dialysis ran as follows – clearly illustrating the quality of life:

> You often feel tired and sluggish. A piece of tubing has been inserted into a vein in either your arm or your leg. This might restrict some of your physical movements. There is no severe pain, but rather chronic discomfort. Two or three times each week you must go to the hospital and spend about 8 hours hooked up to a dialysis machine ... You must follow a strict diet: low salt, little meat, and small amounts of fluids ...

This particular state of health was was assessed for 3 months, 8 years, and life. It is a comfort to know that the utilities of the general public follow what most people would intuitively expect. On a utilitiy scale from 0 to 1, the mean daily health state utilities were 0.62 for 3 months' hospital-dialysis, 0.65 for 8 years of home-dialysis, 0.58 for 8 years with a kidney transplant, 0.56 for 8 years of hospital-dialysis, and life-long home- and hospital-dialysis were at the bottom of the list with 0.40 and 0.32, respectively. Compared with the previous rank-order discussed, it is of interest to note that home-dialysis comes out highest on the list, but here costs were disregarded[32].

The discussion of a broader CBA and CEA perspective has deliberately concentrated on the inclusion of quality of life aspects. Due to space limitations a thorough criticism of human-capital-based CBA will not be given. In passing, it just has to be noted that the issue is not whether life can be valued or not. It clearly can, but whether it is satisfactory to use earnings as a measure of value of life is an entirely different matter. In the author's opinion it is not satisfactory; a willingness-to-pay approach to valuation of life ought rather to be pursued. Another tempting issue would have been to discuss some of the recommendations and conclusions discussed in the Office of Technology Assessment's recent publication "The Implications of Cost-Effectiveness Analysis of Medical Technology". Some of the conclu-

---

31 See Pliskin et al. (1980) and Pliskin and Beck (1976a, b) for slightly different applications of decision theory to chronic renal failure.

32 See Sackett and Torrance (1978) for further description. See Torrance et al. (1973) for a discussion, where the utility function is used in connection with an illustrative CEA involving chronic renal failure.

sions are truisms of the type "this OTA assessment finds that CEA/CBA cannot serve as the sole or primary determinant of health care decision . . ." (Office of Technology Assessment 1980 a). Not many economists have made this claim[33].

Cost Analyses

A cost analysis is distinguished here from CEA by the fact that end-results are not considered, e.g. there is no analysis of cost per life-year gained. Most often the analysts attempt to estimate the cost per dialysis or annual costs. Typical cost studies are the studies by Stewart et al. (1973), Warner and Kalff (1976), Schippers and Kalff (1976), Pearson et al. (1976), and Hoffstein et al. (1976).

The usefulness of cost analyses per se is somewhat limited. They may be useful when trying to estimate the cost side in a CEA provided that a clear cost concept has been employed. This is rarely the case. Most often the perspective of the hospital is taken – and in some instances no distinction is made between real costs and expenditures. In some cases, however, a quasi-CEA approach is taken. Thus Schippers and Kalff (1976) reasoned that it is generally accepted that renal transplantation as a routine therapy for terminal stage renal patients has various medical advantages over chronic haemodialysis. And a comparison of costs of both types of treatment clearly demonstrated a considerable difference that was, also in favour of transplantation. This type of analysis was then used to recommend that transplantation activities ought to be expanded. A clear-cut CEA is definitely to be preferred to this type of analysis.

If cost analyses are to become more useful, the purpose of these studies must be clarified. In this connection the cost concept used will also be made clearer. Some of the cost analyses encountered in this literature review are mere exercises in what many economists scornfully term "book-keeping economics". This can be changed if the above two recommendations are followed.

Conclusions

No far-reaching conclusions will be drawn. It has been shown that relatively many economic evaluations have been undertaken in the field of dialysis. One may wonder whether they have had any impact on the actual course of the development of dialysis. In terms of overall decisions, i.e. the level of resources allocated to dialysis, it is doubtful whether CBAs have had any impact. In this connection it has to be remembered that only two studies have been undertaken. It is notable that in the early phase of the decision process, identified lives call forth substantially greater investment of public resources than statistical lives. Rettig (1976) noted that publicity often includes dramatization of particular identified lives. Thus, in 1965 a Philadelphia physician who was dialysing himself testified before the House Committee

---

33 See Drummond (1981 b) for a useful discussion of welfare economics and CBA in health care. The decision-making approach is discussed as are human-capital-based analyses versus willingness-to-pay principles.

on Appropriations to great effect – a testimony later seen on the NBC TV documentary. Rettig (1976) also noted how the same thing was done in 1971, and that this apparently contributed to the willingness of Wilbur Mills, a Representative, to support a kidney disease amendment to Medicare. All this may sound unduly pessimistic. This is not the case. First of all, CBA and CEA are only inputs to the decision process. Never do they provide necessary and sufficient inputs to a decision – in particular not decisions about distributive matters. Second, there is no doubt that CEAs can contribute to the choice of the most "outcome-efficient" treatments. If they are undertaken on an almost continous level they can function as an effective monitoring device combining end-results and the resource costs associated with the attainment of the specific end-results.

10 Discussion of Paper by Pedersen

W. van Eimeren

Institute for Medical Informatics and Health Services Research, Neuherberg, FRG

The methods of treatment currently applied cannot be regarded as alternatives in the sense that one of them makes the other completely redundant. It also seems to be clear that the largest possible number of transplantations is being advocated and also as much home-dialysis or continuous ambulatory peritoneal dialysis (CAPD) as will then be possible. Because hospital-dialysis will have to continue in any event, the point to be discussed is what would be the ideal mix. Unfortunately, the economic analyses carried out so far have concentrated almost exclusively on a comparative evaluation of the individual methods of treatment. From this it can be deduced – as Pedersen showed very clearly – that at present the important analyses are those that investigate the programme from a comprehensive viewpoint; in the given situation and in view of the high complexity this seems most readily achievable by means of simulation as Pedersen has also indicated in his paper.

Let me now deal with problem areas that I believe have not been thoroughly dealt with. The "society as a whole" and the insurance concept, in the presence of a rare disease with even rarer secondary diseases, seem to me to be the opposite of the approach selected by cost-effectiveness analysis (CEA) and cost-benefit analysis (CBA): it is precisely the rare/high-cost disease against which I want to be insured. Does an isolated study such as that conducted in a CEA and CBA make any sense at all, or should not preference be given to a financing method based on a "mixed calculation"? The equity concept is worthless in the sense of a postulated "common weal", "public interest", or whatever because disease and death are the greatest "dis-equalizers" that one can imagine. On the other hand, we have long weighed some lives against others: in the vaccination programme, for instance, we sacrifice partly drastic side effects and lives to anticipated still worse consequences. The way out would seem to consist of a method of analysis that would strictly separate the insurance from the public interest point of view. The logical consequence would be a system providing basic services on to which specific insurance programmes could be grafted. It would then be up to the different sections of society to decide if and to what extent they are prepared to support "non economic" services that are nonetheless regarded as justified from a public interest perspective. Personally, I would prefer a system that did not pervert the egalitarian principle so far as to forbid someone from choosing an "uneconomic" method of prolonging his life if the persons surrounding him (or he himself) decide to give him the possibility of so doing.

Even if "society as a whole" is considered a realistic concept this does not necessarily lead to false conclusions: disability pensions and sick pay are, in my opinion, not merely a reshuffling of purchasing power, they drastically impair a society's economic capacity to produce and, in my view, are not neutral in social terms.

What must characterize CBA and CEA in an area where alternatives are still very much in a state of flux, i.e. to what extent would CBA, were it taken seriously, change the perspectives, since economically potentially interesting objectives would not be attained at all because temporary "overpayments" are not recognized as such and therefore do not appear as necessary or sound investments?

To examine prevention and therapy jointly would be readily possible only when starting out from prevention: by this I mean to say, to what extent can we do without prevention if therapy is as effective as it is efficient. Setting out from therapy (after, so to speak, the baby has fallen down the well), the problem is given another basis of assessment in the sense of a point made above – that of the solidarity and insurance community. To me, the discussion of Fig. 9.4 seems important because it brings out the following point: therapy can be substituted for prevention. Prevention can be substituted for therapy only after splitting up the interests involved.

In the evaluative discussion it does not appear to me to be certain that the lifestyle of people actually supports the thesis that human beings prefer to live long though unsatisfactory lives rather than short but good lives: a popular poll would not be sufficient to obtain conclusive evidence. Such a poll should also at least provide for the probability that contrary to the thesis people actually live "badly and briefly" or "well and for a long time".

What is a "decision-maker"? An example: costs of hospital confinements are borne by the German health services; even in earlier times 90% of all deliveries took place in hospitals on the basis of "medical interventions". The health services simply took over the costs of the consensus that had long existed between physicians and patients.

Summary of Workshop Discussion

The discussion following van Eimeren's comments on economic evaluation of the different methods of treatment applied in end-stage renal failure focused on a series of important issues.

First, the *question of alternatives* is crucial in the course of cost-effectivite analysis (CEA). One way of defining alternatives would be to compare one procedure, e.g. home-dialysis or continuous ambulatory peritoneal dialysis (CAPD) with another, e.g. haemodialysis in a hospital. Such an approach may be sufficient as a first step. Another and probably more appropriate definition of alternatives, however, would be to compare alternative combinations of treatment once supportive treatment is clinically indicated. One such combination is, for example, from an initial training session at the hospital to home-dialysis to a transplant and back if the graft is rejected. Such a programme could be analysed for cost-effectiveness with another established sequence of steps and perhaps be differentiated for different groups. Such a model would come closer to reality but the analysis would be far more demanding. On the other hand, analyses of isolated procedures do not provide sufficient information to enable decisions to be taken about the most efficient path.

Second, the *quality of life aspect* needs to be taken into account. The patient obviously uses other criteria about the effectiveness (or benefit) of a given procedure and he might value "noneconomic" arguments highly. The patient's attitude towards shorter life with better quality but higher health risks or longer life with medium quality may run counter to the preferences of another decision-maker. Thus, a careful economic analysis at the clinical level should include the preferences of the patient and consider how well they are taken into account by his physician. Nobody in the discussion group thought that cost-benefit analysis (CBA) or CEA should ignore individual client preferences, and there was widespread agreement that life itself should be valued in a more sensible fashion than in the human-capital approach.

Third, the studies considered here are characterized by one important feature: that they have been carried out ex post facto. This means that the decision to implement a procedure has already been taken (as is so often the case in medicine). So actually performing CEA is just a way of looking back, "did we do the right thing?" and "what are we paying for the decision we took?" But one important aspect in the decision-making context is that ex post facto analysis yields information necessary for further decisions on investments for expansion.

It would be injudicious to suppose that physicians who introduce a new procedure are universally cost-conscious. (The degree of cost-consciousness shown by physicians in relation to renal dialysis is untypical because the economic aspect of dialysis therapy has been apparent from the very start.) But there is now a great deal of effort put into making physicians more cost-conscious in most countries and this we should bear in mind. If health economists and epidemiologists can help to develop a frame for evaluation, dissemination of knowledge and insight into the complexity of the problems would be faster.

11 The Epidemiological Evaluation of Active Therapy of Patients with Renal Failure

E. Schmitt and H. Klinkmann

Clinic of Internal Medicine, Rostock, GDR

In any epidemiological appraisal of therapy by dialysis one cannot avoid considering the subject from a wider point of view. No dialysis patient turns up out of nowhere: he passes through a prior phase of renal disease, the final result of which is end-stage renal failure and the need for dialysis. It is desirable that during this phase the patient be subjected to regular treatment at outpatient clinics. The data supplied by such clinics provide an indication of the foreseeable increase in the number of dialysis patients. Furthermore, chronic dialysis treatment is inseparable from the incidence of kidney transplantations. The two methods may be regarded as more or less equivalent: they complement each other and, as part of the *"renal replacement therapy"* concept, form an integral unit.

Estimates provided by a number of authors concerning the annual incidence of *new cases of renal insufficiency* range from 30 to 200 per million population. It is certain, however, that the correct figure is higher than 50 per million, but definite and representative data are difficult to obtain because they are based on such widely divergent sources as, for example, screening tests and dialysis statistics.

To illustrate the manner in which adequate care can be provided for nephrological-urological patients with reduced renal functions during the phase preceding treatment by dialysis we propose to examine, as an example, the intensive kidney dispensary system which over the past few years has been set up very comprehensively throughout the German Democratic Republic. To evaluate dialysis and transplantation in patients suffering from chronic renal failure we use data gathered by the European Dialysis and Transplant Association (EDTA). Concerning so-called acute dialyses in the presence of acute renal failure we refer to the records of the Society for Nephrology of the GDR.

Under the expert guidance of the Society for Nephrology of the GDR and the Working Group for Infantile Nephrology of the Society for Paediatrics of the GDR a network of mobile and static facilities has been created for the purpose of compiling a complete record of kidney patients and their treatment. In cooperation with other internal specialists and general practitioners a nephrologist in each district town is charged with the specialized care of kidney patients. He reserves regular special nephrological consulting hours and has a number of beds on call for his needs at the district hospital. The highly specialized nephrological therapy takes place at a kidney centre, whose services include regular outpatient consulting hours, a nephrological ward, and a dialysis department. A corresponding facility exists for infantile nephrology. On the basis of such a high degree of careful organization it has become increasingly possible to monitor all kidney patients, especially those in an advanced phase of renal disease. As a result, it has been extremely rare in the past 5 years for a patient to have been put on dialysis without prior outpatient treatment. The Society for Nephrology annually reports data from district nephrologists and kidney centres to the Ministry of Health on numbers of patients, broken down by age, primary diseases, and retention data.

Table 11.1 contains figures illustrating the activities of the nephrological dispensaries, taking into account new patients and degrees of retention, listed in comparison with the number of patients placed on dialysis. For ease of comprehension the figures refer to numbers of cases per million population. While the total number trebled between 1975 and 1978, the number of retention cases (creatinine ≧ 5.1 mg/dl) doubled.

Table 11.2 shows the breakdown of diagnoses established for our outpatients. The ratios did not substantially alter between 1975 and 1980.

The breakdown according to age shown in Table 11.3 remained substantially constant between 1977 and 1980. As for Tables 11.1 and 11.2, Table 11.3 does not take into account any infantile nephrological data.

Table 11.1. Nephrological dispensary system in the GDR (number of cases per million inhabitants)

Year	n total	New patients	Creatinine mg/dl		Creatinine at start of dialysis (mean value, mg%)
			1.5–5	≧ 5.1	
1975	965	–	99.7	31.7	9.9
1976	1459	494	125.5	36.3	12.2
1977	1935	480	135.7	41.3	16.7
1978	2205	270	181.1	47.0	14.5
1979	2325	120	199.8	58.0	17.8
1980	2614	289	230.9	62.7	21.0

Table 11.2. Nature of diagnoses at nephrological dispensaries in the GDR

Year	n total	PN (%)	GN (%)	Cyst (%)	Others (%)
1975	16214	57	17.8	4.6	20.6
1976	24523	60.5	14.9	3.6	21.0
1977	32515	60.8	13.5	4.0	21.7
1978	37050	63.2	14.4	4.9	17.5
1979	39057	64.2	16.5	4.2	15.1
1980	43918	60.8	17.2	4.9	17.1

Abbrevations: PN, pyelonephritis; GN, glomerulonephritis; Cyst, cystic kidney

Tabel 11.3. Age distribution for patients with creatinine ≧ 5.1 mg/dl treated at nephrological dispensaries in the GDR

Year	n total	< 50 years (%)	> 50 years (%)
1977	693	51.7	48.3
1978	789	56.1	43.9
1979	675	54.9	45.1
1980	1054	52.2	47.8

The case numbers compiled in Table 11.4 were collated from surveys conducted among selected samples of patients under care at paediatric kidney clinics. Here it should be borne in mind that the staffs of all university clinics, all regional hospitals, and many district hospitals include a specialist in infantile nephrology. Since 1976 no child has been subjected to dialysis without prior nephrological outpatient care. During the same period all children needing dialysis were assigned a fixed place at a dialysis clinic. The number of fresh infantile dialysis cases has been constant over the past 5 years at 0.7 per million of the total population.

Whereas our data on kidney patients are culled from studies covering the GDR alone or from individual studies, we have at our disposal the data on dialysis and transplantations contained in the statistical reports compiled by EDTA. The relevant report for 1980 is based on the data for a total of 107004 patients, of whom 67412 were alive at 31 December 1980. Participants in the surveys were, in addition to the countries of Europe (not including Albania, Rumania, and the USSR), Egypt, Israel, Lebanon, Libya, and Tunisia. About 80% of all dialysis and transplantation centres completed and returned their questionnaires. In 1980 the totals were 1225 returns from 1495 dialysis centres. Since 1970 EDTA has requested a completed questionnaire concerning each dialysis and transplant patient for purposes of computer analysis. This material forms a full history of the therapy of each patient, starting with the initial dialysis and ending with the exitus of the patient. In addition to personal data, the information requested concerns the patient's primary disease, start or change in therapy (haemodialysis, peritoneal dialysis, haemofiltration, transplants, and transplantation data), date and cause of death, occurrence of malignant growths, origin of transplant (cadavers or living donor), cause of transplant

Table 11.4. Children with renal failure in the GDR

Year	n total (dialysis included)	New cases with renal insufficiency n per million populations		New cases with dialysis n per million populations	
1973	52	24	1.4	10	0.6
1974	58	18	1.1	10	0.6
1975	55	21	1.2	15	0.9

Table 11.5. Number of patients in selected countries treated by dialysis and/or transplantation in 1980 (EDTA)

Country	Number per million of population	Country	Number per million of population
Switzerland	259.7	Yugoslavia	76.3
Belgium	233.1	Iceland	75.0
FRG	208.0	GDR	65.3
Sweden	178.1	USSR	40.9
Spain	144.5	Portugal	27.8
Finland	134.6	Hungary	19.7
Eire	99.4	Turkey	3.9

failure, vital statistics such as height and weight of children, progress of rehabilitation, and mode of dialysis/haemofiltration [frequency per week, number of hours per week, type of dialyser, as well as frequency of dialysis after peritonitis and hospitalization of continuous ambulatory peritoneal dialysis (CAPD) patients]. When a patient moves to another place of treatment, a corresponding transfer note is added to his record.

Every year EDTA issues two reports at its congress and as part of the "proceedings" – the "Combined Report on Renal Dialysis and Transplantation in Europe" and the "Combined Report on Renal Dialysis and Transplantation of Children in Europe". The significance of these reports will be illustrated by a number of excerpts from reports from outside the paediatric sector. In all information expressed in numbers per million of population it must be taken into consideration that 10%–20% of all centres failed to return their questionnaires, so that the relative values might actually be greater.

First of all, the total number of surviving patients who were treated by dialysis and/or transplantation is shown in Table 11.5.

In the past 15 years the use of dialysis has increased by leaps and bounds (Fig. 11.1). Today there are about 150000 patients worldwide living with artificial kidneys. Basically, dialysis is indispensable in patients whose kidneys have largely

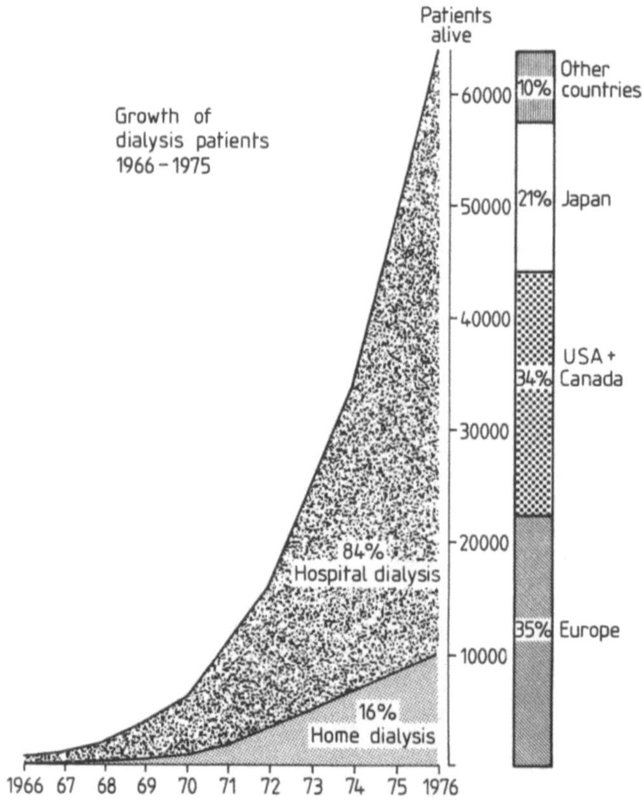

Fig. 11.1. Increase in number of dialysis patients, 1966–1975

ceased to function. If kidney function declines to a point lower than 5% of normal, life becomes fatally endangered. Today the view prevails that there exist no absolute contraindications for dialysis, yet the application of this therapy is questionable in patients of very advanced age or if another illness has a severely negative effect on the patient's short-term prognosis.

The contraindications have been eliminated apace with the advances achieved in the basic material technological development of dialysis. Calculations of the quantitative demand for dialysis facilities may be based on the number of new dialysis cases but only in those countries that provide complete practical coverage of all potential dialysis cases. Table 11.6 summarizes the mean figures recorded over a period of time in EDTA countries optimally equipped with kidney care facilities (Belgium, FRG, France, Israel, Netherlands, Sweden, Switzerland). It is to be assumed that, given the reduction in contraindications under conditions of optimal dialysis care, about 50 new patients per million of population are admitted to dialysis treatment programmes per year.

The records of EDTA also disclose the total number of patients treated by dialysis over a period of several years. As a result of the process of technological improvement as well as of the concentrated development of specific therapeutic procedures, this number quadrupled between 1972 and 1980. However, no quantitative examinations of the incidence of patient numbers alone suffice to determine the number of successfully treated renal failures. In Europe there were, according to the EDTA report, 12394 patients with functioning transplants in 1980, in other words, 111 persons per million of population had survived treatment by dialysis.

In the EDTA area both the figures of patients living with transplants as well as the number of transplants performed per year are rising: in 1972 there were 22.0 patients per million of population on dialysis therapy, in 1975 this figure was 46.3, and in 1980 it was 89.0 (mean EDTA figures). The annual rate of increase in the number of renal transplant patients is approximately 10% (Fig. 11.2).

Dialysis procedures (including CAPD, haemofiltration, and haemodiafiltration) have greatly improved the rehabilitation quota in comparison with 14 years ago, notwithstanding the steady rise in average age. Whereas in 1965 only 76% of dialysis patients were capable of regular work, this figure attained 88% in 1979 (Table 11.7). For patients with transplants the ratio is reported to be as high as 93%. Dialysis therefore has succeeded not merely in ensuring survival but, due to its ability to encourage social integration, also guarantees an acceptable quality of life.

Of major interest is, in addition, the information indicating the cumulative survival rate of patients (after transplantation) under differing therapeutic conditions

Table 11.6. Number of patients newly admitted to dialysis programmes (mean figure from seven "fully developed EDTA countries")

Year	Number of patients per million of population
1972	19.3
1974	26.4
1976	34.0
1978	36.6
1980	45.6

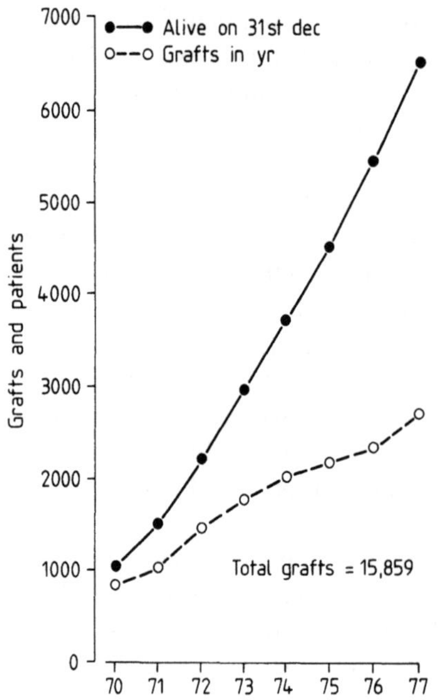

Fig. 11.2. Number of patients living with transplants and number of grafts performed in Europe, 1970–1977 (EDTA region)

Table 11.7. Ability to work and incapacity to work according to type of dialysis

	Total		Dialysis	
			TC	HD
1965	AW	76%		
	IW	24%		
1979	AW	88%	80%	92%
	IW	12%	20%	8%

Abbreviations: AW, ability to work; IW, incapacity to work; TC, treatment centre; HD, home-dialysis

or in comparison with other diseases (e.g. heart failure or carcinoma). By 1978 it emerged, for instance, that treatment by dialysis or transplantation had a probability of survival comparable with that for patients with myocardial infarction or carcinoma of the breast (Fig. 11.3.).

Home-dialysis or transplantation of kidneys from a living donor (LD) show the best results, although it must be considered that the patient sample is selected by optimum criteria: the average age of LD patients is, at 29 years, quite low; patients receiving cadaver grafts have an average age of 36 years; home-dialysis patients are on average 4 years younger than patients treated at dialysis centres and rarely suffer from severe parallel or secondary diseases that may have a negative influence on their prognosis (cf. Fig. 11.4; also Fig. 11.6).

Also of interest to the clinician are data obtained from EDTA records concerning differences in the progress of transplant results over a given period of time. The

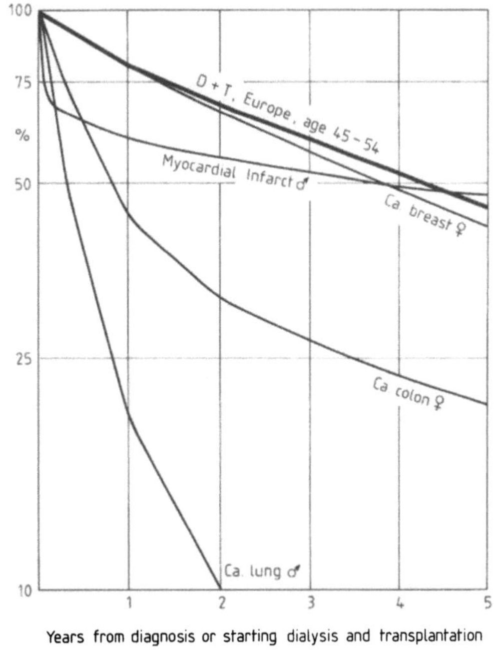

Fig. 11.3. Survival rate for end-stage renal disease with dialysis and transplantation as compared with myocardial infarction and cancer. *Ca.*, cancer; *D+T*, dialysis and transplantation

Table 11.8. Transplants and dialysis therapies in selected countries (numbers of patients per million population). (EDTA 1980)

	Total patients	Deaths	Patients with functioning transplants	Transplants in 1980
Switzerland	259	163	88	23.0
France	228	186	30	9.4
FRG	208	177	18	6.7
Denmark	202	102	94	20.4
Sweden	178	83	90	22.7
UK	127	69	56	16.9
EDTA total	117.6	84.0	21.6	6.6

comparisons are based on transplantations performed in the periods from 1973 to 1975 and from 1976 to 1978. The transplant survival rate improved by an average of 9%, patient survival by 8%. Substantial differences exist between individual countries with regard to the ratio of kidney transplantation (Table 11.8). Whereas Switzerland, Denmark, and Sweden have achieved high scores in their overall performance in the area of "renal replacement" through a major share of kidney grafting, dialysis is prevalent in France and the FRG. The reason for the low incidence of transplants in these countries may lie in the large proportion of elderly dialysis patients or even in practical difficulties encountered in finding people prepared to act as donors. For the pronounced prevalence of dialysis one may even suspect materialistic motives. But Table 11.8 demonstrates that it should be quite feasible to pro-

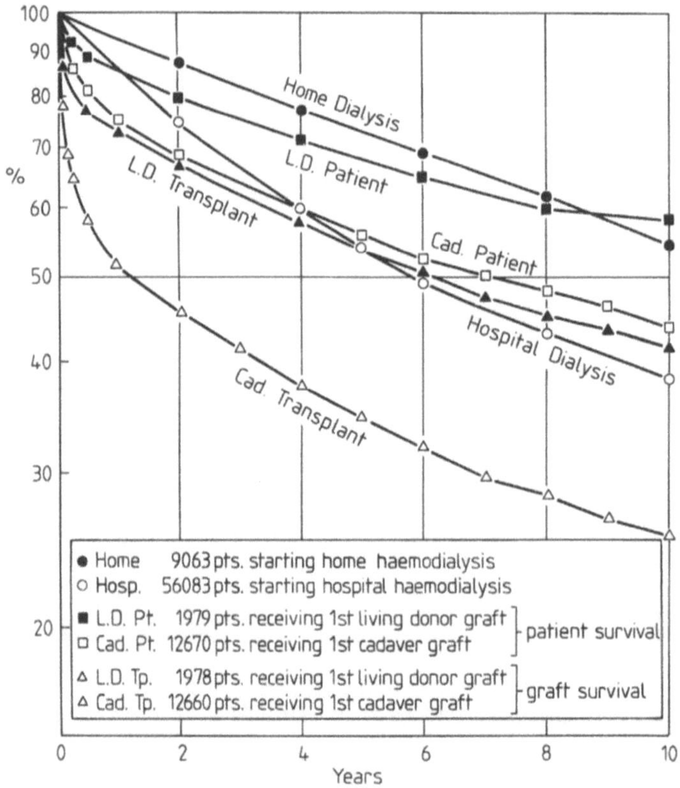

Fig. 11.4. Survival of patients with renal dialysis treated at home and in hospitals. Graft survival of transplants of different origins

vide the means for submitting 20–23 patients per million population to treatment by transplantation per annum.

As indicated above, the expansion of the dialysis capacity has been accompanied by a decline in the number of (previously arbitrarily established) contraindications. This applies particularly to the increasingly open-ended upper age-limits. It is reflected also in the case frequency occurring within specific age-groups of all patients registered with EDTA (start of dialysis) in a comparison of 1974 with 1979 (Table 11.9).

It is to be assumed that the increase in dialysis capacity is of particular benefit for older patients. This may be deduced from a comparison of the evolution of the case frequency within certain age-groups over a period of time – in this case from 1975 to 1978 – in comparison with the total number of dialysis patients in 1978. Whereas in France, the FRG, and Italy more than 50 patients per million inhabitants are cared for by dialysis, the corresponding figure for the United Kingdom is 4 per million.

Figure 11.5 shows the potential of identifying the modes of therapy applied, at the last count, to 67412 patients over a period of 8 years. With respect to the total number of patients and the rate of increase, treatment at dialysis centres (hospital haemodialysis) continues to be in the lead ahead of home haemodialysis (HD) and

Table 11.9. Percentage of case frequency within specific age-groups

Year	Age (years)		
	15–34	35–54	>55
1974	30	51	19
1979	22	43	35

Table 11.10. Number of new patients of the 55–64 and 65–74-year-old age-groups who started dialysis treatment from 1975 to 1978 compared with the total number of dialysis patients (numbers per million inhabitants, EDTA)

	France Age (years)		FRG Age (years)		Italy Age (years)		UK Age (years)	
	55–64	65–74	55–64	65–74	55–64	65–74	55–64	65–74
1975	59	32	50	18	49	22	10	1
1978	69	57	71	50	70	52	23	4
Dialysis patients total	133		117		120		52	

home peritoneal dialysis (PD). Of interest is again in this connection the case frequency within defined age-groups with regard to different therapeutic methods. Whereas PD is preferentially used on older patients and very frequently in home dialysis (increasingly CAPD, see below) in the over 55-year-old age-group, the middle age-groups predominate in the area of HD (Fig. 11.6).

Most transplant patients are less than 55 years of age. But clear differences exist between younger patients who receive transplants from living donors and older patients who are given cadaver transplants. Information is also otbainable concerning haemofiltration patients. According to EDTA statistics for 1980 there were 893 continuous and 1420 occasional haemofiltration cases. Continuous patients ranged from 0.8% (Italy) to 4.2% (FRG) of all HD patients. This confirms the earlier assumption that the number of haemofiltration patients was unlikely to exceed 10% of total dialysis cases. Interesting discrepancies were evident between various countries during a study of home dialysis (Table 11.11). The table shows the percentages represented by home dialysis patients in the overall number of dialysis patients. With a total of 64% the United Kingdom ranks far ahead of all other countries. Leading positions are occupied also by Switzerland, France and the German Federal Republic. In the area of CAPD the United Kingdom, jointly with Switzerland, ranks ahead of all other countries. In both countries 5.5% of all dialysis cases are treated by CAPD.

The following selection from available data on primary renal diseases may be instructive. In contrast to the pessimistic outlook expressed concerning the possibility of treatment by dialysis of diabetic nephropathy as recently as 10 years ago, the number of new patients starting dialysis rose steadily from 124 in 1973 and 183 in 1974 to 847 in 1980, so that on 31 December 1980 some 1920 diabetics were alive under dialysis treatment. Regarding so-called phenacetin kidneys – drug nephropathy, analgesic nephropathy (in 1980 a total of 1488 patients were registered) – interesting regional differences existed a listed in Table 11.12. In this connection Switzerland

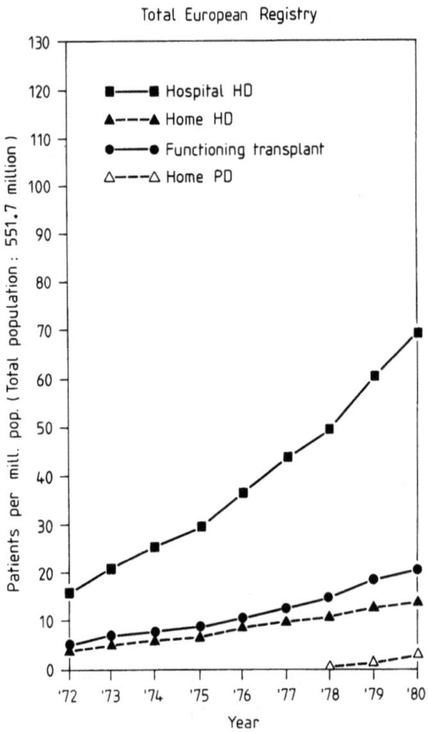

Fig. 11.5. Cumulative number of patients under dialysis and number of patients with functioning transplant

Table 11.11. Percentages of home dialysis patients of the overall total of dialysis patients

Country	Percentage	Country	Percentage
U.K.	64	Italy	14
Switzerland	27	Spain	8
France	22	Yugoslavia	0.4
FRG	19	GDR	0

has the best number among all countries. It is conceivable that because of Switzerland's record the number of patients in need of dialysis expands, which in turn may be a reason for this country's prominent status in the area of dialysis and transplantation.

In addition to end-stage renal insufficiency there are several reasons why dialysis therapy should be applied, including acute kidney failure in urgent need of dialysis, exogenous intoxications, psoriasis, and schizophrenia. Regarding the diagnoses referred to, EDTA provides data only concerning psoriasis. It was found that in 1980 a total of 150 psoriasis patients (including 50 with normal kidney functions) were dialysed at 99 dialysis centres. In 30%–50% of the patients the psoriasis condition appeared to have been alleviated as a result of dialysis, but these results are not regarded as definitely established and further study is considered indispensable. On the subject of schizophrenia, no specific data are available, apart from some material submitted at symposiums.

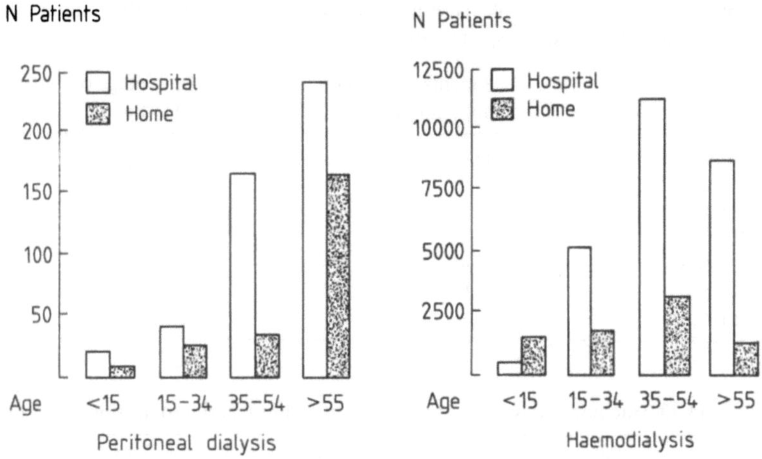

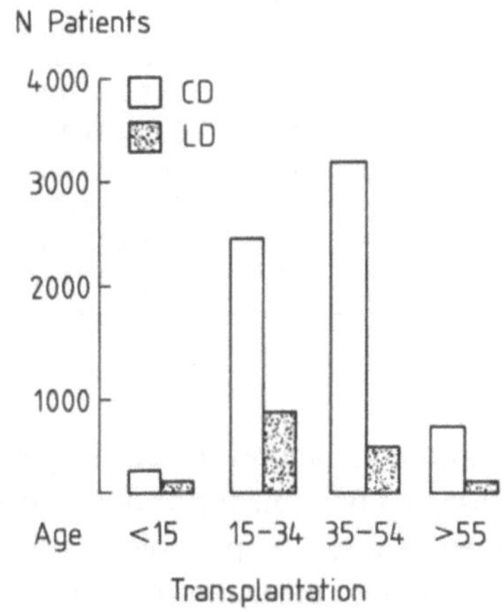

Fig. 11.6. Case frequency within age-groups of haemodialysis and peritoneal dialysis patients and patients with functional transplants (European Dialysis and Transplant Association 1978)

For information concerning "acute dialysis" in the event of acute kidney failure or intoxication we depend on statistics published by individual countries. The Society for Nephrology of the GDR has for years compiled data on all acute dialyses. The results are contained in Table 11.13. Despite a 2.5-fold increase in the total number of dialysis treatments between 1975 and 1980, the number of acute dialyses has remained constant. From this figure it is possible to assume a requirement for 32 dialysis cases per million population. In the event of acute kidney failure an average of 4.2 dialyses per patient is needed for intoxications, an average of 1.8 per patient.

Concluding Remarks

The statistical reports issued by EDTA may be regarded as models of comprehensive and useful reporting for purposes of accurate evaluation. They provide infor-

Table 11.12. Share held by phenacetin kidneys (analgesic nephropathy) amongst the primary diseases of all dialysis and transplant patients

	Patients per million population	Percentage of all patients
Switzerland	44.6	18
Belgium	26.0	11
Denmark	11.5	6
FRG	7.7	4
Netherlands	6.4	4
Uk	1.6	1
Europe	2.7	2

Table 11.13. Haemodialysis in cases of acute renal failure and intoxication in the GDR

Year	Patients		Dialysis		Deaths	
	Total	No. of intoxications	Total	No. of intoxications	Acute renal failure	intoxications
1975	550	285 = 46.9%	1532	426 = 27.8%	169 = 30.7%	34 = 20.1%
1976	486	201 = 41.4%	1622	303 = 18.7%	155 = 54.4%	31 = 16.1%
1977	507	203 = 39.9%	1828	428 = 28.4%	145 = 47.4%	30 = 14.8%
1978	541	187 = 34.6%	1944	322 = 16.6%	212 = 39.2%	31 = 16.6%
1979	495	164 = 33.1%	1645	282 = 17.1%	170 = 51.4%	26 = 15.3%
1980	617	261 = 42.3%	2006	370 = 18.4%	171 = 48.0%	44 = 16.9%

mation on the prevalence of significant medical developments, such as primary disease and possible forms of therapy and their longer term evolution. They enable the identification of possible trends and the analysis of health care strategies. Even much more difficult problems than those touched upon in the present paper – epidemiological data relevant to specified themes were obviously emphasized – have been dealt with as far as has been feasible. Thus it has been possible to monitor several different forms of therapy by dialysis and transplantation on the basis of a substantial number of cases. However, a severe deficiency persists in the epidemiological coverage of renal failure patients prior to therapy by dialysis. In this context the organization established for the nephrological ambulatory care of kidney patients in the GDR in cooperation with the Society for Nephrology may serve as a model for an efficient system for the exchange of relevant information.

A prerequisite for the operational efficiency at the level of both national and international information exchanges certainly consists, on the one hand, of a specialized organization and, on the other hand even more urgently, of the willingness of every individual nephrologist and urologist to perform the tedious chores of completing the questionnaires involved in the task. This readiness should be especially expected in the case of those physicians who as medical specialists are active exclusively in particular medical activities and already feel that they can benefit by the results of such collated data relevant to their specialized professions.

12 Discussion of Paper by Schmitt and Klinkmann

G. Stoddart

McMaster University, Hamilton, Canada

I will summarize the main points of Schmitt's and Klinkmann's paper and react to it as a nonexpert. I might say that I feel particularly qualified to do the latter since I am neither a nephrologist, an epidemiologist, nor even a biostatistician! Consequently, I shall take my cue from White's opening remark and attempt, at least, to ask some of the right questions.

The paper presents selected European Dialysis and Transplantation Association (EDTA) statistics on the number of end-stage renal failure cases under treatment and additional data on the incidence of renal disease from the records of the outpatient kidney clinic system of the GDR. The picture that emerges is as follows:

1. Based on clinic data, estimates of the incidence of end-stage renal failure range from 30–200 per million population of which 1.4 per million cases are children.
2. Again, based on GDR data, the number of new cases of infantile dialysis is 0.7 per million.
3. There is considerable international variation (European Dialysis and Transplantation Association 1980) in the number of patients on dialysis or transplantation, ranging from 4 per million in Turkey to 260 per million in Switzerland.
4. The number of dialysis patients in Europe and North America grew approximately by 35% between 1966 and 1976; mean EDTA figures indicate that the number of dialysis patients per million quadrupled from 1972 to 1980; the number of patients on hospital dialysis has grown considerably faster than the number on home dialysis (when North America and Japan are added to EDTA countries).
5. The approximate annual incidence of new dialysis cases is 50 per million in countries with fully developed facilities.
6. Transplantation is growing at an annual rate of approximately 10%.
7. Significant international differences exist in the ratio of transplantation to dialysis (e.g. France very low; Denmark, Sweden, and Switzerland very high) and the proportion of dialysis provided at home (e.g. 64% in the UK compared with effectively 0% in GDR and Yugoslavia).
8. England exempted, the proportion of all EDTA-registered patients that are over 55 years of age nearly doubled between 1974 and 1979.

Reactions to the Paper

My first reaction to these interesting statistics selected by the authors is that the EDTA is to be commended on its data collection and monitoring. More of this type of activity is to be encouraged in other clinical areas. I would agree, however, that we must look at both renal disease and treatment in order to establish the epidemiology; it would be misleading to focus entirely on the incidence of dialysis/transplantation simply because these are the statistics available. In this respect I wonder if we might not be able to obtain a more precise estimate of incidence of renal disease (however defined) than the range provided in this paper. Can we make use of mortality data in this regard, for example? And, do we have any idea of what the "steady state" stock of dialysis patients might be? This would seem critical if current policy is to accommodate future needs.

Even supposing that the usual epidemiological data on aetiology, incidence, and prevalence were improved, one is tempted to question how such data fit into the overall synthesis of epidemiological, clinical, and economic evaluation. In this regard I should like to offer a conceptual framework which I at least have found useful in thinking about this subject in the past. The framework, illustrated in Table 12.1, is defined by the answer to two questions: (1) is there a comparison of alternatives involved? (since comparison is a necessary condition for evaluation); (2) are both costs and consequences considered? (since examination of both inputs and outputs is a necessary condition for economic evaluation). With reference to this matrix, I would suggest that the provision of basic epidemiological data such as incidence, prevalence, and natural history of disease is an important initial step in developing a macrounderstanding of the costs and consequences of a condition. As such, I would place these data in the upper left-hand quadrant of the chart, in cells no. 1 and no. 2. It is important, in fact essential, however, to have sound clinical trial results on alternative interventions. These results fall into one specific cell of the matrix, cell no. 5. Only on the basis of such clinical evaluation can we proceed to

Table 12.1. A framework for merging clinical and/or epidemiological data with economic evaluation

Is there comparison of two or more alternatives?	Are *both* costs (inputs) and consequences (outputs) of the alternatives examined?			
		No		Yes
		Examines only costs	Examines only consequences	
	No	① PARTIAL APPRAISAL (Basic epidemiological data) Cost description	② Outcome description	③ PARTIAL APPRAISAL Cost-outcome study
	Yes	④ PARTIAL APPRAISAL Cost analysis	⑤ Clinical trials Outcome analysis or effectiveness evaluation	⑥ FULL APPRAISAL (Economic evaluation) Cost-minimization analysis (CMA) Cost-effectiveness analysis (CEA) Cost-utility analysis (CUA) Cost-benefit analysis (CBA)

economic evaluations using cost-effectiveness analysis (CEA) and cost-benefit analysis (CBA), as shown in the lower right-hand quadrant.

In this respect, I should note that I think it is important to have population-based clinical trial results, because once the trial is over the economist's job is often just beginning. Frequently, the question then to be answered is "what would the cost and benefit array look like if we altered the health care delivery system on the basis of these results?" To the extent that trial results pertain to selected patients, or even "average" patients, they may not be generalized to the "marginal" cases likely to be encountered when the intervention is diffused.

Having drawn this chart to set the stage, my main reaction is to ask whether our epidemiological and clinical data on outcomes are adequate to go forward with economic evaluation. For example, from the paper it is possible to tell the percentage of patients surviving a given number of years on dialysis or transplant. Can this be reformulated as an average survival time, thus providing an estimate of life-years gained for the average patient? Do we know enough about long-term survival to have confidence in such an estimate if it is provided? Again, I pose these as questions: I certainly do not profess to have answers. Further, is survival itself an adequate measure of outcome for renal therapy? The authors suggest that due to quite successful rehabilitation (over 90% of patients able to work in home dialysis), dialysis "guarantees an acceptable quality of life". Given the rather extensive list of psychological costs encountered in Pedersen's paper I seriously question this. And I ask, can we adjust outcome measurement, either in clinical trials or on a population basis, to reflect quality of life? I do not know if early attempts along this line will ultimately prove successful. But I think we must try.

I should also like to mention one or two reactions to the existing state of clinical evaluation of dialysis therapy. First, it seems to me that what we require is not comparison of alternatives *modes* of therapy so much as comparison of alternative *pathways* (through perhaps several modes) for patients. In this regard, I wonder if I might ask the clinicians in the group to comment on the optimal clinical path (and contraindications to it). Second, I should like to ask whether new developments in renal therapy (e.g. continuous ambulatory peritoneal dialysis) are being subjected to clinical trials, and if not why not? Finally, although the authors do not discuss in detail the subject of prevention, I think we should examine it, since it obviously affects significantly the epidemiological, clinical, and economic evaluation. Are there any prospects for prevention? If not, is the concept of postponement referred to in Bergström's paper something to be seriously investigated?

Summary of Workshop Discussion

The dicussion following Stoddart's comments on Schmitt's paper confirmed that:

First, we do not have sufficient *epidemiological information* about the various conditions that result in end-stage renal failure. An estimated incidence lies in the range between 100 and 200 patients/year/million population with end-stage renal disease (based on mortality rates), with considerable variations among countries. But what are the dynamics of the patient population over time? Is it approaching an equilibrium and, if so, what will be the eventual size of the patient pool? From there we could start to predict how many patients would benefit from active treatment. In Sweden, an estimated figure was 88 patients/million population/year but this was in the 1960s. Comprehensive recent figures are lacking.

Second, the approximate data on *incidence of new dialysis* cases per year of 50 patients per million population gives the impression that an excellent technology is terribly under-utilized. Although the growth in the number of patients on dialysis has been quite substantial there are considerable differences between countries in the number of patients under treatment – 4 per million in Turkey, 260 per million in Switzerland (European Dialysis and Transplant Association 1980). Financial considerations seem to be a prime determinant of these numbers.

Third, a further aspect to consider is the *prediction* of the number of patients suitable for treatment in the future, for example, in the UK estimates are of 340 patients per million population by the year 2000. The trend, however, depends on the development of renal disease and – of course – also on progress in technologies.

Fourth, important features pointed out in Schmitt's paper and in the discussion are the *international differences* (1) in the extent of home dialysis versus hospital dialysis, ranging from 64% of the patients in the UK to close to zero in the German Democratic Republic and Yugoslavia; (2) in the level and the growth rate of continuous ambulatory peritoneal dialysis (CAPD); and (3) in the ratio of transplantation to dialysis, which is very low in France and very high in Denmark, Switzerland, and Sweden.

With this as a background the question was: do we have sufficient information to go forward and perform an economic evaluation? Here the economists were concerned about the *lack of epidemiological data on outcomes*. It seems that we would need more information about the quality of life at various points in the course of dialysis treatment or after transplantation. Schmitt suggested that – based on reports from the European Dialysis and Transplant Association (EDTA) – dialysis and transplantation guarantee an acceptable quality of life with a chance of survival time comparable with myocardial infarction or breast cancer. In contrast, Pedersen's paper (see pp. 128–129) focuses on the discomfort, the pain, the anxiety, the displacement, and the social costs that occur both in patients and in families as a result of being on these treatments. In the light of these differences in perspective social output data are really a prior issue to economic evaluation. Is there a methodology for getting there? With a suitable instrument at hand for this type of analysis one could perform trials on the optimum mix of treatment modes.

According to one participant it would be useless (at this conference) to try to develop some sophisticated method to evaluate the quality of life when we already know that the quality of transplantation is far better than the quality of any kind of dialysis. In Europe, the average rate of kidney transplantation is 6.6 patients per million population, with a maximum in Scandinavia and Switzerland, each of which have 22 patients per million population. The best way to improve quality of life is to encourage those countries with low transplantation rates to develop their transplantation programmes. In view of the fact that suitable organs may not be available for transplantation within reasonable time one participant vigorously argued that one should keep in mind that most patients on dialysis increase their quality of life independently of the type of treatment.

13 Macroeconomic Evaluation of Kidney Dialysis

F. F. H. Rutten

University of Limburg, Maastricht, Netherlands

Introduction

Medical technology plays a decisive role in the development of health care consumption. One estimate is that 50% of the increase in hospital care cost is due, directly or indirectly, to medical technology (Gaus 1976). Aaron (1981) points at the dual role of medical technology nowadays:

> On the one hand medical technology that existed until recently made relatively cheap the collective decision to treat health care as a right to which the usual canons of the market allocation and distribution were not allowed to apply. On the other hand recent changes in medical technology make the continuation of that traditional approach very costly. These changes in technology have led to world-wide interest in medical cost containment; but they have forced (or soon will force) a popular reexamination of attitudes toward health care delivery in most developed countries and will probably lead to important changes in the role of government in financing and regulating the delivery of health care.

This statement shows in a nutshell the formidable problems faced today. It also suggests that ultimately choices will have to be made by policy-makers at government level. In this paper we will see how macroeconomic analysis may augment policy-making, focusing on the treatment of end-stage renal disease (ESRD) by haemodialysis.

Before turning to this basic question we will briefly consider dialysis and establish the specific details of this type of treatment that are relevant to our discussion. First, dialysis is life-saving. There is only one alternative to dialysis, which is transplantation. In some cases, however, transplantation fails and patients have to be placed on dialysis again. This procedure may be repeated; in Europe 101 third transplants were reported between 1972 and 1976 (European Dialysis and Transplant Association 1976). The second observation is that dialysis is very costly: the costs vary from about US $10000 to US $17000 for home-dialysis, about US $21000 to US $25000 for dialysis at a free-standing outpatient facility, to more than US $25000 per patient annually at a hospital facility (Evans et al. 1981). A third observation is that technology is only gradually advancing.

The so-called Burton report (Burton 1969) predicted in 1967 that in the late 1980s dialysis would not need to be applied on a large scale any longer due to large successes of the treatment and the prevention of primary kidney disease. This turned out to be much too optimistic. Finally, one may observe that the number of ESRD cases is relatively small. From these few observations one may conclude that in the case of renal dialysis a life-saving medical treatment is being provided to a relatively few number of beneficiaries at a very high cost to society. Therefore, the issue with respect to ESRD treatment concerns the basic choice between scarcity on one hand and the priceless value of life on the other (compare Rettig 1981).

In this paper we will address the following four issues associated with macroeconomic evaluation of dialysis: (1) the assessment of benefits and costs of dialysis to society; (2) the determination of the scope of variables to be taken into account in a macroeconomic evaluation of dialysis; (3) the identification of relevant criteria for choosing between alternative policies; (4) the relevance of evaluative studies for policy-making. In the next section we will sketch the macroeconomic impact of dialysis, providing figures on the costs per case and the number of cases treated in various countries. We will also shortly discuss different methods of calculating the indirect costs and benefits of dialysis. In the section "Macroeconomic Evaluation of Dialysis" we consider this topic in general, while one particular study on the evaluation of the ESRD programme of Medicare is looked at in detail in the penultimate section. The final section deals with a number of policy issues and concludes our paper.

The Macroeconomic Impact of Dialysis

The Direct Costs of Dialysis

The direct costs of dialysis should include expenditures for treatment, research, training of medical manpower, and investment in medical facilities. Most available data refer to the average charge for dialysis or the total running costs incurred for dialysis. It is usually assumed that these figures more or less include the items mentioned above; in other words physicians' fees include investment in training and the prices of medical equipment represent research embodied in the equipment. In this paragraph we will review the development of direct costs of dialysis in a number of countries (Office of Technology Assessment 1980b; Evens 1981).

In the United States Congress passed legislation (Public Law 92–603) in September 1972 extending Medicare benefits to virtually all ESRD patients who were not employees of the federal government or covered by Veterans Administration benefits. Medicare covered 80% of a patient's medical expenses. In January 1974, shortly after the introduction of the Medicare ESRD programme, 10300 patients were receiving dialysis. Currently, there are more than 50000 dialysis patients in the United States, indicating a remarkable growth. The cost of the programme exceeded $1 billion in 1979, the cost of dialysis averaging about $30000 per case annually. The United States accounts for approximately one-third of all patients in the world receiving dialysis. In Canada about 11200 dialysis patients were counted in 1978. Europe accounts for another one-third of all patients receiving dialysis. In the United Kingdom 2946 patients were on dialysis in 1978. France counted 7096 dialysis patients in 1977, West Germany 7000 patients in 1978 (about US $30000 to US $52000 per dialysis annually), the Netherlands 1465 patients in 1980 (about US $30000 per dialysis annually), and Sweden 602 patients in 1978.

In Table 13.1 the treatment of ESRD patients by country and year is presented. These data suggest that most countries have reached levels of patients receiving treatment that are close to, or exceed, 100 per million population. The United States and Japan are far beyond this point, with the United States having something closer to 200 dialysis patients per million population and Japan exceeding 200 (Office of Technology Assessment 1980b).

In most countries there is a development towards treating more patients by dialysis. An important stimulus is the start of social programmes providing necessary funds, as for instance the ESRD programme of Medicare. Rettig et al. (1981) estimated that Medicare annual benefit payments would exceed $3.4 billion in 1990 and $4.5 billion in 1995 (incurred basis). Furthermore, they estimated that in 1980 3.7% of all Medicare benefit payments would be allocated to ESRD treatment. In other terms, 3.7% of all Medicare benefit payments go to 50000 ESRD beneficiaries and 96.3% to the other 23 million aged enrollees. This illustrates the contribution of dialysis treatment to the concentration of medical expenditure–relatively few people consume a large percentage of medical care, compare with Lecomte (1977). For the United Kingdom the European Dialysis and Transplant Association (1976) estimates that the dialysis population will reach 340 patients per million population sometime after the year 2000, about five times its level in 1976.

Benefits of Dialysis

In the classic literature (Rice 1966; Rice et al. 1976; Cooper and Rice 1976) the economic cost of illness is measured in terms of direct costs for treatment and the indirect cost or loss in output due to disability (morbidity) and premature death (mortality). These are the cost to society rather than to sick individuals or their families. The measurement of these indirect costs can be done in various ways. The "hu-

Table 13.1. Treatment of ESRD patients by country and year (per million population). (Office of Technology Assessment 1980)

	New patients (on dialysis or with a functioning transplant)		Total patients (on dialysis or with a functioning transplant)		
	1975	1976	1975	1976	1978
Japan	–	–	–	140	222
US	–	–	–	123–129[a]	164–206[a]
France	30.3	29.1	102.2	125.0	133[a] (1977)
Canada	30.3	31.4	–	121.1	–
West Germany	29.6	30.8	87.7	105.0[b]	114[b]
Netherlands	18.9	21.4	90.2	108.5	–
UK	14.5	15.1	62.0	71.2	92
Australia	–	–	–	–	77[a]
Ireland	–	–	41.5	50.0	–
Sweden	28.7	28.7	85.4	99.3	73[a]

[a] Dialysis only
[b] Estimate

man-capital" approach, which considers a human person as human capital for production, has been used frequently in these studies. There are, however, other approaches to valuing a life, including explicit statements of value by individuals or the "willingness to pay". Another major category of indirect costs, which is difficult to quantify, is that of pain and suffering of the individual and the burden of illness on the family. Also the opportunity cost of the patient's time can be a relevant cost-item.

Treatment by dialysis decreases the indirect costs of ESRD. Because dialysis is life-saving, the most important benefit is the number of life-years saved. An important aspect of the valuation of life-years saved concerns the quality of life when undergoing dialysis. Compared with transplant patients, dialysis patients have a lower rehabilitation rate. In fact, several aspects of the quality of life may suffer under dialysis. Klarman et al. (1968) estimated that the difference in quality of life for transplant and dialysis patients could be quantified by giving an extra weighting of one-quarter to years gained with a transplant. Ludbrook (1981) argues that "for an individual patient, the higher risks involved in undergoing transplantation mean that life expectancy is reduced. To the extent that the decision to accept a transplant is voluntary and fully informed, this indicates a revealed preference for life with a functioning graft". Ludbrook expresses, however, some doubt about the assumption of voluntarily acceptance of a transplant in the light of shortage of dialysis facilities. In summary, it is clear that life-years saved as benefits of dialysis should be somehow corrected for quality. Furthermore, since the quality of life may vary between different patients undergoing the same treatment, this correction may be rather complex when summing up total benefits for a particular dialysis programme and is likely to be dependent on the target population of the programme.

The Aggregation Problem

The emphasis in this paper is on macroeconomic evaluation. Assuming therefore that benefits and costs of individual treatment can be adequately estimated, the problem remains how to value a programme for treating a number of people for a certain disease; in other words what social value should be ascribed to life-years gained (corrected for quality) for a number of individuals. A simple postulate for aggregating benefits is that a year of healthy life is to be regarded as of equal intrinsic value to everyone, irrespective of age, sex, etc. (see Williams 1981). This aggregation rule has been used frequently (for instance Torrance 1976) and allows for simple aggregating numbers of life-years saved over individuals. Williams, however, argues that a relaxation of this postulate might be proper and that an additional year of healthy life expectation could be regarded as of differential intrinsic value according to age and/or sex of the beneficiary. Furthermore he points out the fact that

> A disproportionate amount of attention has been paid to be eliciting of relative values from individuals, and to comparison of these relativities between individuals, but very little to eliciting people's views about how the valuation of one person should be weighed with those of another in order to reach a set of social values.

If this line of thought is followed, a number of other problems msut be solved before relative values can be used in a macroevaluation. Williams mentions four problems, the most important being the selection of those people in the community whose judgement is asked with respect to evaluation of life-years saved with regard to different individuals. The other problems concern the issue of time-preference and risk-aversion (whether it should or should not be accounted for in the evaluation procedure), and the problem of possible "false signalling" by respondents in order to manipulate the outcome to their own advantage. Given the fact that patient selection in the case of ESRD treatment has great importance, the ideas of Williams might prove to be very relevant for further development of evaluation studies in this field. Relaxation of the egalitarian principle might be necessary in view of the limitation of resources. This, of course, involves complex ethical questions.

Macroeconomic Evaluation of Dialysis

Specification of Alternative Programmes

Before discussing the specification of alternative programmes for ESRD treatment it is essential to point out the uncertainty that exists with respect to progress in medical technology. As we already mentioned in the first section of this paper, the prediction of medical technological development in the late 1960s prevented the Burton committee (Burton 1969), which stood at the cradle of the Medicare ESRD programme, to foresee what burden on the economy the programme would place in the long run. It will be obvious that improvements in transplant techniques or better prevention of graft rejection will influence the evaluation of dialysis programmes. But also improvements in certain dialysis techniques may influence the evaluation of different modes of dialysis to a large extent (compare recent developments in peritoneal dialysis). Furthermore, in discussing alternative programmes of dialysis we assume that the programmes are run efficiently; some evidence is provided that a more intensive usage of existing equipment could reduce the costs at the microlevel. Below we shall consider different modes of dialysis, criteria for patient selection, and the choice between dialysis and transplantation.

Haemodialysis might be done in a hospital, in an independend outpatient facility, or at home. Another form of treatment, peritoneal dialysis, is becoming more common (in Japan 0.7% in 1978, (Office of Technology Assessment 1980). Most patients start with dialysis in the hospital and may transfer to home-dialysis when they have shown to be able to carry out the dialysis process. Costs associated with these different forms of dialysis may differ as we have already illustrated in the first section, with home-dialysis being considerably cheaper than dialysis in a hospital or outpatient facility. As is indicated in Table 13.2, the percentage of dialysis patients receiving treatment at home differs substantially between different countries.

According to an Office of Technology Assessment report (OTA 1980):

> Several countries have policies to encourage more home dialysis. In the UK, the goverment pays for special housing or plumbing requirements, over and above the more strictly medical components of the service. The US recently revised its

reimbursement policy, which had paid a larger proportion of the costs for centre dialysis than home dialysis, in an attempt to remove financial reasons for favouring centre dialysis. West Germany's sickness funds decided in the early 1970s to pay the full costs of home dialysis for the same reason. France has guidelines limiting the maximum number of dialysis centres in a region; home units are specifically excluded from this limit to encourage their use.

Another way in which programmes may differ is the criteria used for selecting new patients. Inspection of the figures in Table 13.2 suggests that selection criteria in England are more strict than in some other developed countries (compare British Medical Journal 1978). Assuming that patients are currently selected according to their suitability for treatment, it is worthwhile noting that expansion of facilities for ESRD treatment means a relaxation of selection criteria. Ludbrook (1981) shows that the marginal treatment costs per life-year saved would go up from £3000–/£5000 (1976/1977) to £5000–£6000 if more patients not medically suitable for transplantation were accepted. Further, if patients who are unsuitable for home-dialysis or transplantation were accepted, then the marginal cost of treatment would be £7000 to £11000 per life-year saved. This indicates that a strong relation exists between selection criteria for new patients and the marginal costs of dialysis treatment. Furthermore, this evidence suggests that relaxation of selection criteria might conflict with policies towards promotion of home-dialysis; in other words the allocation to different treatment facilities should be in agreement with the characteristics of the target-population of the programme.

The choice between transplantation and dialysis is a matter that lies somewhat outside the scope of our paper. It is difficult, however, to evaluate dialysis treatment without considering transplantation. Transplantation is not only the main alternative for dialysis, but the two are often combined in the treatment of one ESRD patient. Ludbrook (1981) analyses three overlapping treatment processes: hospital-dialysis alone; mostly home-dialysis and periodic hospital-dialysis; and finally hospital-dialysis, home-dialysis, and transplantation. Using transition probabilities, describing the chance of transition from one state to the other (Markov-model), the average costs of the three treatment packages are calculated. The results indicate that the first package is considerably more expensive than the second or the third, the last being cheapest.

Table 13.2. Percentage of dialysis patients receiving treatment at home by country in 1976. (OTA 1980)

Country	Percentage
UK	65.5
Canada	33.4
West Germany	27.5
Sweden	25.6
US	23.7
France	13.8
Netherlands	10.2
Japan	0.6
Ireland	0.0

Criteria for Macroeconomic Evaluation

The macroeconomic evaluation of a major treatment programme should ideally include (compare Williams 1981): (a) changes in total resources used for the provision of the treatment (direct cost); (b) changes in gross domestic product (GDP) (indirect cost of illness); (c) changes in total resources used by patients and their helpers (opportunity cost); (d) changes in health status of the target-population. As we have seen in the previous section, it is likely that the marginal costs of dialysis will increase when the programme is extended and less suitable patients are elected for treatment. With respect to the changes in GDP, calculated on the basis of the human-capital approach, one may hesitate to give this item full weight in the analysis especially where "a community can afford to carry a significant proportion of 'unproductive' people" (Williams 1981), Furthermore, one should be aware that extending the life of ESRD patients may provoke additional costs for society in the form of social security disability (or other) benefits given to ESRD patients. The estimation of changes in health status of the target-population as a result of applying the programme is obviously the most difficult part of the evaluative analysis. In estimating these changes some correction should be made for the quality of life-years saved. Finally, a social evaluation of the life-years saved, corrected for quality of life, is necessary to estimate programme benefits to society.

Assuming that all ingredients mentioned above are available, the social benefits and the net economic costs may be compared for alternative programmes, selecting those with the highest benefit/cost ratio with all values properly discounted. In reality, however, the necessary information for this ideal approach is seldom available and more ad hoc ways have to be chosen. Many studies have concentrated on calculating the net costs of 1 life-year saved, taking into account direct costs and benefits (sometimes life-years saved adjusted for quality, future earnings of surviving patients included). Ludbrook (1981) provides an overview of results of cost-benefit studies in terms of costs per life year saved (Table 13.3). These results certainly show a clear picture and are in agreement with Ludbrook's results mentioned in the previous section of our paper. When ranking a programme for public policy purposes these values should be compared with those of other programmes providing prevention or treatment for other diseases or providing services other than health services, when extending the analysis to the whole public sector.

Table 13.3. Costs per life-year saved (from previous studies). (Ludbrook 1981)

Study	Hospital-dialysis	Home-dialysis	Transplant and dialysis	Transplant and dialysis adjusted for quality of life
Klarman et al. (1968)	$11600	$ 4200	$2600	$2200
Buxton and West (1975b)	£ 4720	£ 2600	–	–
Stange and Summers (1978)	$27600	$17800	$15000 to $18000	–

Detailed consideration of study of cost-benefit analysis goes beyond the scope of our paper. The paper will instead discuss in detail a recent evaluative study of the Medicare ESRD programme, emphasizing the macro-aspects of an economic evaluation.

The ESRD Programme of Medicare

Evaluation of the ESRD Programme of Medicare

In this section we consider a study that provides an example of a thorough evaluation of a large programme for dialysis treatment. This study by Rettig et al. (1981) was prepared for the Office of Demonstrations and Evaluations of the Health Care Financing Administration in Washington and provides an account of the first 5 years of the Medicare ESRD programme. Furthermore, in the report the actual impact of the programme after this 5-year period is compared with the initial policy objectives of the programme and an explanation for observed divergence from originally intended goals is provided. Special attention is given to the role of government, its possibilities and limitations. Our approach will be to attempt to evaluate this evaluative study by identifying useful elements, which allow for policy relevant conclusions.

Research Method

As is set out in pages 8–10 of the study report emphasis was on thorough data collection from both documents and interviews with individuals. Many details with respect to the planning and implementation of the programme are provided in the final report because, as the authors believe, "implementation research needs good descriptive accounts, because the empirical detail can point to more general categories of analysis, and because lessons that may have eluded us may be seen by others from the empirical data we have provided". The many data and details are presented against a global conceptual framework, which describes the implementation of a federal programme, such as the ESRD programme, in five steps: agenda setting, policy formulation, implementation, termination, and finally, monitoring review and evaluation. These respective steps were divided into different subphases, which were also described in detail for the ESRD programme by the authors. Their eye for detail makes the report very informative, but confronts the person evaluating the study at the same time with problems in identifying major issues in implementation, in generalizing findings, and in summarizing lessons for policy-making.

Implementation of the Programme

The legislative history of the ESRD programme was very brief and the legislative start of the programme caught many by surprise. The text of the amendment (section 299 I) did convey the basic intent of Congress, but great authority was delegated to the Department of Health, Education, and Welfare (HEW) Secretary on all other matters. For instance "the silence of the statute on home dialysis meant that reimbursement policy was constrained by the regulations and policies for durable medical equipment, which introduced financial disincentives for this treatment form" (Rettig et al. 1981). Rettig et al. point furthermore to the uncertainty that the statute left with respect to matters of medical review, minimum utilization rates, and planning and financing of ESRD networks. This has hampered the implementation process, especially since new legislation only arrived in 1978. Rettig et al. argue that legislative authority may be complemented by regular oversight hearings, in which Congress can exert more continuing and constructive influence over implementation.

Further, Rettig et al. identified two basic sources of problems at the delivery system level:

> First differences of opinion exist within the medical community about the relative desirability of transplantation versus dialysis, center dialysis versus home dialysis, dialysis reimbursement rates for different institutional settings, the function of networks and the kind of data to be collected.

When the policy system does not resolve these conflicts a divergence of the programme from original objectives is possible. The second problem is that the patients, who acquire much knowledge about their chronic condition, have not been recognized as an important information resource about the performance of the ESRD programme. On matters of quality of care Rettig et al. suggest that "systematic access by the government to patient opinion could be very useful. But the development of patient access mechanisms requires an explicit policy commitment and a strong policy system to supervise implementation".

Cost-Containment

In Table 13.4 a comparison of current and constant dollar average ESRD programme benefit payments per patient is provided for the period 1974–1978. „The two deflators set lower and upper limits to ESRD programme inflation under the assumption that inflation has affected the ESRD programme at least as much as the entire economy but no more than medical care in general" (Rettig et al. 1981). From the figures in Table 13.4 it may be concluded that programme costs are rather stable.

Table 13.4. Comparison of current and constant dollar average ESRD programme benefit payments per patient, 1974–1978. (Rettig et al. 1981)

Calendar year	Average annual enrollment	Average benefit payments per patient		
		Unadjusted	Adjusted by CPI Index	
			All items	Medical[a]
1974	19000	$14895	$12842	$13368
1975	27000	$16667	$13111	$13111
1976	35000	$17086	$12771	$12257
1977	41000	$18463	$13049	$12073
1978	47000	$20149	$13255	$12170

[a] Consumer Price Index medical care subindex value

A number of factors are responsible for the moderate development of the cost per person of the programme. First, there was a general screen on facility reimbursement of outpatient maintenance dialysis (maximum of $150 per treatment), which turned out to be rather effective. A second measure was to restrict payments to physicians supervising the dialysis process. It was suggested that a fee for service reimbursement was proper only when an identifiable service to the patient was performed, e.g. the patient goes into shock, experiences severe chest pains. Instead a monthly payment was given to physicians, which depended on the frequency and complexity of the physicians' services and ranged from $112 to $240. Both measures were not accepted directly at the delivery-system level and a number of cases on these matters were treated in court, but they certainly provided effective incentives for cost-containment.

As was already mentioned in the previous section, in the first years of the programme there was a clear disincentive for home-dialysis as financing of equipment for home-dialysis was difficult. Furthermore:

> Physician fee arrangements were especially adverse to home dialysis: where centre physicians could receive a portion of the facility 'overhead' for general patient supervision, no matter how distasteful the arrangement, physicians with home patients were deprived of even this compensation (Rettig et al. 1981).

These negative effects of reimbursement policy for home-dialysis required new legislation, which was introduced in 1978 after 5 years of "sharp political conflict at every stage of the process". Rettig et al. conclude:

> Reimbursement issues are at the heart of health financing programmes. These issues are highly complex and, because the outcomes of policy decisions are so significant, intense conflict surrounds them. Initial policy sets the controls that govern for relatively long periods of time, partly because this policy creates vested interests that then set political limits on learning from experience. High level competence is required to articulate policies consistent with Congressional intent and the general public interest, both in the early policy planning and in later policy modifications (Rettig et al. 1981).

Conclusion

Rettig et al. draw a number of relevant conclusions from their study. We will mention a few:

Government intervention through reimbursement seems more effective than through organization of delivery of services

Where cost-containment requires an explicit preference for one type of treatment, like home-dialysis, policy will be harder to establish and its effects are more likely to be marginal

Whether formal medical review can improve the quality of care is an empirical question not likely to be answered for several years

The ESRD programme benefited from sound early policy decisions but subsequent policy guidance was ambivalent on both organizational and data issues, to the programme's detriment

Effective implementation requires a constant communication of policy to the administrative and delivery system

Congress may insure effective implementation of a programme through regular hearings in which issues of implementation are addressed

Many conclusions of this study indeed have general relevance for policies with respect to implementing large public programmes. From an economic point of view a number of interesting observations were made concerning the possibilities of containing the cost of such programmes. Above all, the study provides a clear insight into the complexity of implementing large public programmes and stresses the necessity of cooperation between different disciplines in tackling problems related to planning and implementing a programme like the Medicare ESRD programme.

Policy Issues and Conclusions

Government policy with respect to health technology can be described in terms of a four-level hierarchy (Russell 1979). At the first level a government may actively promote research and adoption of new technologies. Then, it may intervene to encourage greater efficiency in the production or use of a technology. At the third level of the hierarchy the benefits of medical technologies are questioned and tested, and finally a government may reach a point where its objective becomes to limit the diffusion of technologies to a level that strikes a balance between the benefits to be gained and the costs of achieving them. In the recent report of the Office of Technology Assessment (OTA 1980) it is suggested that most developed countries have not moved beyond the second level of hierarchy, but that developments will quickly bring countries to consider questions related with levels three and four. In fact, our paper has mainly dealt with problems in the last categories and with problems of implementation at a macrolevel. The present economic recession will probably increase the need for evaluative studies of this kind.

From our global review of evaluative studies a number of observations can be made that have relevance for policy-making. First, it was concluded that the treatment of ESRD patients by renal dialysis should not be considered separately from transplantation. Several studies showed that the introduction of transplantation into the treatment package is cost-effective. This suggests that efficiency of treatment of patients can be increased by carrying out more transplant operations or by reducing the waiting time for a transplant, in other words by reallocating resources away from dialysis treatment towards transplantation. A number of constraints have to be relaxed in order to reach this higher level of efficiency, such as the shortage of kidneys and the availability of operating facilities. One effort to remove these barriers is international cooperation, as for instance in Eurotransplant, which is an international nonprofit-making organization in which dialysis centers, tissue typing laboratories, and transplantation centres cooperate. Notwithstanding the good results of this organization, the number of patients on the Eurotransplant list waiting for transplants continues to increase – from 2581 in 1979 to 2865 in 1980. This last phenomenon is also due to the fact that the total number of donors reported shows no substantial increase – 856 in 1979 and 860 in 1980 (Eurotransplant 1980). More resources should be allocated to improving cooperation between doctors working in casualty departments and intensive-care units and to the promotion of donor cards (or other means of obtaining donations). Finally, international cooperation can reduce the number of so-called mismatched transplants. It has been shown that transplant centres which are still using primarily their own kidneys, have much higher numbers of mismatches per transplant (Eurotransplant 1980).

Our second observation was that home-dialysis is less costly than other forms of dialysis treatment and that peritoneal dialysis appears to be promising for further increasing the efficiency of treatment and the quality of care. Given the large differences in the percentage of patients dialysed at home, reallocation of resources in the direction of these forms of treatment seems possible and could contribute considerably to the efficiency of dialysis treatment. From the evidence considered in this paper we conclude that the provision of clear incentives to physicians, consumers, and others in the health care field towards these more efficient forms of dialysis is crucial for improving programme efficiency.

The provision of "right" incentives may be promoted by allowing for profit firms to enter the market for dialysis services. Lowrie and Hampers (1981), the last being chairman of the board of National Medical Care (NMC) – a profit-making company – argue that the success of the ESRD programme in controlling costs is largely due to the creation of a system of incentives that involves physicians in the medical marketplace. The proft-making firm NMC now owns 120 proprietary dialysis centres, where physicians share profits and take responsibility for the management; 17% of all dialysis patients in the United States are treated in those centres. Given their large share of the market it seems worthwhile to do further research to determine the magnitude of their contribution to cost-control and to see whether private enterprise (compare Egdahl et al. 1979) really can provide solutions to the problems associated with efficient operation of dialysis centres.

Thirdly, the findings in this paper stress the economic relevance of patient selection. Extension of a treatment programme to a larger population-group may lead to considerably higher marginal costs of treatment. Furthermore, it may alter opportunities for the promotion of home-dialysis or transplantation as new patients may be less suitable for these more efficient forms of treatment. But the relation holds also the other way round in the sense that the economy may influence selection in future. It might be that explicit priorities have to be set with respect to the individuals to be selected for treatment. The ideas of Williams (1981) as described above may be helpful in tackling this difficult problem. Further, one may observe that the present system in most countries is haphazard in the respect that there are few instances in which society chooses whether to use a particular technology and to what extent diffusion should take place (compare Leveson 1978). Choices are made implicitly in planning and reimbursing medical services and facilities and explicitly in the actions of individual patients and physicians. In case of technology with exceptionally high costs for relatively few beneficiaries (as ESRD treatment), public programmes using this technology may be based on clear principles set by parliament, but often explicit statements concerning the factors to be used in patient selection are lacking. Individual clinicians have to decide which patients should be selected, a burden which should not be delegated. Guidelines should be developed at high administrative levels to monitor patient selection and these guidelines should be the subject of thorough public debate.

Our fourth issue concerns the degree and type of government involvement in implementing a public programme for ESRD treatment. In the previous section we quoted a conclusion drawn by Rettig et al. (1981) stating that government intervention through reimbursement seems more effective than through organization of delivery of services. More generally one may conclude that the financial arrangements with respect to health care programmes should incorporate incentives for efficient allocation of resources. Moreover, depending on the specific structure of a health care system, government planning and regulation or even public supply of services may contribute to the attainment of this objective. But evidence, reviewed in this paper, suggests that the latter form of government intervention requires a high degree of administrative competence and a good information system allowing feedback to administrative levels. One example of successful government intervention is the establishment of a network of dialysis centres in the United Kingdom in the mid-1960s, which was directly supervised by central government and gave Britain a leading position in Europe with respect to the provision of this service at that time.

A final and central point in our discussion remains, however, the problem of determining the appropriate level of resources to be allocated to the treatment of ESRD patients. Assuming that there is a fixed budget for the health care sector the ideal approach to this problem seems to be to compare alternative ways of allocating resources to health care programmes on the basis of some criterion that involves costs and benefits of a particular programme to society. Lack of information and research capacity will prohibit a development along the lines of this ideal approach for some time to come, but we may attempt to get as close a possible. In the meantime, careful analysis of existing programmes can certainly complement our knowledge, as our discussion of the analysis of the Medicare ESRD programme in the previous section shows, and may help us in improving the efficiency of existing programmes.

14 Discussion of Paper by Rutten

J. Bergström

Huddinge University Hospital, Sweden

In my discussion I will start briefly summarizing the main points of Rutten's paper. I will then comment on some specific questions. In his introduction, Rutten made three important points that are relevant for the further evaluation: (1) dialysis is life-saving; (2) dialysis is very costly; and (3) technology is only gradually advancing. In his paper Rutten thoroughly reviews the macroeconomic impact of dialysis with figures for direct costs and gives data on growth of programmes in diffferent areas of the world. The most obvious benefit of dialysis is the number of life-years saved – but it should somehow be corrected for poor quality of life. Relaxation of the egalitarian principle that healthy life is of equal intrinsic value to everyone may be necessary in view of the limitation of resources, which involves complex ethical questions.

Alternative programmes are specified and it is concluded that the cost associated with different forms of dialysis may differ with hospital-dialysis being the most expensive and home-dialysis considerably cheaper, which is reflected in several countries having policies to encourage more home-dialysis. Although not considered within the scope of the paper the choice between transplantation and dialysis is discussed and it is concluded that programmes that combine dialysis and transplantation are less expensive than programmes of dialysis without transplantation. A review is given of the end-stage renal disease (ESRD) programme of Medicare in USA and it is concluded that government reimbursement seems more effective than private funding for providing effective care.

In the last section government policy is described in terms of four levels of hierarchy. A government may: (1) actively promote research and adoption of new technologies; (2) encourage greater efficiency in the production and use of a technology; (3) question and test the benefits of medical technologies; and (4) eventually seek to limit the diffusion of technologies to a level that strikes a balance between the benefits to be gained and the costs of achieving them. It is expected that developments will quickly bring countries to consider questions related to levels 3 and 4, i. e. levels that may impose limitations of growth of existing programmes and development of new programmes.

It is concluded that: (1) renal dialysis should not be considered separately from transplantation; (2) incentives should be towards home-dialysis and inexpensive forms of peritoneal dialysis and that right incentives should be promoted by allowing for private enterprise; (3) patient selection should be restricted and based on clear principles set in parliament, but individual clinicians have to decide which patients should be selected; (4) the financial arrangements with respect to health care programmes should incorporate incentives for efficient allocation of resources; (5) the final and central problem remains how to determine the appropriate level of resources to be allocated to the treatment of ESRD patients. Assuming that there is a fixed budget for the health care section the ideal approach to this problem seems to be to compare alternative ways of allocating resources to health programmes on the basis of some criterion that involves costs and benefits of each programme to society.

I will start my discussion by briefly commenting on some of the points with emphasis on the medical point of view since I am myself a clinician and, as it happens, I have the largest dialysis programme in Sweden and am also committed to research on the treatment of end-stage renal failure. My first point concerns a basic question: is dialysis really as costly as it appears? As pointed out by Rutten, when extending the analysis to the whole public sector, cost estimates for ESRD programmes should be compared with those of other programmes providing preventive treatment against other diseases or providing other health services. Data can be given showing that in Sweden the annual costs of dialysis are of the same magnitude as annual costs for other chronically ill patients (senile dementia and other debilitating diseases) requiring inpatient supervision by medical personnel, i.e. patients who are not at all rehabilitated in contrast to the majority of dialysis patients who work full-time or at least part-time. Comparison can also be made between the costs of dialysis and programmes providing other public services outside the health field (e.g. defence expenditure) in comparison with which dialysis costs are trivial.

The second question I would like to raise concerns the relevant cirteria for choosing between alternative policies. Continous ambulatory peritoneal dialysis (CAPD) was recently developed as an alternative to intermittent dialysis treatment. CAPD is a form of self-dialysis requiring no expensive machines, only bags with sterile fluid which the patient changes four times a day, leaving the fluid in the abdomen for 4–8 h. CAPD has shown a very rapid growth especially in Great Britain where financial limitations severely restricted the development of hospital-haemodialysis. Even if CAPD is still not established as an acceptable method for long-term treatment and is only marginally less expensive than haemodialysis, reimbursement policy favours this form of treatment (CAPD is prescribed as a drug). I would also like to emphasize further the close connection between dialysis and renal transplantation. They should never be considered independently of one another, but always looked upon as one treatment system where each method complements the other. They are not competitive alternatives.

In recent years transplant results show that long-term survival with cadaver transplantation is comparable with hospital dialysis and that living donor transplantation affords the best treatment available both with regard to expected survival and rehabilitation. Results of transplantation are markedly better in centres that perform a large number of operations per year than in centres with few transplants. Looking at the world statistics, it is evident that both Switzerland and Denmark, which have the highest figures for ESRD patients alive on active treatment, have a very high proportion of transplanted patients, thus being able to run their total programmes at a considerably lower cost than say, the USA, France, Italy, and Japan, where transplantation is rarer. Measures that could increase renal transplantation may be:

1. An integrated national policy of supporting the development of transplantation units of sufficient size, provided with adequate backup from immunologists, nephrologists etc.
2. Continuing information to health authorities and patients about benefits and potential hazards of renal transplantation as compared with dialysis treatment taking long-term results into consideration
3. A reimbursement system for physicians and patients that does not favour dialysis over transplantation
4. Inter-centre collaboration on the harvesting of kidneys, tissue typing, transfer of kidneys etc. aiming at a higher efficiency level than the present one
5. Legislation to facilitate transplantation from living donors and the harvesting of viable kidneys from cadaver donors

The final point I would like to discuss is the growth of technology and its enonomic impact. It is true that this growth is gradual. However, scientific and technical development do have great impact. Dialysis times have been shortened, patients experience fewer side effects and long-term medical problems are better mastered than in the early days of chronic dialysis. Introduction of CAPD, which in the long run may turn out to be the treatment of choice both from medical and economic points of view for the majority of patients requiring long-term dialysis, is a result of these scientific and technical achievements. However, a matter of concern is that *existing* medical knowledge is not utilized. One of the major risk factors in the aetiology of ESRD is chronic abuse of an analgesics containing phenacetin. In countries where such drugs can be bought over the counter, analgesic nephropathy is one of the leading causes of end-stage renal failure, whereas in countries where these drugs have for 20 years or so been available only on prescription, new cases of end-stage renal failure due to analgesic nephropathy are rare. Another example is conservative treatment of end-stage renal failure with protein-restricted diets and amino acids or keto acids. This form of treatment has the potential to extend the period prior to starting the patient on dialysis. In about one-third of all patients with chronic renal failure such dietary treatment may postpone the start of dialysis by an average of 8 months. This would reduce the total costs considerably, especially if such a programme were combined with an effective programme of renal transplantation.

Summary of Workshop Discussion

In the final discussion of this workshop, after Bergström's comments on Rutten's paper, the following important points were made:

First, if we are discussing in terms of costs and benefits it is obvious that about 50% of the adult chronic dialysis patients work and all of them can at least be at home and have some sort of meaningful life.

Second, if we look at long-term survival, transplantation is the best choice but it is dialysis that enables patients to survive prior to receiving a well-functioning transplanted kidney.

Third, countries with a low ratio of functioning transplants pay much more for their end-stage renal programmes than countries with a developed transplantation policy. The consequence is that it is important to reach an integrated national policy to support the development of transplantation units of sufficient size. There should be inter-centre communication with regard to harvesting kidneys, aiming at a higher efficiency level than the present one (in Sweden 30% of all transplantation is through living donors!).

Fourth, research potential is not used to its full extent with regard to optimizing dialysis/transplantation programmes so as to minimize the time on dialysis. One procedure is postponement of dialysis with an appropriate diet, combined with an efficent transplant-action programme. In addition, more effort should go into possible preventive measures against development of end-stage renal failure. Furthermore, there was a claim in the literature that profit-making firms in the US were extremely efficient in setting up dialysis centres (200000 patients on dialysis), showing that management can play an important role in the overall cost-effectiveness.

Any discussion of optimal treatment patterns should include discussions of the *size* of a specific programme since that will have an impact on the cost-benefit ratio. Once the form and size of "the best programme" have been established the question remains how to promote the idea in order to be successful in obtaining its goals. Possible incentives to different people concerned in the health care system and feedback information both from patients and from lower organizational levels to higher organizational levels were discussed.

One participant remarked that although with respect to the chronic debilitating illnesses we have probably reached a population equilibrium, with respect to dialysis the patient pool is still growing. Therefore, the point about trying to keep costs down by adapting the mix of treatments is an important one. In this connection it was interesting to hear in a recent European conference on dialysis that most clinicians agreed that a breakdown of about one-third of patients on hospital dialysis, one-third on home-dialysis, and one-third with transplants was a good mix. Continuous ambulatory peritoneal dialysis could eventually be considered in 10% to 30% of patients. In this workshop, however, there was a consensus that there ought to be a deliberate policy of trying to increase the proportion on transplantation from existing levels in most countries.

If one looks at the economic situation the clear logic at step is to find systems both to promote transplantation and to promote really coordinated goal-directed research by improving the existing technology.

Part III

Cimetidine

15 Clinical Evaluation of Cimetidine with Special Reference to Socioeconomic Effects

A. Walan

Linköping University

From the advent of this century to the beginning of the 1960s there was an increase in the prevalence of peptic ulcers. It is a matter of dispute whether there has been a decrease during recent decades and especially during the last few years. The prevalence of peptic ulcer disease in 50-year-old men and women has been found to be between 10% and 15%. The incidence in men between 50 and 60 years of age and without a previous peptic ulcer history has been found to be about 3%. The incidence of peptic ulcers in patients with a previous known ulcer disease is harder to evaluate partly because it is dependent on the length of time the patient had the previous active ulcer and also on the attitude to treatment among physicians and surgeons as medical or surgical treatment can substantially decrease the incidence of recurrences as we shall see. In Sweden about 3%–4% of men between the ages of 32 and 60 years are absent some time every year because of dyspepsia and in about one-third of cases the cause of the dyspepsia has been found to be due to or related

Table 15.1. Healing of duodenal ulcers, endoscopically proven

Author	No. of patients		No. of patients after 4 weeks		Healing (%) after 6 weeks	
	Cim	Plac	Cim	Plac	Cim	Plac
1. Albano et al. (1978)	78	79	72	34		
2. Bank et al. (1976)	19	19			86	42
3. Barakat et al. (1979)	16	18	69	44		
4. Blackwood et al. (1976)	21	21			62	19
5. Bodemar and Walan (1976)	30	14			90	36
6. Dobrilla et al. (1978)	15	15	80	40		
7. Figueroa et al. (1979)	13	16			92	43
8. Gilsanz et al. (1979)	27	31			60[a]	45[a]
9. Gray et al. (1977)	20	20	85	28		
10. Hentschel et al. (1979)	44	47	73	32		
11. Hetzel et al. (1978)	43	42			84	38
12. Mazure et al. (1980)	17	19			82	50
13. Multicenter trial[b] (1979)	134	46	66[a]	28[a]		
14. Semb et al. (1977)	20	20	85	60		
15. Ubilluz et al. (1919)	14	14	93	27		

Abbreviations: cim, cimetidine; Plac, placebo

[a] Healed ulcers and complete disappearance of erosions

[b] Bardhan KD et al (1979) Comparison of two doses of cimetidine and placebo in the treatment of duodenal ulcer: a multicenter trial, Gut 20: 68–74

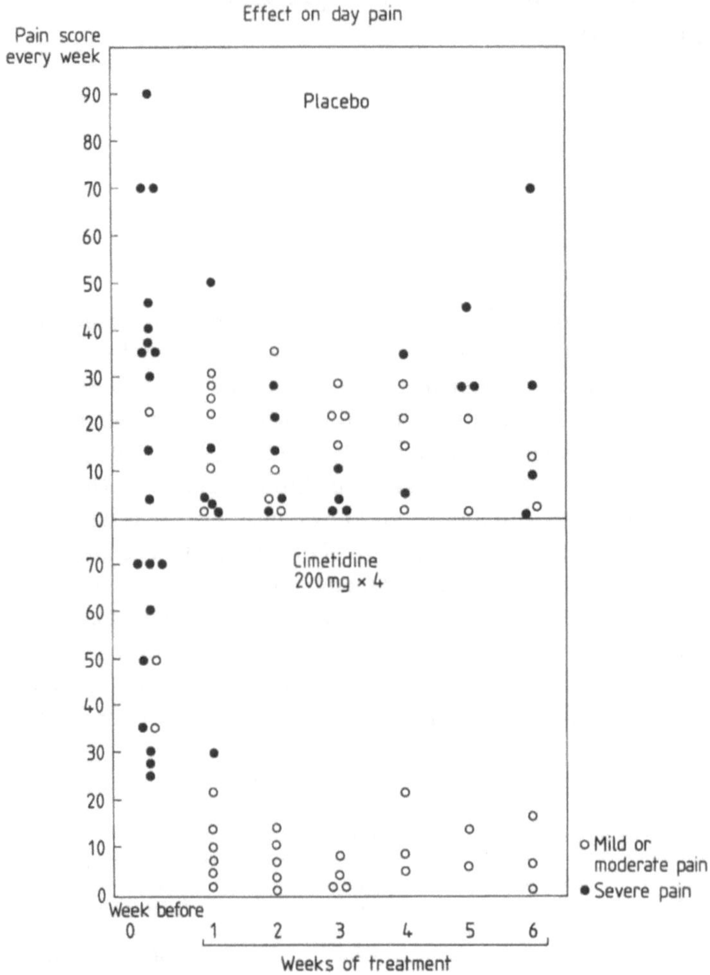

Fig. 15.1. Individual data on pain score per week during daytime immediately preceeding and during 6-weeks treatment with placebo or cimetidine in patients with active peptic ulcer

to peptic ulcer disease. In patients where an active peptic ulcer has been found the mean absence – at least in the recent past – was rather stable at about 40 days per year. These figures give a rough impression of the prevalence, incidence, and socioeconomic impact of peptic ulcer disease in a Scandinavian community before the introduction of cimetidine.

When the histamine H_2 receptor antagonist cimetidine (Tagamet) was first described in 1975 no drug had at that time been shown to accelerate healing of active peptic ulcers located in the duodenal bulb. Since then the many trials performed all over the world (Table 15.1) have clearly shown that cimetidine effectively promotes healing of active duodenal ulcers. The healing rate after treatment for 4–6 weeks with cimetidine (mean 79%, range 60%–92%) is much greater than after placebo (mean 38% range 19%–60%). Cimetidine is also very effective in alleviating symp-

Table 15.2. Number of pain-free days and nights per patient during treatment with cimetidine ($n = 39$) and placebo ($n = 33$)

	Preceding Week	Week 1	Week 2	Week 3	Week 6
Days					
Cimetidine	1.6	4.9	6.3	6.6	6.7
Placebo	1.5	2.8	3.1	4.6	5.5
P	NS	0.001	0.001	0.01	0.01
Nights					
Cimetidine	3.9	6.6	6.9	7.0	6.9
Placebo	3.1	5.6	5.0	6.3	6.5
P	NS	NS	0.001	0.02	NS

Table 15.3. Mean number of days with pain and hours with pain during treatment with cimetidine ($n = 60$) and placebo ($n = 28$)

	No. days with pain		No. hours with pain	
	Cimetidine	Placebo	Cimetidine	Placebo
1st period (1–9 days)	4.3	7.1	11.9	31.5
2nd period (10–19 days)	2.3	5.3	5.1	21.5
3rd period (19–27 days)	1.9	4.9	3.4	21.0
Total period	8.5	17.3	20.3	74.0

toms from active peptic ulcers, which is exemplified by one study in Fig. 15.1. Patients in this study had significantly fewer attacks of ulcer pain both during the day and night during treatment compared than the placebo group (Fig. 15.1).

The same rapid increase in the number of pain-free days and nights in patients with an active ulcer who were treated with either cimetidine or placebo is shown in Table 15.2 (Hetzel et al. 1978). In another study Gudmand-Høyer et al. found that not only the number of days with ulcer pain were significantly fewer during treatment with cimetidine than with placebo but also that the duration of this ulcer pain was much less in the cimetidine group (Table 15.3).

Our experience is that most patients with symptomatic active ulcers become symptom-free during the 1st week of treatment with cimetidine and that only a few patients have any remaining symptoms at the end of the 2nd week of treatment. This great symptomatic improvement in ulcer symptoms caused by cimetidine is found not only in clinical trials like these but also when the drug is used in ordinary clinical practice. As stated earlier patients with active peptic ulcer often have to stay at home from work because of ulcer symptoms. As cimetidine relieves these symptoms the working capability of patients is improved during ulcer healing (Table 15.4). These figures derive from the first studies with cimetidine when we did not know that cimetidine would reduce symptoms so fast. Today only a small minority of patients with an established duodenal ulcer need be absent from work after the 1st week and many are not absent at all. It was thus shown early in the first studies on cimetidine prescribed for healing an active ulcer that the symptoms were

Table 15.4. Percentage of patients (number in brackets) who needed to be off work for more than half of the week during ulcer-healing treatment with cimetidine or placebo. (Ricardo-Campbell et al. 1980)

	Preceding week	Week 1	Week 2	Week 7	Week 8
Placebo	81 (26)	65 (26)	46 (26)	27 (20)	25 (8)
Cimetidine	76 (37)	35 (37)	25 (36)	8 (24)	9 (11)

markedly and quickly alleviated, that there was small risk of complications of peptic ulcer disease during treatment with cimetidine, and that few patients needed to be absent from work.

Maintenance Treatment

The next question was whether long-term treatment with cimetidine could decrease the incidence of recurrences, which was known to be high soon after a period during which an active peptic ulcer had been present. There are now a great number of controlled studies on the effect of maintenance treatment with cimetidine in patients with chronic duodenal or gastric ulcer disease (Tables 15.5, 15.6). The results are unequivocal with a pronounced decrease in recurrences with or without symptoms during continuous treatment with cimetidine. In our own long-term study on 68 patients with chronic recurrent peptic ulcer disease the patients were treated with either cimetidine (32 patients) or placebo (36 patients). The clinical results with socioeconomic consequences will be reported in more detail. The results with regard to recurrences are similar in most other maintenance studies. We therefore believe that our results are representative also for the socioeconomic consequences, although information on absenteeism and other socioeconomic effects in other studies is either sparse or not presented at all.

Recurrences

During the year on maintenance treatment recurrences were observed as follows: in the cimetidine group there were five patients with one recurrence each and one patient with two recurrences: in the placebo group there were 18 patients with one recurrence and 12 patients with two recurrences. All recurrences were confirmed by endoscopy. When recurrence occurred an open course of cimetidine, 1 g/day, was given for 6 weeks and at the end of that time patients were either readmitted to the double-blind trial or underwent surgery.

Table 15.5. Summary of results of long-term trials of maintenance treatment with cimetidine or placebo in duodenal ulcer

Reference	Number of patients		Cimetidine dosage	Duration of treatment	Relapse rate			
	Cimetidine	Placebo			Cimetidine		Placebo	
					With symptoms (%)	Without symptoms (%)	With symptoms (%)	Without symptoms (%)
Bardhan et al. (1979)	29	31	400 mg × 2	6 months	14	7	58	10
Berstad et al. (1979)	23	24	400 mg at night	12 months	9	0	58	8
Blackwood et al. (1978)	21	24	800 mg at night	6 months	14	10	50	38
Bodemar and Walan (1978)	19	23	400 mg × 2	12 months	16	0	61	17
Dronfield et al. (1979)	20	22	400 mg × 2	6 months	25	–[a]	73	–[a]
Gray et al. (1978)	26	30	400 mg at night	6 months	27	0	80	0
Gudmand-Høyer et al. (1978)	26[b]	25[b]	400 mg × 2	12 months	12[c]	–	80[c]	–
Hansky et al. (1980)	20	20	400 mg × 2	12 months	5	0	80	20
Mekel (1978)	26	14	400 mg × 2	12 months	8	8	100	0

[a] Endoscopy if symptoms appeared
[b] X-ray-proven ulcers
[c] Relapse assessed symptomatically without X-ray or endoscopy

Table 15.6. Results of maintenance trials of cimetidine in gastric ulcers

Author	Number of patients	Durations of treatment (months)	Daily dosage	Percentage remaining healed		
				Cimetidine	Placebo	Significance
Jensen et al. (1979)[a]	19	12	800 mg	100	44	$P<0.025$
Machell et al. (1979)	25	11	1000 mg	82	14	$P<0.002$
Kang et al. (1979)[b]	31	12	800 mg	100	56	$P<0.02$

[a] Relapse defined on symptomatic grounds without endoscopic confirmation in all cases
[b] Asymptomatic patients not submitted to follow-up radiology/endoscopy

Complications

No patient in the cimetidine group had any complication but four patients in the placebo group had complications in the form of bleeding during the trial. Three of these four patients were the only patients who required admission to hospital except for elective operation during the trial.

Surgery

During the year one patient on cimetidine and 15 patients on placebo were operated on because they had two recurrences or because of severe symptoms of the first recurrence.

Absenteeism Before and During Maintenance Treatment

Most of the patients in this study were suffering from a severe ulcer disease. Quite possibly they are not representative of patients with peptic ulcer taken at random from a population. Many of the patients had been off work due to their illness during each of the 3 years preceding the start of our study (Table 15.7). Both the number of patients spending time away from work and the number of days per period off work increased yearly, probably reflecting an increase in the severity of the disease. Absenteeism during the 6 months immediately preceding the study period is, however, not included in the figures in Table 15.7 (almost all of the patients in both groups had some time off work during this half-year due to dyspeptic symptoms of active ulceration). To heal their ulcers most patients received a short course of treatment with cimetidine, 1 g/day. Only a few of them had any remaining symptoms after 2 weeks of treatment.

Table 15.8 indicates the reasons for the absence from work during the year on maintenance treatment. All 23 of the patients in the placebo group who took time off work during the year had endoscopically proven reulceration. A total of 769 of these days represents the periods when the patients were receiving cimetidine to heal a recurrent ulcer, resulting in a mean time of 24 days per recurrent ulcer and a median time of 20.5 days. The median value is probably more relevant for the effect

Table 15.7. Days off work and workers off work in the 3 years preceding the 1-year maintenance study (1973–1975) and during the study year itself (1976–1977)

	1973		1974		1975		1976–77	
	Patients off work	Days off work per patient off work	Patients off work	Days off work per patient off work	Patients off work	Days off work per patient off work	Patients off work	Days off work per patient off work
Placebo ($n = 36$)	14	Mean; 24.1 Median, 11	19	Mean, 43.7 Median, 24	24	Mean, 48.1 Median, 41	23	Mean, 52.0[a] Median, 44[a]
Cimetidine ($n = 32$)	10	Mean, 24.4 Median, 15.5	14	Mean, 36.2 Median, 27	15	Mean, 39.9 Median, 42	1	79

[a] Days off work during double-blind placebo treatment and during open cimetidine treatment for healing of recurrent ulcer. Days off work awaiting surgery are not included

Table 15.8. Absenteeism from work during the 1-year maintenance trial

	Patients off work	Days off work without recurrence during double-blind treatment	Days off work awaiting surgery	Days off work with recurrence during open cimetidine treatment	Total days off work
Placebo ($n=36$)	23	428	208	769	1405
Cimetidine ($n=32$)	1	59	0	20	79

Table 15.9. Clinical outcome of 1 year's treatment and 2-year follow-up

	Placebo $n=35$[a]	Cimetidine $n=31$[a]
Asymptomatic or with only mild symptoms during 3 years	6 (17%)	16 (52%)
Bleeding ulcers		
Before trial	11	17
During 1-year trial	4	0
During 2-year follow-up after trial	1[b]	1[b]
Candidates for surgery at start of the trial	13	11
Referred for operation		
During trial	15	1
After trial	7	6[c]
Total number of patients operated on during 1-year trial and 2-year follow-up	22 (63%)	3[c] (10%)

[a] At the start 36 and 32, respectively. One patient from each treatment group stopped treatment during the trial

[b] Both patients developed bleeding ulcers after they had been asymptomatic for 1 year after the end of the trial

[c] Two patients were operated on after the trial; four preferred continuous long-term treatment with cimetidine

of the ulcer per se as some patients were off work even though their recurrent ulcer became asymptomatic. Some of the patients with recurrences in the placebo group were also off work for a total period of 428 days with peptic ulcer symptoms but without a recurrence seen at endoscopy at that time. The 15 patients referred for surgery were off work for 208 days awaiting surgery. This makes a total of 1405 days off work due to recurrent ulcers with symptoms, symptoms without a recurrent ulcer, and waiting for surgery.

In the cimetidine group, however, only one patient was off work with a recurrence and he was also absent for another period when no recurrence was seen at endoscopy. The number of patients off work thus decreased from 15 during the year preceding the trial to one during maintenance treatment, while the number of patients absent from work in the placebo group was unchanged (23 patients) compared with the preceding year (24 patients).

What Happens After Long-term Treatment with Cimetidine Is Stopped?

We followed up the patients from our 1-year maintenance study, described earlier in this paper, for 2 years after the conclusion of that trial. Table 15.9 shows their clinical history during this time. When moderate or severe symptoms developed after the trial, they were well controlled by short courses of treatment with cimetidine or, in three patients, with almost continuous treatment.

During the 1-year trial we regularly performed control endoscopies on all patients. After the trial period was completed we did endoscopies only on patients with symptoms, so we have no reliable information on the relapse rate after treatment was stopped. However, the results presented in Table 15.9 suggest that the severity of chronic peptic ulcer disease is favourably influenced by 1 year's treatment with cimetidine, and that this influence continues even after treatment is stopped. Many of the patients had had more than two episodes of bleeding ulceration before treatment; during the trial none of the patients in the cimetidine group had a bleeding ulcer, compared with four in the placebo group. Fifteen placebo patients were referred to surgery because of two recurrences during the trial or because of the severity of symptoms at their first recurrence, whereas only one patient from the cimetidine group was so referred.

In the 2 years after the trial, one patient from each group developed a bleeding ulcer, each was 1 year after discontinuing treatment; each had bleeding ulcers before the trial and the patient in the placebo group had a bleeding ulcer during the trial. When reulceration occurred during the 2-year post-maintenance period, both patients were referred for surgery; the patient from the cimetidine group, however, refused surgery and was given a rather short course of treatment with cimetidine. Seven patients from the placebo group underwent surgery during the 2 years after the trial, compared with two from the cimetidine group. Three other patients from the cimetidine group fulfilled the criteria for surgery but refused operation. Thus over the entire 3-year period from the beginning of the maintenance trial until 2 years after its end, 3 of the 32 patients from the cimetidine group were operated upon (four more were considered candidates for surgery but preferred cimetidine treatment) compared with a total of 22 of the 36 patients from the placebo group.

Cimetidine as an Alternative to Surgery

In the previous study several patients were considered to be candidates for surgery before entering the trial and they fared well on maintenance treatment with cimetidine. We have therefore started a trial with the aim of comparing continuous treatment with cimetidine with selective proximal vagotomy (the standard operation for duodenal ulcer) in patients who were considered candidates for surgery by themselves, the physician, and the surgeon.

Eighty-three patients with severe chronic ulcer disease were randomized for selective proximal vagotomy (40 patients) or for maintenance treatment with cimetidine, 400 mg Noct. (400 mg bi daily schedule continuously after the first relapse). The study is still continuing, so the following figures are preliminary results. The patients are seen every 3rd month and endoscopy is performed every 6th month and at the occurrence of peptic ulcer symptoms. Completeness of vagotomy is assessed by modified sham feeding and insulin tests. Of the 40 operated patients, one (a 64-year-old woman) died a few days after the operation from a pulmonary embolus; 39 have been followed-up after operation for a median time of 21 months. Of these, 11 patients have until now developed new ulcers mostly with only mild symptoms. Three more patients have had other postoperative complaints, such as vomiting, which sometimes interferes with working capacity, possibly for several months. All patients were, of course, off work at the time of operation, mostly for not less than 1 month.

Forty-three patients were randomized for continuous treatment with cimetidine. They have been followed-up for a median time of 23 months. Recurrences have been observed in 20 patients. At the occurrence of a relapse the patients were offered operation or continuous cimetidine (400 mg bi daily schedule) treatment; six patients preferred operation. The majority (80%) of the patients who were initially considered candidates for surgery have had no recurrence. There was one mild recurrence that did not interfere with working capability. The study is still in progress with the intention of discontinuing cimetidine treatment after 3 years with further follow-up for as long as possible in the hope that the intensity of the disease will decrease with time. This is because in general practice it has been found that there seems to be a peak in the severity of peptic ulcer disease and 10–15 years later the disease seems to resolve itself (at least in those patients who have not been operated on). Whether this finding is relevant for the present group of patients will be evident within the next 10–15 years.

16 Discussion of Paper by Walan

M. F. Drummond

University of Birmingham

In studying the evaluation of cimetidine my main interest is: what can we learn from the way the evaluation of cimetidine is being handled that will help us with the next drug to come along of this character? So although I will be talking briefly about some of the results and how economists might use them, I have also in my mind this more fundamental methodological problem in the evaluation of new technologies.

Following a short discussion of the prevalence of peptic ulcer disease and its economic burden in terms of work-days lost, Walan gives a very clear and succinct summary of the results of clinical trials comparing cimetidine with a placebo. He argues that the results of such trials show the following:

1) Cimetidine administered for relatively short periods (4–6 weeks) promotes the healing of active duodenal ulcers (the healing rate being checked endoscopically)
2) Cimetidine administered over a similar length of time reduces the amount of ulcer pain experienced by patients
3) When given as a long-term maintenance treatment (up to 1 year), cimetidine reduces the recurrence of ulcers. This in turn reduces the necessity for surgery during the course of treatment and the number of work-days lost
4) Although information on relapse rate after the cessation of long-term treatment is less reliable, it appears that after a 2-year follow-up the ulcer experience of the treatment group is no worse than that of the placebo group. This means that the difference in ulcer experience observed during the course of treatment is maintained
5) Cimetidine is being compared with surgery (selected proximal vagotomy) in a current study. (All those admitted to the trial were originally considered to be candidates for surgery.) Interim (23 months) results show that 80% of the cimetidine-treated patients have had either no, or one mild, recurrence and no interference with working capability. The study is still in progress and issues still to be investigated include what happens when cimetidine treatment is discontinued after 3 years. It is thought that quite a long-term (10–15 years) follow-up would be beneficial

In judging the paper from an economist's perspective, I find the following three issues of interest. They are linked to one another.

Can economic evaluators build on the results of the clinical trials concerned? Reliable information on the medical effectiveness of therapies is of crucial importance to economists. Therefore, one would need to be confident that clinical trials have been conducted in a manner that clinical epidemiologists and biostatisticians would find satisfactory. Some of the trials described are certainly properly randomized controlled studies but it would be useful to know more in general about the selection of patients for admission to clinical trials, the methods of control, the numbers required for statistical purposes, and the variables measured (e.g. what side effects are recorded?). It may be that Walan has confined his interest to controlled trials in this instance. Nevertheless, I understand that in the early stages of the development of new technologies many trials are uncontrolled and I would welcome some discussion of the role of such trials and the influence they have both on future research and the spread of the new technology.

Quite apart from the reliability of the medical information generated in clinical trials it is useful to explore whether other information important for subsequent economic analysis is routinely collected. In the case of the studies reported here we are fortunate that socioeconomic information, such as number of days absent from work, has been recorded. Also dosages can give us an indication of the cost of treatment although there are other factors, such as physician time and patient time, that are important. One additional item that economists would like recorded is the associated health service resource use, such as visits to the family physician, home care, or hospital treatment. On a more complex level economists would like information relating to patients' functioning over and above their ability to work. (This information could then be used in the construction of health status indices).

Finally, there is the problem of the generalizability of the results of small-scale clinical evaluations. What factors should economists consider when trying to generalize from the results of such clinical studies? One thing that is often mentioned to me is that in the research setting the results obtained are a best estimate of the likely impact on health, in that in a trial one has enthusiastic and meticulous health care workers which one may not always have when that therapy diffuses more widely.

How does the clinical evaluator's formulation of the problem differ from that of an economist? The line of enquiry outlined in Walan's paper seems to me to be completely respectable from a clinical point of view. First, one investigates the *efficacy* of cimetidine administered over short periods with particular attention to side effects and dosage levels. Then one can go on to investigate long-term effects and its comparison, in terms of *effectiveness,* with alternative patient management strategies. An economist would have a different, perhaps complementary, research agenda. Given a perspective of wanting to maximize the benefit from the use of scarce health service resources, he would be interested in the likely changes in clinical practice and their resource impact. This would lead him to consider issues such as:
What are the clinical indications for the use of cimetidine? (are these confirmed ulcers or just ulcer-type pain?)
What are the alternative acceptable patient management strategies? These might *not* include placebo, but may include antacids, other H_2-receptor antagonists and surgery. (There are presumably a number of options within the surgical alternative itself.)
How is the new technology likely to diffuse into the health system and what is the implied change in resource costs (up or down)?
Given the time to undertake decent clinical studies, what happens to clinical practice in the meantime? What is the likely extent of cimetidine prescription by family physicians in *inappropriate* cases?

So I think economists would require some discussion of the clinical indications for the use of this technology. The main thing I missed from the paper relates to the fundamental question: what do we really mean by clinical evaluation? Is there some discussion of this in the early stages of a launch of a new therapy? How precise can we be even before the drug is launched as to how it is going to be used? It seems to me from the United Kingdom experience that we can make some pretty good guesses about how family physicians will behave. They will just use the new drug as yet another way of keeping people happy in their consulting rooms, and use it for a much wider range of conditions than it has been evaluated for in the kind of clinical trial setting that Walan has described.

How and when should economists be involved in the evaluation process? At present I am not sure that I can provide an answer to the question I have posed. However, it does seem to me that:

The involvement of economists should be phased in some way. That is, as more clinical evidence is produced, economic issues need to be introduced progressively

The rate of economists' involvement should in some way be related to the projected rate of diffusion of the technology

I think economists would be interested in how the new technology is likely to diffuse into the health system and whether the implied change in resource costs is up or down. For example, one might have a very cost-effective procedure, that is, a new procedure which is cost-effective compared with existing ones. However, costs could still rise in total because the new procedure might open up therapy to a much wider group of patients. Also, any gains that could be made in resource terms from the correct use of a new cost-effective procedure might of course be wiped out by inappropriate use of the new procedure or therapy. And linked to that point, given the time that is needed to undertake decent clinical evaluations – and remember Walan was suggesting about 10–15 years to obtain really good evidence on some (though not all) aspects of the new study that he is mounting – what happens to clinical practice in the meantime?

It strikes me that it is not only economic evaluation that people take no notice of. There are many examples of people not taking notice of medical evaluation either. I like the story from Frederik Mosteller who said it took the British Navy something like 250 years to recognize the impact that vitamin C might have on scurvy. And so there may be many procedures that persist even though good evidence has been or is being generated that they are worthless.

One area I would like to explore is: what can we do to feed more research-type thinking into everyday clinical practice? How can people who conduct controlled clinical evaluations influence clinical practitioners who are going to be using some of the new therapies even during the time some of the medical evaluation is being carried out. Things come to mind like consensus development programmes, or what they call "model health care programmes" in Scandinavia. Moreover, this is an area we ought to study with cimetidine because the diffusion of drugs is harder to manage than the diffusion of equipment in that government (especially in countries with a national health service) could make a ruling that only certain places should have scanners, whereas a new medicine can be prescribed freely by many family physicians throughout the country.

Summary of Workshop Discussion

It was generally agreed that cimetidine has brought about a radical change in the treatment of duodenal ulcer: (1) it removes pain within a matter of days; (2) administered for relatively short periods of around 4–6 weeks it promotes the healing of active duodenal ulcers and appears to heal 80% of ulcers within this period of time; (3) it reduces the necessity for hospitalization and surgery during the course of the treatment; and (4) it reduces the number of workdays lost. Cimetidine has been evaluated more than most new drugs.

What worried some members of the discussion group about some of these trials were the tests of cimetidine against placebo, which seemed to one expert to be very close to being unethical. The main reason for comparing cimetidine with placebo at the time these investigations were started in summer 1977 was that there was no therapy that had been shown to be *effective in ulcer healing*. It is true, and has been reported in several studies, that antacids given seven times a day, 30 ml each time (about 210 ml a day – this varies in different studies), gave approximately the same healing rates. But the *side effects of the antacids* (mainly diarrhoea) occurred at a rate of about 30% and therefore it was not possible to continue the trials. In studies against other forms of therapy (anticholinergic) cimetidine has been found to be more effective. Of course one could test cimetidine against an ordinary pain reliever. Antacids in short-term treatment for symptomatic relief only might be equally effective provided the patient carries around a bag full of antacids so as to be able to take them roughly every hour or so. However, it is quite obvious that this sort of treatment, in order to be equally effective, has to be carried out in such a fashion that the patient is apt not to do it correctly. For this reason cimetidine is a better drug not only because of its new mode of action but because it is also an easier drug to work with: the patient usually takes it the way it is prescribed.

A very controversial area of dicussion proved to be the relapse rate after short-term treatment and the effect of cimetidine as a long-term maintenance treatment. Although all the evidence shows that short-term treatment does not affect recurrence rates whatsoever, some information on relapse rate after stopping long-term treatment gave the impression that patients on cimetidine relapsed earlier than patients on antacids combined with rather small doses of anticholinergic drugs as maintenance therapy. The data are not conclusive and must be interpreted with caution. If different treatments are differentially effective in producing healing because one drug – let us say cimetidine – is more effective in healing the difficult cases, then including the cimetidine-healed patients biases the pool towards those who are more prone to develop recurrence. This is a theoretical argument but one that is worth keeping in mind.

An important result that was extensively debated, was the effect of cimetidine on surgical practice. Information on the immediate effect on the rate of surgery was presented from a well-documented nationwide study from the Netherlands, which showed a large impact on the number of operations both in the case of gastric and duodenal ulcer with a very sudden decline in the rate of vagotomies and partial gastrectomies performed for duodenal ulcer (Figs. 16.1–16.4).

There is no doubt that surgery for duodenal ulcer (partial gastrectomy and va-

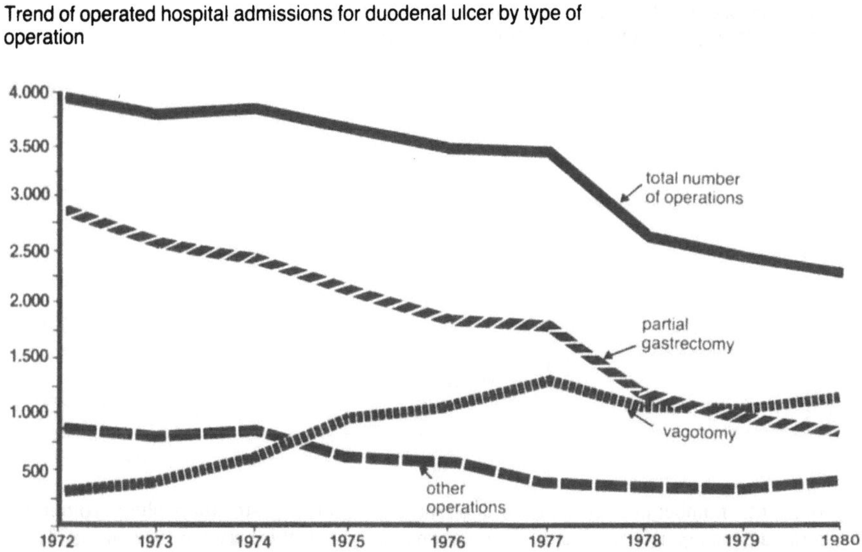

Fig. 16.1. The development of the number of operated patients for duodenal ulcer in the Netherlands; it shows a drop in the total number of operations following 1977 as compared with the previous development from 1972 to 1977. The graph also demostrates the replacement of partial gastrectomy by the vagotomy technique during the course of the 1970s

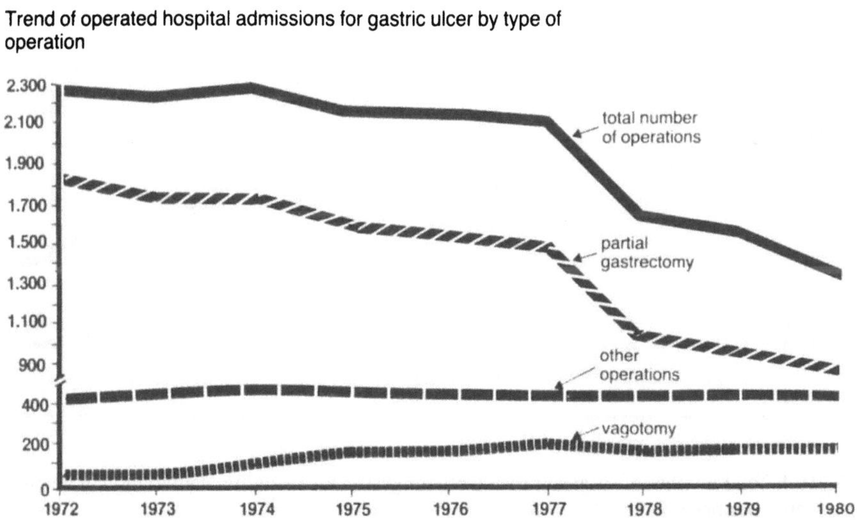

Fig. 16.2. The development of the total number of operations for gastric ulcer; it shows a drop following the introduction of cimetidine in the Netherlands in 1977

gotomy) has fallen since the advent of cimetidine. But it is important, too, to emphasize that in some countries (e.g. in the UK) the operation rate was falling before cimetidine came along and the critical question is whether cimetidine has accelerated an already existing trend and to what extent. Obviously it would be desirable to

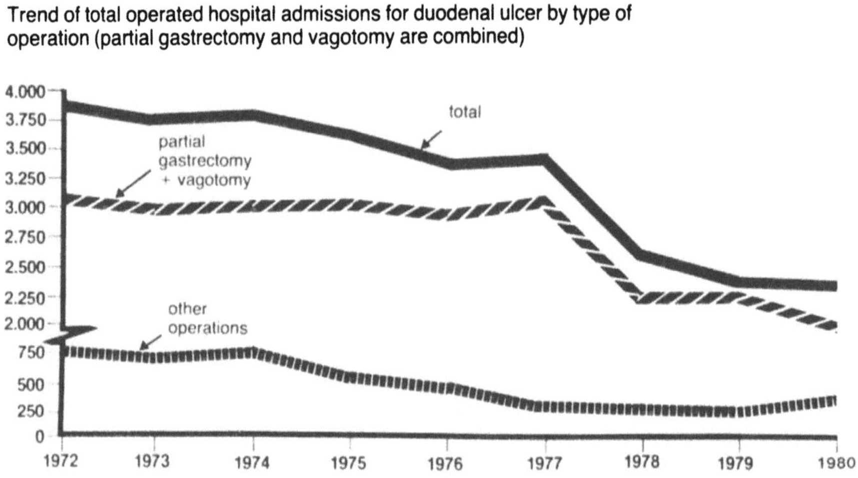

Fig. 16.3. Total number of operations for duodenal ulcer (partial gastrectomy plus vagotomy) in the Netherlands; the reported number of interventions was quite stable between 1972 and 1977 (around 3000 per annum). Between 1977 and 1978 a drop below 2500 was observed that represented a reduction of over 20%. The decline is statistically very significant

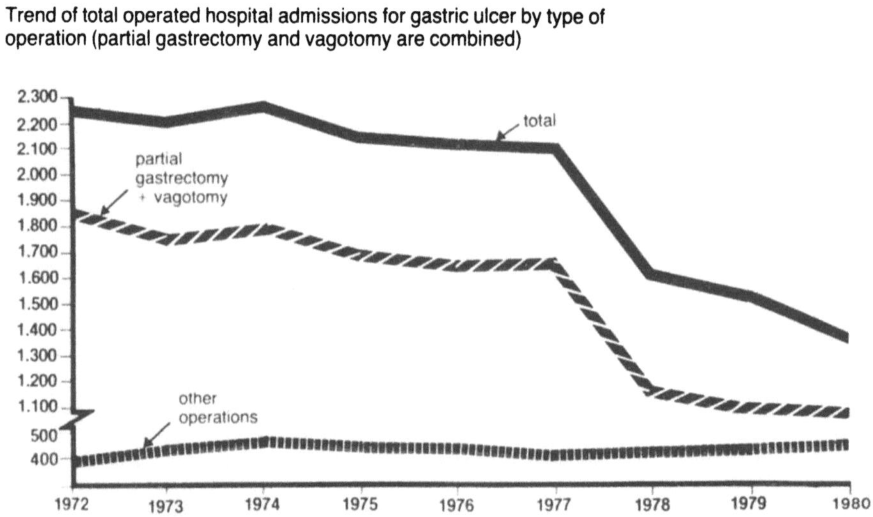

Fig. 16.4. Total number of surgical procedures for gastric ulcers in the Netherlands; here an analagous drop has been observed

study a group of patients originally considered to be candidates for surgery and offer them either an operation or the tablet. Thus far, this has not been done, but it might well be suggested that surgery is simply doing the same thing as cimetidine, namely reducing the maximal acid secretion by hopefully about 70%. Why should it be any more successful than H_2-receptor blockers? In a hospital unit in Glasgow over 600 patients randomly allocated to truncal vagotomy plus two different types of drainage procedures were compared with 52 patients on cimetidine: after analysis of at least 2 years the results in the latter group were just as good as the previous experience with surgery in the pre-cimetidine era.

According to a patient-management strategy followed by one participant in a highly industrialized area in the UK (80% of the patients working in the steel and coal industry), three-quarters of the patients with proven duodenal ulcer are selected for intermittent treatment with cimetidine and one-quarter receive drug maintenance therapy or surgery. In the first 3 years of this practice there was about a 15% drop in surgery: a later reduction in surgery of about 80% was observed. Patients are closely followed-up; some may undergo a silent asymptomatic relapse, but the symptomatic relapse rate on cimetidine appears to be very low. The problem – of course – is whether patients who take these tablets for several years and do not heal will eventually develop higher complication rates. Experience thus far seems to suggest that this is not the case. If one compares a group of patients that had never taken the drug but underwent surgery immediately with a group of patients who had taken cimetidine but the drug failed to be effective, the postoperative recurrence rate is the same.

17 Economic Approaches to Evaluating a New Medical Technology: The Drug Cimetidine

B. A. Weisbrod

University of Wisconsin-Madison

Introduction: Why Evaluate a New Medical Technology?

The objectives of this paper are to show: (1) why, and under what conditions economic evaluation of a new technology (health or other) may be useful; (2) what alternative evaluation approaches are available; (3) how those approaches have been applied to the case of one new technology, the drug cimetidine; and (4) what obstacles there are to improving the quality of economic evaluations. Economic evaluation of a drug involves both conceptual and empirical issues. Many of these issues arise in any economic evaluation. The evaluation of technological changes in health care (such as the use of a new drug) has many unusual dimensions, but we should not lose sight of the broad framework of evaluation within which it fits.

Why is evaluation needed for a new technology? The entire market system is a complex system for evaluating economic activities. In a private market economy, a producer's profitability is a measure of the firm's private success, and profitability is also a measure of its overall economic success (allocative efficiency) if the prices it pays for resources and the prices it receives for its output reflect the values of these goods to the resource owners and consumers. These values may or may not be reflected accurately in market prices, depending on whether, for example, consumers are well informed about the usefulness of the new and old technologies.

A considerable literature has grown up concerning the conditions under which a firm's self-evaluation of the profitability of some change (e.g., production of a new drug) does or does not coincide with a society-wide perspective on the desirability of that change. Most of this literature involves the search for sources of "private market failures" – when private and social costs, or values, diverge, so that the "invisible hand" cannot be relied upon to guide economic activity (Musgrave and Musgrave 1980, pp 54–74; Weisbrod 1978, chap 3). Some of this literature also includes the concept of "equity" in the social evaluation. Are the results of the economic change "fair" (Musgrave and Musgrave 1980, pp 85–105; Wolff 1979; Weisbrod 1979)? There are several reasons to believe that when a new medical technology such as cimetidine is involved, the private profit calculus deviates materially from the social desirability calculus. For one thing, extensive government regulations constrain private behavior – from controls over approval of new drugs (by the Food and Drug Administration in the US) to controls over their use (under Medicare and Medicaid in the US). A second reason, overlapping with the first, is the presence of "distortions" that tend to cause prices confronting consumers to diverge from real costs. I refer particularly to widespread private and public "insurance" for health care. Such insurance often makes access to a new medical technology free to a patient, or, at least far below real cost; this is true for drugs as well as for such expensive new technologies as renal dialysis, coronary bypass surgery, and the computerized tomographic (CT) scanner. The insurance broadens access to all persons, not simply to the affluent, but it causes not only patients, but also physicians, hospitals, pharmaceutical firms, developers of new technologies, and others to be less sensitive to high costs than would otherwise be the case (Goddeeris and Weisbrod 1980).

Given these distortions, there are reasons to question the presumption that the private marketplace – and its private profitability signals – is an appropriate mechanism for social evaluation. Some alternatives should be sought. The next section deals with the nature of these alternatives.

Evaluation Approaches

How "best" to evaluate a new medical technology such as cimetidine depends on the objective. Following a brief survey of alternatives, I shall illustrate some of them by actual evaluations of cimetidine.

Social Benefit-Cost Analysis

The economist's idealized evaluation framework is a comprehensive one that attempts to identify and to quantify all of the desirable consequences (that is, the "benefits") and the undesirable consequences (the "costs") of a new technology, to determine which is greater. The new technology under consideration must necessarily be compared with some alternative, or "counterfactual", which is often the preexisting technology, but others may be selected – for example, a placebo. Benefits and costs are typically defined in terms of what individuals are willing (and, implicitly, able) to pay either to obtain the benefits of the new technology or to avoid its costs. "Willingness to pay" is defined as economic demand, so that the intensity of anyone's linking of the new technology is gauged by what he or she would pay to obtain it; thus, economic demand reflects both the strength of preferences and the distribution of wealth. Just as with the private market for any good or service, a poor person with intense feelings may have less demand than a wealthier person with more moderate feelings about the new technology. As commonly used, the benefit-cost analytic framework is, in effect, an attempt to simulate the information that a smoothly functioning competitive private market would generate.

Both mechanisms for evaluation – the private market and benefit-cost analysis – must deal with the question of whether the consumer is sufficiently well informed about the new technology and its alternatives to evaluate it. If not, then the theoretical concept is not the *actual* willingness-to-pay, whether manifest in the private market or in the econometric estimates of the benefit-cost analyst, but what the *hypothetical* consumer would pay if he or she were well informed. Such estimates are typically very difficult to make.

The dependence of willingness-to-pay on the distribution of wealth has led to much debate over whether this is, or is not, a problem with which benefit-cost analysis should attempt to deal. Those who deny that distributional considerations should be dealth with in a benefit-cost analysis rely upon the private-market analogy; this market's evaluation process makes no attempt to adjust for any distributional considerations; whatever is the wealth distribution that generates consumer demands, these economic demands are taken as satisfactory measures of value (Harberger 1971).

Yet it can be argued that when social policy issues are at stake – such as in the areas of education, welfare, and health – it would not be appropriate to evaluate a program as having only small benefits simply because its beneficiaries were poor and, therefore, had relatively low economic demands. This position leads to the explicit inclusion of "distributional weights" in benefit-cost analysis – adjustments for effects of the income distribution on evaluation. If, for example, benefits to some particular groups of people are a goal of the program, benefits accruing to them may be given a greater weight than benefits accruing to others (Weisbrod 1969). Such an evaluation approach attempts to make use of a social, or society-wide, perspective. The issue of whether to deal explicitly with income distributional matters highlights the underlying social orientation of benefit-cost analysis.

Budgetary Analysis

When a government agency undertakes an evaluation, it often uses a different approach. It is likely to be preoccupied with those benefits and costs that are incurred by the agency and in a monetary form. For example, if a new technology could be expected to increase costs to a particular agency while decreasing costs to another agency or to private individuals, the decreased costs might be omitted from the first agency's evaluation. This is often the case, and when it occurs it leads to the same types of planning failures that occur in private markets – the disregard of "external" effects. A health-planning agency, for example, might evaluate a new drug negatively if that drug were more expensive than those already available, even if a variety of favorable effects were realized by consumers and, indeed, by other government agencies. In short, agencies often engage in incomplete benefit-cost analyses – or what I term here *budgetary* inflow-outflow analyses.

A budgetary analysis may differ from a social benefit-cost analysis in two ways. (1) An agency's budgetary analysis *excludes* benefits and costs that are not manifest in money flows. Thus, for example, a saving of lives – which would be a benefit in the social analysis – might be omitted because there is no associated flow of funds. Even monetary benefits and costs are often excluded if they do not accrue to the agency performing the analysis, as when one governmental unit's efforts to reduce on-the-job accidents reduces medical care demands on another unit. (2) A budgetary analysis *includes* sums that would be omitted from a social analysis because they reflect transfers, not real social benefits or costs. In one recent benefit-cost analysis of alternative means for treating the mentally ill, it was noted that a substantial portion of the "experimental" program's budgetary cost was for meals and lodging, and since those costs would be incurred by someone, whether or not the treatment program was involved, this "cost" was a transfer, not a social cost (Weisbrod 1981).

The budgetary analysis, although it omits effects that do not appear as changes in money flows and includes money flows that represent transfer payments – benefits or costs to one group being offset by corresponding, offsetting, costs or benefits to another group – does capture important benefits when they take the form of reduced expenditures. Thus, if a new technology improves patients' health, so that there is less need for surgery or other physician attention, the resulting reduction in medical care expenditures is a benefit that will appear in a budgetary analysis (Geweke and Weisbrod 1982b).

Economists' preference for a social perspective notwithstanding, government agencies will continue to pursue budgetary analyses. Facing a budget constraint and, generally, not being rewarded for benefits or reduced costs that appear elsewhere in the economic system nor being penalized for reduced benefits or increased costs that occur elsewhere, each agency's suboptimization will lead to collectively nonoptimal results. This is one factor contributing to the soaring growth rate of health-care expenditures, up from 3.5% of the gross national product (GNP) in the US in 1929, to 4.5% in 1950, 7% in 1970, and over 9% today.

Economic evaluation is only one area in which inappropriate incentives produce inefficient and inequitable economic behavior. One hypothetical, though realistic, example of how an agency's budget perspective can lead to socially inefficient decisions may be instructive. Consider a state Medicaid official in the US confronting the question of whether to include a new drug on the list of drugs approved for reimbursement. The new drug is more costly than substitute therapies, but it is far more pleasant to take and is more effective in that it leads to a better quality of life for the patient. The official, facing a budget constraint but with no incentive to be concerned about patients – either their satisfaction or quality of life – chooses to deny approval of the new drug. The outcome would be different, however, if the drug could be demonstrated to reduce the amount of, say, surgery, which would also be a drain on the agency budget.

Cost-Effectiveness Analysis

The terminology used in economic evaluation is often confusing. In one recent study "benefit-and-cost analysis" was coined "to encompass both cost-effectiveness and cost-benefit (or benefit-cost) analyses" (Fineberg and Pearlman 1981a). Another term, "risk-benefit analysis," appears to be similar to cost-effectiveness analysis (defined below), as applied in the health area. "Risks" and "benefits" are defined in terms of a nonpecuniary measure of output, with costs other than "risks" of adverse outcomes being measured in monetary terms. "Cost-benefit analysis is broader than risk-benefit analysis because risks are only a part of the total costs" (Ricardo-Campbell 1980).

In any cost-effectiveness analysis, the costs of achieving some particular "output" in alternative ways are compared. In the health area the concept of "output" that is increasingly used is "quality-adjusted life-years." Whereas, in general, no attempt is made to place a value on such a year, the implication is that its importance is equal for people in a "similar" state of health. In any event the output concept is clearly distinguishable from the willingness-to-pay basis for output assessment.

When a social benefit-cost analysis is undertaken, analysts frequently find that the outputs, or benefits, are considerably more difficult to quantify and to evaluate in monetary terms than are the costs[1]. In the case of a new drug, for example, how

1 Analytically, there is no distinction between a benefit and a cost, since "benefits" can be negative

should we quantify and value better health, reduced anxiety, and longer life? While economists have examined these questions conceptually and have also developed estimates of such hard-to-measure-and-value benefits, the difficulties are considerable (e.g., Mishan 1971; Jones-Lee 1976; Zeckhauser 1975). As a result, these forms of benefit are often omitted or simply mentioned (US Department of Health, Education, and Welfare 1966); sometimes they are dealt with explicitly but are not valued, so that the analysis includes both monetized and nonmonetized magnitudes (Weisbrod 1981).

Given the problem of valuing benefits, an alternative is to concentrate on the costs, leaving the determination of benefits to others – such as the "political process." "Cost-effectiveness analysis" does this; it poses the evaluation-analytic problem as follows: What is the cost of achieving a particular outcome by each of a variety of means? Once the "particular outcome" is stated, the problem becomes a search for the lowest-cost solution. What is the least-cost way of maintaining a specified number of combat-ready military aircraft, given the alternatives of having more new planes, fewer new planes but more replacement parts for any disabled planes, or fewer new planes and fewer replacement parts but more mechanics to make repairs? What is the least-cost way to "save" a given number of lives, given such alternatives as to increase the number of influenza vaccinations, increase the number of chest X-rays to detect lung diseases, or increase the amount of Coast-Guard protection for pleasure sailors? What is the least-cost way to treat an ulcer patient – with antacids? cimetidine? surgery?

More than a decade ago the US Department of Health, Education, and Welfare published a report containing a table of predicted "Costs per Death Averted, 1968–1972," which reported that the federal government spent $ 87 on automobile seat-belt-usage programs per death "averted," $ 6400 on programs to reduce smoking (and lung cancer) per death averted, and $ 42944 on colon-rectum cancer detection programs per death averted. While such numbers are interesting and certainly thought-provoking, their policy relevance can be questioned on many grounds, only one of which I want to deal with here.

Is a "death averted" (or an ulcer patient treated) an appropriate output unit? That is, should public policy in the health area be directed to allocate resources so as to minimize the cost of such an "output" (or an ulcer patient treated)? The answer is no, for several reasons[2]. (1) A death averted (or ulcer patient treated) is not a homogeneous good; does it make no difference, for example, how long-lasting the outcome is? (2) Some diseases are causes of pain and suffering but not death; thus, an allocation of resources that focused solely on deaths would erroneously disregard, for example, arthritis. (3) The cost per death averted (or per patient treated) may depend on the magnitude of the effort – that is, on the number of deaths averted or persons treated; as between two health programs, one might cost twice as

as well as positive, as can "costs". A negative benefit – that is, an adverse effect – is equivalent to a (positive) cost. In common parlance, however, costs are thought of as the resources that are expended on the project and benefits are the outcomes; the statement that benefits are more difficult to measure is thus a view that outcomes are more difficult to measure than are resource costs.

2 To the credit of the report that presented the numbers, most of the following issues were, at least recognized.

much per unit of output (say, death averted) at one scale of effort, while the relative cost could be quite different, and even reversed, at a larger or smaller scale.

This brief summary of some of the problems with cost-effectiveness analysis illustrates that "there is no such thing as a free lunch." One cannot escape the problems (costs) of defining and measuring benefits without facing a new set of problems. It may be easier to determine which alternative approach is least costly once someone else has specified the outputs or objectives, but great pains are required to ensure that the specification of outputs does not inadvertently bias choices. Averting deaths (however that is exactly defined) is surely a worthy goal, but if a policy based on that goal were to disregard diseases that brought much pain and suffering but few deaths it would surely be inappropriate and economically inefficient.

There is no easy solution to these difficult problems of identifying and valuing benefits and costs comprehensively. We can, however, be aware of the nature of the problems, thus reducing the likelihood that the "simplifying" assumptions of analysts – not to mention their oversights and outright errors – will go unrecognized. Table 17.1 shows the variety of evaluation approaches that may be used. The idealized benefit-cost analysis is society-wide (cell i). Cost-effectiveness analysis is, typically, less comprehensive and from a narrower perspective, such as a particular government agency (cell b)[3].

We turn next to a review of the quantitative work evaluating the new drug technology, cimetidine. The various studies differ in both evaluation perspective and comprehensiveness.

Evaluations of Cimetidine: A Review

Culyer and Maynard (1981) undertook a cost-*effectiveness* analysis of cimetidine. They asked, in effect, this question: If duodenal ulcer problems are to be treated in one of two ways – by surgery or with cimetidine – which is less costly? They do not evaluate the alternative of no treatment at all. Neither do they evaluate alternative treatment therapies such as antacids. They are aware of these alternatives, and they also recognize that "a complete evaluation should take account of the benefits as well as the costs". The justification for the more restricted cost-effectiveness approach is simply that it is often as far as one can realistically, or persuasively, go because of data problems.

Culyer and Maynard recognize yet another qualification noted in the preceding section, that outputs (effects) of the alternative treatment approaches may not be the same, so that: "The least cost method may therefore not be the one which should be chosen, especially if higher-cost methods produce more beneficial outcomes for patients."

The fact, discussed in the previous section, that an economic evaluation may be quite different depending on the perspective of the evaluator, is also recognized by

3 Under some conditions, a budgetary analysis is the equivalent of a cost-effectiveness analysis. This is the case when (1) the alternative therapies being compared have "equal" results, and (2) all budgetary inflows and outflows measure real costs (outflows) and real benefits (inflows). These conditions, however, do not generally hold.

Table 17.1. A typology of evaluation approaches

Perspective	Comprehensiveness		
	Budgetary analysis	Cost-effectiveness	Social benefit-cost
Government agency	a	b	c
Government generally	d	e	f
Society	g	h	i

[a] The scale (a to i) measures the comprehensiveness of evaluation approaches carried out from the perspectives of given units. Thus the most comprehensive evaluation would be a benefit-cost evaluation from the perspective of society in general

Culyer and Maynard. The question of whether a new technology such as cimetidine is "worthwhile" can be examined, they note, from the standpoint of the National Health Service, the public sector as a whole, or society generally (see Table 17.1). While they do not say so explicitly, Culyer and Maynard proceed to take a society-wide perspective in their cost-effectiveness analysis. That is, they attempt to be broad in their (social) *perspective*, but only partial in their *comprehensiveness* (examining only costs, not benefits). In terms of Table 17.1, they focus on cell h.

Notably, their social perspective encompasses forms of costs for which there are no associated market prices – for example, time costs to patients for obtaining treatment and costs of death from surgery. At the same time, the social perspective leads them to exclude such transfer payments as social security, which would have entered a governmental budgetary analysis, as we noted above.

Deciding on an evaluation perspective is a crucial matter, but the methods used to estimate specific forms of benefits and costs are no less important to the outcome of the evaluation. The cost of hospitalization, for example, is far from ambiguous. Culyer and Maynard, in estimating costs of surgical treatment of duodenal ulcers (DU), present several average costs per case, calculated in different ways. When based on average cost per day for all acute hospitals and the average number of days of hospitalization for DU surgery patients, a cost of £615 per case is derived; when a multiple regression model is used to distinguish between types of cases, the estimate for a DU surgery patient fell by nearly one-third to £419; and when there was direct observation of staff time employed to treat a DU surgical patient at a particular hospital, the resulting estimate was £386 per case (Culyer and Maynard 1981, p6).

That hospital "costs" depend on the evaluation approach used was recently shown in another study of the costs of treating mental patients. It highlights the systematic omission in hospital cost calculations of real social costs that the hospital does not pay (Weisbrod 1981). Specifically, there were omitted costs of the land on which publicly owned hospitals are located and understated costs of capital depreciation resulting from the use of depreciation accounting based on historical rather than replacement costs.

Culyer and Maynard included among the forms of costs they estimated not only hospital costs but the patient's loss of earnings during the period of surgery-related hospitalization. Depending on which of two alternative assumptions they used re-

Table 17.2. Estimated cost per case of vagotomy and cimetidine in the UK

	Cost per case of vagotomy (surgery) and cimetidine	
	Lowest estimate	Highest estimate
Vagotomy	£1180	£16370
Cimetidine	£1010	£ 1240

garding the difference in days lost from work if surgery or cimetidine therapy was employed, they derived savings from cimetidine treatment that were even greater than the savings in hospital costs (£584–£974 per case). Of particular importance is their inclusion of unpaid housewives' time. The loss of housewives' productivity associated with surgical treatment is a real cost to the economy, but because it is not reflected in explicit payments it is often overlooked in expenditure-oriented evaluations. It is noteworthy that work time lost due to peptic ulcer disease varies substantially among countries. An ulcer patient with "active symptoms" is off work for an average of 12 days (per year) in the US, 35 days in Italy, and 45 days in the Netherlands (Bodemar et al. 1979). The potential absenteeism cost savings from successful treatment vary accordingly.

Culyer and Maynard acknowledge that they did not "measure the costs of pain, etc., nor of the hidden costs falling on the families of patients, nor of other costs falling on primary care services, local authority services, etc." (Culyer and Maynard 1981, p 6). Nevertheless, they did estimate the costs of "case fatality," the value of lives lost because of surgical treatment. These costs were estimated using three alternative theoretical approaches, which produced a very wide range of estimates: £230, £340, and £15000 per case. The latter figure, which is derived from another author's estimate of £3 million per death avoided, is characterized by Culyer and Maynard as the "conceptually superior" method (Culyer and Maynard 1981, p 8). The £15000 per case for the higher case-fatality cost of surgical treatment is enormously more important quantitatively than the other costs they estimated. At the same time, it is notable that even using their lowest figure for the cost of a fatality the treatment by cimetidine was less costly than was surgery.

When Culyer and Maynard compare their various estimates of the greater cost of surgery with estimates of the cost of a cimetidine regimen lasting from 20 to 35 years they find the results shown in Table 17.2.
Since the authors prefer the risk-avoidance basis for estimating the cost of deaths from surgery, and since that approach leads to by far the highest cost estimate in the table, their conclusion is that "we have little hesitancy in judging the drug treatment to be substantially less costly than surgery for DU where the choice is clinically acceptable (Culyer and Maynard 1981, p 9).

These calculations assume that surgery and cimetidine are alternative ways to produce a particular output; this is the cost-effectiveness approach. The "output" is, implicitly, a DU patient who is no longer troubled by the DU. Unless the two therapies, however, are essentially equivalent in this respect, the comparative-cost estimates are of little or no value for economic planning. The authors acknowledge that their study is not a cost-benefit study, but is "a *cost-effectiveness* study in which the unit costed has been the case." Only when the difference in benefits between the two therapies in their effects on patient welfare is essentially zero can "the results reported ... be considered as decisive."

There are reasons to wonder about how reasonable it is to assume that the outputs or benefits are virtually the same for the two therapeutic approaches. One issue is whether cimetidine substitutes for surgery or only postpones it. Insofar as the latter is the case, Culyer and Maynard's estimates overstate the cost saving from cimetidine. As one writer put it, to the extent that cimetidine only postpones surgery the question arises as to whether "those patients would have been better off if surgery had been advised at a much earlier stage."[4] And since the enormous bulk of that saving came from the risk of mortality from surgery, it is of considerable importance to determine the extent to which cimetidine substitutes for, and the extent to which it only postpones surgery. It is really not enough to note – parenthetically at that – "(for example, whether the drug may, for some patients, only *postpone* the necessity for surgery is not at present known.)" (Culyer and Maynard 1981, p 8).

In a study published before the Culyer and Maynard paper, there was some evidence that cimetidine is not 100% successful in eliminating the need for surgery for ulcer patients (Bodemar and Walan 1978); that is, for some patients it only postpones surgery. During a double-blind trial lasting only 1 year, 1 of 32 patients receiving cimetidine was referred for surgery, and even though this was a far lower proportion than the 15 of 36 placebo patients who required surgery (a difference significant at the 0.0005 level). The point is that for some patients cimetidine does not substitute for surgery. This is not to deny the possible value of postponement, since postponement of costs is an economic benefit (the value of which depends in part on the interest rate). However, the full cost-saving estimated by Culyer and Maynard applies only when the "postponement" is permanent. Otherwise, short-term savings may disappear over the patient's lifetime. If it were possible to distinguish patients by the probability that cimetidine would be a permanent substitute for surgery (or by the expected duration of postponement of surgery), then the Culyer-Maynard estimates would apply to the extreme group; other, smaller cost-savings would be found for populations in which varying durations of cimetidine-caused postponement of surgery were expected.

Other costs omitted by Culyer and Maynard are the pain associated with surgery and its aftermath and the inconvenience of permanent drug maintenance. The former are costs of surgery; the latter are costs of cimetidine therapy. Pointing out these omissions is not a means of fault-finding; rather it is simply a reminder that any economic evaluation is incomplete, whether because of data unavailability or theoretical complexity.

The Culyer-Maynard paper has a number of significant methodological and substantive lessons to offer. For one, it helps us to focus on the importance of specifying precisely the question to be answered in a program evaluation. They sought to determine the actual relative costs of cimetidine treatment compared with surgical treatment, not – what I would have preferred to ask – whether the new medical therapy, cimetidine, can be expected to *reduce* the average cost of treating DU cases. It is this latter question that is relevant to the policy issue of whether cimetidine should or should not, on economic grounds, be substituted for surgery. In any event

4 Wulff, quoted in Fineberg and Pearlman 1981 a.

the policy analyst must recognize that depending on the exact question being asked, the form or the analysis and the nature of the data needed will generally differ.

There are several other noteworthy aspects of the Culyer-Maynard paper. (a) They deliberately attempted to resolve uncertainty by using quantitative estimates that "favored" the surgical approach, in order to see whether even with such a systematic bias the cost of cimetidine treatment still would turn out to be lower than the cost of surgery. This is a useful approach, especially when combined with sensitivity analysis to determine whether the ranges of cost estimates for the alternative treatment approaches overlap substantially.

Apart from their overall quantitative findings, Culyer and Maynard showed that (b) only some of the social costs of either treatment approach fall upon government – the budgetary impact on the National Health Service (NHS) – while some fall on patients or other parties. Consequently, for example, because the cost of mortality falls upon the patient, surgery can appear to be the cheaper alternative to the NHS even if it is more costly from the social perspective, which includes the costs to patients (Culyer and Maynard, p 10). This illustrates the difference between the perspective in rows 1 and 3 of Table 17.1, and specifically the difference between cells a and h.

(c) Another point that the reader carries from the Culyer-Maynard study is the enormous handicap under which any economic analyst must labor when required to do retrospective analysis. Clearly, the economic evaluation should "be designed at the same time as the clinical part of the exercise, and data to be collected *pari passu*" (Culyer and Maynard 1981, p 10). Otherwise, selection bias regarding who does and who does not receive the new technology can seriously contaminate the evaluation – a point also emphasized by Geweke and Weisbrod (1981), to be discussed below.

Two examples of the feasibility of integrating economic analysis with clinical trials are the studies by Ricardo-Campbell et al. (1980) and Bodemar and Walan (1978) of days of work lost by patients receiving cimetidine compared with those receiving a placebo (note that the counterfactual comparison here is not surgery). In connection with the double-blind randomized trials of cimetidine, it was found that cimetidine was significantly more effective than a placebo in reducing work time lost among ulcer patients. Unfortunately, no comparison was made with surgery or other therapies in either study, nor was there any attempt to place a monetary value on the work time lost. In the case of DU patients, the realistic alternatives to cimetidine include antacids, anticholinergics, and surgery – not placebos. The importance of Ricardo-Campbell's and Bodemar and Walan's studies, therefore, is less their findings than their demonstrations of the feasibility of studying economic variables such as work time lost through random assignment of patients.

The limitations of comparing cimetidine with a placebo treatment are uppermost in the thinking and work of Geweke and Weisbrod, who have attempted to evaluate cimetidine relative to other therapies currently in use. This work is examined later in this paper.

The recent paper by Fineberg and Pearlman (1981b) reviews a number of economic studies of the *cost* of ulcer disease. It should be noted that study of the total costs of any disease – regardless of the perspective, the comprehensiveness of the work, or the quality of the estimates – itself tells us nothing regarding the economic efficiency of using cimetidine or any other therapeutic approach. The key question for the purpose of making resource-allocation decisions is: How much would total costs be reduced, and benefits increased, by using one specific therapy rather than another?

Thus, from any of the economic-evaluation perspectives discussed above, the real issue is not whether cimetidine is "effective" – relative to a placebo or even relative to an alternative therapy such as antacids, anticholinergics, or surgery – but how its *relative* effectiveness compares with its *relative* costs, viewed (ideally) over the patient's lifetime. Evidence of the kind presently obtained from clinical trials – involving comparisons with placebos, and even then not examining costs – is only one component of an economic-evaluation process.

It is clear that the effectiveness of cimetidine relative to a placebo is less germane to economic evaluation than its effectiveness relative to alternate therapies. Alternate therapies have been in widespread use; they are replaced, to at least some extent, by cimetidine. Consequently, the economic evaluator wishes to know: (1) how much *more* effective cimetidine is than these other therapies; (2) how great the "value" is of the additional effectiveness; and (3) what the *differential* cost is. The evaluation analysis focuses on "marginal" behavior – *changes* in benefits and in costs. It is worth noting that a new medical technology that is *less* effective than another therapy would pass an economic-efficiency evaluation (e. g., a benefit-cost test or a budgetary test) if it were sufficiently less costly than the alternative therapy with which it is being compared.

The earliest effort to evaluate the likely impact of the introduction of cimetidine on the social costs attributed to DU was carried out by Robinson Associates (1978). In this study, 23 of the physicians who conducted clinical trials of cimetidine for the Food and Drug Administration were asked to describe in detail their drug-treatment regimens for various types of DU patients with and without the availability of cimetidine. They were asked to evaluate both regimens according to the following criteria: frequency of repeat episodes, frequency of patient visits to physician, likelihood and frequency of hospitalization, likelihood of surgery, frequency of diagnostic X-rays and endoscopies, amount of missed work, and likelihood of death from ulcer complications. These estimates were then combined with information from secondary sources of indirect and direct costs of various forms of treatment, and cost reductions resulting from the availability of cimetidine were computed for each type of DU patient. The physicians were also asked to estimate a "penetration" rate for cimetidine – the proportion of each type of patient that would be treated with cimetidine when the drug would be used by most of the physicians in the US who would eventually do so. The study estimated a reduction of $ 645 million, or 29%, in US health care costs for DU. The drug cost component was estimated to increase by 40%, but decreases in all other components were predicted.

According to Fineberg and Pearlman (1981 a, pp 55–57):

> The Robinson Associates analysis substantially overstates expected savings from cimetidine. Considering the exaggerated baseline costs of ulcer disease assumed in the analysis, the incomplete spectrum of patients included, and the distortion introduced by the method of calculating mean percentage reductions in costs, the estimated $ 645 million savings are probably two to three times too

large. Potential bias introduced by the selection of physician informants would increase the magnitude of that overestimate.

Geweke and Weisbrod, in a set of three papers (1981, 1982a, b), directed attention to the effects of cimetidine on budgetary expenditures. They emphasize both the incompleteness of their analyses relative to the social benefit-cost perspective and the partial justification for focusing on expenditures: "The question of whether a particular medical input – drug or otherwise – causes medical expenditures to increase or decrease has obvious policy relevance, given the current political emphasis on 'cost containment.'"

Geweke and Weisbrod compare the budgetary expenditure approach with the full social benefit-cost approach. They point out that the focus on budgetary analysis represents a simplification of the benefit-cost framework, in which benefits from a new technology consist only of reductions in costs and, indeed, reductions in only those costs that are reflected in explicit payments for health resources.

The Geweke-Weisbrod studies are the first published efforts to use panel data to trace DU patients over time in order to determine differences in expenditures and resource-use patterns for specific patients treated with different therapies, including cimetidine. They evaluated cimetidine from a government budgetary perspective, utilizing data from the Medicaid programs in the states of Texas and Michigan. They were able to follow identifiable patients for periods of 2–3 years, noting the level and nature of their medical care expenses for hospitalization, physicians, drugs, etc., distinguishing between those treated with and without cimetidine. Because they studied people in real (although nonexperimental) settings, they were able to compare expenditures for patients who were treated with antacids, anticholinergics, surgery, or combinations of therapies but excluding cimetidine. Comparing expenditures of DU patients taking cimetidine with those receiving other therapies would seem to be more meaningful than a comparison with a placebo group.

One dimension of costs of treatment that is often overlooked in the evaluation process is the inconvenience, discomfort, and risk of a treatment mode to the patient. This is potentially important for two reasons: (1) These costs are real, although not reflected in an expenditure of money, and they may vary markedly among alternative treatment measures. Use of large quantities of antacids seven or eight times each day, for example, is clearly less convenient than taking a single cimetidine pill three or four times per day, and having surgery is clearly more anxiety-producing and dangerous than is the taking of antacids or pills. (2) These differences in convenience, etc., can affect compliance with physician recommendations. A patient simply may not take the prescribed large quantities of antacids, whereas he or she may comply much more fully with instructions for the easier-to-take cimetidine. The comparative effectiveness (and benefits) of various therapies thus depends not on their success under ideal experimental conditions but under real living conditions.

Geweke and Weisbrod note that in many controlled experiments in the health area the only groups compared are those in which the new technology (e.g., cimetidine) is used by either all persons (the "experimental" group E_1) or none (the "control" group C). But this gives a distorted picture of the actual utilization that can be expected. Thus, they suggest the addition of a third group, E_2, one for which the new technology is available but is utilized only some of the time, depending on provider judgements, as would be the case in the real world. Clearly, the more interesting experiment is a comparison of groups C and E_2.

The critical evaluation question, regardless of which of the perspectives discussed above is taken, is how treatment with cimetidine *changes* outcomes – benefits, costs, expenditures, health state, etc. – compared, not with placebo treatment nor with nontreatment, but with the variety of treatments that actually would occur in the absence of cimetidine. This is what Geweke and Weisbrod attempted to do.

The major problem with which Geweke and Weisbrod wrestled is potential "selection bias." In an idealized experiment, which they describe, DU patients would be assigned randomly to treatment with cimetidine or with other therapies. In fact this has not been done.

Thus, they are concerned about the possibility that those DU patients who have used cimetidine may be *systematically* different from those not receiving it, for example, in terms of severity of illness or need for surgery, and/or the physicians prescribing cimetidine may be better informed, not only about cimetidine's availability but about other aspects of medical care, so that their patients would have better treatment, and different benefits, costs, and expenditures, from the patients of their less-informed counterparts. Geweke and Weisbrod attempted to adjust for selection bias in a variety of ways. The one they judge to be most useful involved a multiple regression analysis in which DU patients' disease severity – measured by history of days of hospitalization for DU and prior expenditures for DU treatments – was controlled (in a statistical sense) in order to estimate the effect on medical-care expenditures of utilizing cimetidine[5].

While this work utilized data for both Texas and Michigan, the authors regard the Michigan data as preferable, both because of its larger sample size and its better quality (more complete data on diagnosis). Their empirical work began with the accounting records for all Michigan Medicaid recipients for the full calendar years 1977 through 1979. Information for each recipient is organized by claim, and for each claim there are one or more lines describing in some detail the nature of the treatment and the amount billed, whether to Medicaid or another party. For each individual, basic demographic information and dates of Medicaid eligibility are available. For physician and hospital claims there is always an associated primary diagnosis and in some cases a secondary diagnosis. The lines for hospital claims specify procedures undertaken and the associated dates but do not segregate drug billings from other charges. Medicaid drug claims originate with pharmacists and include all prescription, generic and over-the-counter drugs billed to Medicaid. Dates filled and amounts billed are available in all cases. From these massive data, file records were assembled for those 2850 individuals who (a) were continuously eligible for Medicaid over the 3 years, and who (b) had at least one primary or secondary diagnosis of DU during the period.

5 The equation $y = b_o + b_1 x_1 + b_2 x_2$ where x_1 is total health care expenditures related to duodenal ulcer treatment, and x_2 is days of hospitalization for duodenal ulcer, in the 2nd through 8th month preceding the "intervention" date; y is one of several kinds of expenditures – on drugs, hospitalization, and physicians – following the intervention date. Separate estimates were made for the groups E (cimetidine) and C (noncimetidine). The estimates of predicted expenditures for the two groups were then compared for specific values of the x_1 and x_2 variables.

Table 17.3. Expenditures per case, groups E and C, assuming mean values of presample hospitalization, 1 day, and presample expenditure for duodenal ulcer, $ 60 ($x_1 = 60$, $x_2 = 1$)

Type of Expenditure	Expenditure (US dollars)		t statistic
	C control group	E experimental group	
Month 1			
Cimetidine	0.00	25.07	–
Other drugs	2.98	2.78	0.78
Hospital	557.69	24.02	12.08[c]
Physician	92.94	29.18	9.82[c]
Total expenditure	653.60	81.04	12.29[c]
Months 2–6			
Cimetidine	0.00	19.15	–
Other drugs	4.01	5.31	–2.48[b]
Hospital	24.65	51.82	–1.47
Physician	12.43	15.74	–0.74
Total expenditure	41.09	92.02	–2.44[b]
Months 7–12			
Cimetidine	0.00	10.14	
Other drugs	2.95	3.77	–1.69[a]
Hospital	19.70	21.56	–0.10
Physician	3.80	13.37	–2.34[b]
Total expenditure	26.45	48.84	–1.13
Months 1–12			
Cimetidine	0.00	54.36	–
Other drugs	9.93	11.86	–1.87[a]
Hospital	602.04	97.40	9.62[c]
Physician	109.17	57.65	5.78[c]
Total expenditure	721.14	221.26	8.91[c]

[a] Significant at 10% level
[b] Significant at 5% level
[c] Significant at 1% level or better

When the actual average values for the previous period (months 2–8 prior to the intervention) were utilized in the statistical analysis – $ 60 per person for health-care expenditures on DU treatment and 1 day of hospitalization for DU care – the regression results are as presented in Table 17.3. To a rough approximation, the results in Table 17.3 may be summarized by pointing out that except for the comparison in month 1, group E – the cimetidine users – shows higher expenditures for other drugs, hospitalization, and physician visits than does the control group, C (although the differences for the highest-expenditure class, hospitalization, are not significant). The greater expenditures for C than E in month 1 are attributable to the nature of the intervention of group C. For one-third of the C sample, the intervention consisted of hospitalization or a physician visit rather than a digestive-disorder drug claim; hospitalization always entails greater expenditures than a monthly drug regimen, and a physician visit often does. It is, therefore, not surprising that this control group displays much higher expenditures in the 1st month than does the cimetidine group E.

The numerical comparisons reveal a less obvious point as well: the month 1 disparity is so great that it overwhelms the difference for the total of the following 11 months. When the 12 months following the intervention date are taken as a whole, per capita expenditures for group E are far lower, only 30% of those for group C. The differences are statistically significant over the whole range of the independent variables.

It might be contended that the comparison of actual expenditures of the C and E groups provides a biased result. Geweke and Weisbrod considered, therefore, the possibility that the appropriate comparison should be based not on the actual expenditures of the groups but on what their expenditures would have been in the idealized, random-assignment case.

It seems plausible that the new technology, cimetidine, has been used as most new medical technologies are used – sometimes substituting for higher-expenditure technologies (e. g., surgery) and sometimes for technologies that involve lower expenditures. This does not imply that such a new technology is being used inefficiently any more than the drilling of a "dry hole" implies that the oil driller was inefficient. If geological knowledge were sufficient to determine with certainty the presence of oil, or if medical knowledge were sufficient to determine with certainty which particular therapy was least costly (given the effectiveness), then all error could be avoided. In realistic situations, however, decision-makers confront the familiar dilemma involving type I and type II statistical errors. In the case of cimetidine this means that if the new technology were to be employed only when it was virtually certain to substitute for more costly surgery, the result would be an inefficiently low utilization rate for cimetidine. Even when it is not certain that surgery can be avoided permanently by the use of cimetidine, the key issues are the probability and duration of postponement. As the estimates in Table 17.3 indicate, hospital and physician costs associated with surgery ("C" column) are indeed very large compared with the average costs of cimetidine therapy ("E" column). Efficiency calls for the use of average, expected values, of the type in Table 17.3; the state of knowledge necessitates probabilistic statements about outcomes.

Because of these uncertainties, Geweke and Weisbrod also estimated expenditures for alternative control groups. This work may be summarized as follows: Suppose that in the absence of cimetidine therapy, interventions would have consisted of a fraction, d, of drug therapy and the balance, $1-d$, of other kinds of therapy, including surgery. Suppose further that with the introduction of cimetidine, a fraction, m, of the nondrug interventions (surgery and physician visits) would be shifted to cimetidine. This implies that cimetidine decreases surgery and physician visits from what they would be with previously available drugs. These suppositions, combined with their estimates in Table 17.3, enabled Geweke and Weisbrod to estimate the total per patient expenditure levels for various values of m. With cimetidine available, the average 12 month total expenditure level per patient, for *all* patients (not just those using cimetidine), was estimated to equal $\$772-\$613 \times m$. If m exceeds 0.084 – that is, if cimetidine reduced the need for surgery and physician visits by 8.4% or more – then the 12-month expenditure level after the introduction of the new drug would be expected to be lower than that which would have prevailed without it, \$ 721. The latter figure is the average, 12-month expenditure for all patients using other drugs (which are relatively inexpensive) and having surgery (which is far more expensive than cimetidine). The expenditure effect of cimetidine thus depends on the degree to which it substitutes for the lower or the higher cost alternatives.

Outside evidence suggests that the appropriate value of m is much larger than 8.4% – that is, cimetidine can be expected to reduce DU surgery by more than that figure. A recent study of the incidence of surgery for DU, before and after the introduction of cimetidine, estimated that surgery was reduced 39% by the introduction of the new drug (Wylie et al. 1981). Taking $m = 0.39$ as an initial estimate, Geweke and Weisbrod obtained an aggregate per patient 12-month expenditure level of $ 534 with the introduction of cimetidine, compared with $ 721 without it. The new drug was thus estimated to have reduced expenditures over a 1-year period by 26%.

The reduction in DU surgery attributable to cimetidine is a critical matter. Fineberg and Pearlman analyzed data on ulcer surgery over time, and concluded that an "unexpected" decline in ulcer surgery occurred in 1978, the year cimetidine was introduced in the US. The sharp decline of ulcer surgery – some 11000–26000 fewer procedures (about 12–30% fewer) than a trend extrapolation predicted – was especially noteworthy because there was no decline in abdominal surgery in general. Even if the effect of the new drug on the frequency of surgery was only half the 39% estimate by Wylie et al. and even if it was at the low end of the range estimated by Fineberg and Pearlman, the drug reduces expenditures on DU substantially.

Whichever approach Geweke and Weisbrod considered, the empirical results show that treatment with cimetidine is an expenditure-reducing alternative compared with previously existing therapeutic interventions (other drugs and surgery). It is, obviously, not expenditure-reducing in those cases in which costly surgery would *definitely* never be required and previously existing drugs would suffice, but the knowledge required to make this distinction, and hence to avoid "dry holes," is not available. The extent to which the use of cimetidine reduces expenditures depends on the extent to which it substitutes for surgery, on the one hand, or more conventional low-cost drug therapies on the other. There is an optimum pattern of cimetidine usage and it is at neither the extreme of indiscriminate usage for all peptic ulcer patients, nor at another extreme, such as usage restricted to extremely severe cases for which surgery is otherwise imminent.

While one of the approaches used by Geweke and Weisbrod shows the new technology to reduce DU expenditures by some 70%, and the other approach estimates the reduction at a smaller but still substantial 26%, they emphasize that unless the probability of surgery being required is very low – 8% or lower – even our more conservative approach predicts expenditure savings attributable to cimetidine. They also reiterate that while they examined only the *expenditure* implications of cimetidine therapy, the "nonmarket" effects – the advantages to patients from avoiding the pain, anxiety, and risks of surgery – are also relevant.

Lessons and Concluding Comments

Many of the problems confronting economic analysts of any new drug technology would be avoidable at relatively low cost if economic evaluation were built into the randomized clinical trials. In its absence, economists have been forced to make assumptions about the expected usage of the new drug (or other new medical technology) – specifically whether users and nonusers constitute random or biased samples from the population of DU patients. Because concern exists that selection-bias does contaminate results, statistical corrective measures have been employed. These measures would be unnecessary if the needs of evaluation had been taken into account at the time of clinical trials.

Whatever the source of data, economic evaluation can proceed from a number of perspectives. From an overall economic-planning point of view, a social benefit-cost analysis is clearly preferable to either a cost-effectiveness or a budgetary analysis. Concerns about conceptual purity should not blind us, however, to the purpose of any evaluation – to facilitate intelligent decision-making. If the issue is whether or not to allocate more resources toward utilization of some new technology, it makes little or no difference whether it is 50% or 500% more efficient than its alternative, for even the lower figure indicates a socially efficient change. Thus, for example, the omission from an evaluation of the greater convenience of using cimetidine compared with antacids or surgery is of no consequence if – or insofar as – the other variables considered already show an excess of benefits over costs for cimetidine therapy.

There are advantages and disadvantages of the various evaluative approaches. Briefly, the point is that alternatives to an all-encompassing benefit-cost analysis have been developed for a reason – because it is costly to obtain data. When the costs and benefits of undertaking a more comprehensive benefit-cost analysis are considered it may turn out that a conceptually less desirable alternative is actually preferable. The variety of evaluations of cimetidine and their several shortcomings point to the important trade-offs between comprehensiveness, practicability, and cost of the study. Incomplete information, both about short-term and even more about long-term effects of a new technology, combine with difficult value-laden problems of how to place monetary values on pain, suffering, and life itself, to make the evaluation of health-care technologies enormously complex. A "useful" evaluation – since it will inevitably be incomplete – should: (1) make clear the nature of its shortcomings; (2) not hesitate to present nonmonetary, quantitative measures of costs and benefits, leaving it to the user to decide upon their importance relative to other consequences; and (3) understand, and make clear to the nonprofessional reader, that attempts to state benefits and costs in money terms do not reflect a morbid preoccupation with money – far from it – but simply the unavoidable need to make the varied effects of a new technology commensurable with each other. To judge the "desirability" of a new technology we need somehow to add all its favorable effects and its unfavorable effects to find which total is greater.

In the case of cimetidine, the clinical evidence of its effectiveness *compared with a placebo* is of little relevance for an economic evaluation seeking to determine whether the drug's favorable effects and costs make it superior, in value terms, to the alternatives it would replace. Placebos are, in general, not among the realistic alternatives. A variety of economic assessments have been undertaken. Each is incomplete. Each has theoretical shortcomings. Yet the evidence is growing that this new medical technology is more than worth its cost (as measured by its price).

The evaluative studies for cimetidine have contributed not only to knowledge about the economic evaluation of that drug but also about the problems of, and the opportunities for, making such evaluations of other medical innovations. Building economic evaluation into the process of random-assignment clinical trials is a high priority, as is the expansion of random assignment to groups utilizing nonplacebo alternatives. In addition, increased consideration should be given to monitoring of costs and benefits after a drug is marketed (along lines utilized in the Geweke-Weisbrod studies) as part of a continuing process of approval and evaluation of new medical technologies.

We have much to learn about how to blend theoretic ideals with feasible methods, and learn we must. The stakes are high – for private innovators, the research community, government agencies, and the society at large.

Acknowledgements. I thank A. J. Culyer for helpful comments on an earlier draft of this paper and Jerald Schiff for research assistance.

18 Discussion of Paper by Weisbrod

A. Sonnenberg, A. Fritsch, and G. S. Sonnenberg

University of Düsseldorf

The Economic Evaluation of Medicine: a Medical Point of View

Approaches of Evaluation

The background to the economic and medical evaluation of health care technologies could be summarized in two questions: How can the output of medical care be evaluated? How can the share of national resources devoted to health care be reduced? A new medical technology can be evaluated by medical measures, by economic measures, or by measures considering both spheres simultaneously (Figure 18.1). A medically better but more expensive technology is the most complicated case to be valued, since medical benefits must be weighted against increased expenditures, and both spheres, namely economic and medical, are involved.

Different approaches of medical and economic evaluation of new technologies have been developed as described in Weisbrod's paper. For analyses at the economic level we have costing studies (von Haunalter and Chandler 1977; Almy 1979; Sonnenberg et al. 1982a; Fineberg and Pearlman 1981a and b); cost-effectiveness analyses (Culyer and Maynard 1981), and expenditure analysis (Geweke and Weisbrod 1981). Though in principle the same approaches also apply to the medical level, physicians restrict their analyses most often to benefit or cost analyses. These types of analysis are the essence of all clinical trials. A cost-benefit analysis with a social perspective, which weighs medical benefits against their social costs, is the most comprehensive type of calculus. The benefits and the costs, however, are difficult to define, the benefits are difficult to value (see Sonnenberg and Blum 1982; Weisbrod's paper, this volume), and we have to calculate with distorted prices.

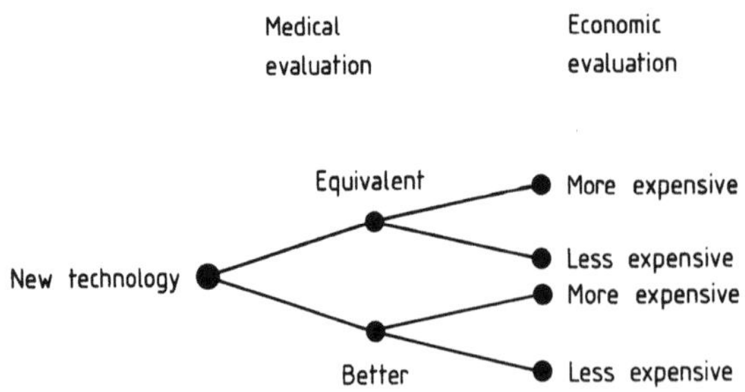

Fig. 18.1. Approaches to the evaluation of a new medical technology

Problems in the Economic Evaluation of Medicine

Even when physicians and economists use identical terms they may mean different things. In a medical cost-benefit analysis death always means a loss. In some economic analyses (for example, those using the human-capital approach) death may mean a gain when it happens at the age of retirement. Physicians use monetary costs of absenteeism and hospitalization primarily to describe the severity of the disease and the drawbacks of therapy (Sonnenberg and Hefti 1979; Sonnenberg et al. 1982b). To the economist, costs due to absenteeism depend on the rate of unemployment and the income of the absentee; hospitalization is an additional cause of expenditure.

There are several reasons for distorted prices in the system of health care (Abel-Smith 1980). Medical research is partly paid by health care money. Permanent positions of hospital staff prevent the reduction of personnel and of hospital beds if they are no longer needed. Government regulations constrain private behaviour. Since many hospitals are run on government money, no competition among physicians and hospitals develops regarding the most effective therapy at the lowest price possible. On the contrary, physicians authorize the use of expensive resources as if they had no cost at all. This behaviour is reinfored by a medical ethic according to which everything that is possible should be done if it is likely to help the patient. The market price of, for instance, duodenal ulcer includes costs that arise from moderate to severe malpractice. The insurance system and the social health care system isolate the patient from any concern about costs. The system of social care lends itself to abuse (Marcus 1974). Figures 18.2 and 18.3 illustrate these last two points. Figure 18.2 portrays an increase in days off work per 1000 members of the AOK (the biggest certified health maintenance organization in Germany). It serves 42%

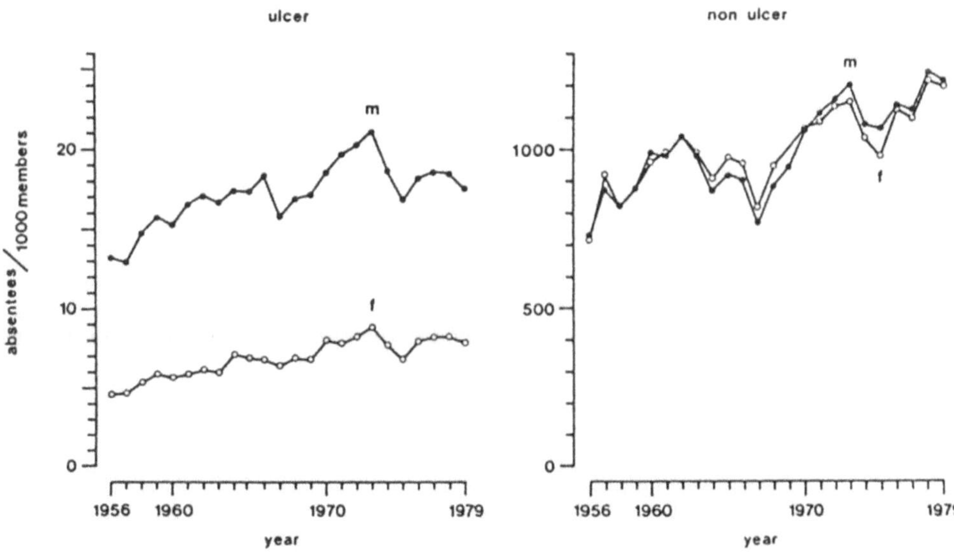

Fig. 18.2. Days off work per 1000 male and female members of the AOK

of all workers and employees in the FRG, i.e. 10 million people (Bundesverband der Ortskrankenkassen 1957–1981). Under German health legislation, there has been a steady rise in subsidies to the sick. Since 1970 any sick worker or employee is granted unrestricted payment during the first 6 weeks of illness. In general, every change in the benefit structure has been followed by a further rise in absenteeism. Although the incidence and prevalence of peptic ulcer have not changed in the FRG (Sonnenberg et al. 1982c), the numbers off work through peptic ulcer increased by more than 50% between 1956 and 1979. The pattern of absenteeism over time is parallel in the ulcer and nonulcer patients. The falls due to the recessions of the German economy in 1967 and 1975 can easily be detected in the ulcer and nonulcer curves. In the ulcer and nonulcer group, there is a parallel decline in the average length of absenteeism. Since the number of absentees increased during the same period, this change means that a growing fraction of the patients was on sick leave for shorter periods of time. The economic recessions of 1967 and 1975 also appear on the two graphs of Fig. 18.3. In times of recession the average length of absenteeism decreases, because those patients who would otherwise be on sick leave for short periods fear losing their jobs and decide to stay at work.

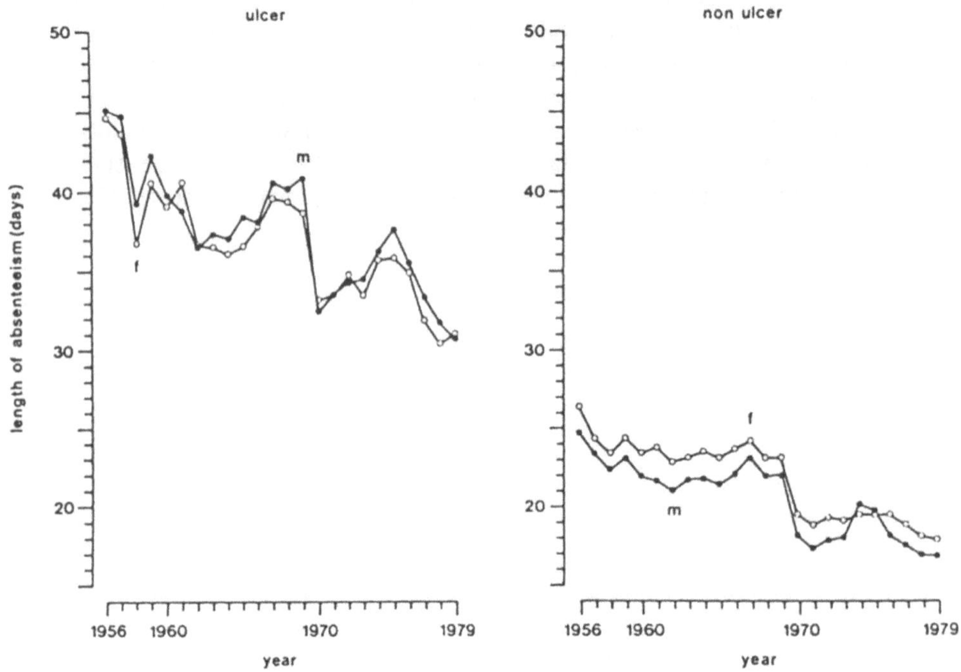

Fig. 18.3. Length of spells off work among male and female AOK members

The Inevitable Rise in Health Care Expenditure

The drug cimetidine is a relatively simple case to evaluate because from a medical point of view it is better than its therapeutic alternatives (Sonnenberg et al. 1981) and strictly economic analyses reveal, as has been seen, that it is also less costly. Would we still prescribe cimetidine were it more expensive than its alternatives? H_2-blockers are not only one of several alternatives to treat duodenal ulcer, but also – at the moment – the best. They have well-defined and well-understood pharmacological actions, few side effects, high efficacy in duodenal ulcer healing and prevention, they cause less harm than surgery, and the intake is easier than that of antacids. We would probably still prescribe cimetidine even if the economic analyses had shown cimetidine to be more expensive than its alternatives.

Apart from cimetidine, we have seen an enormous increase in medical efficacy during the past few years. New drugs have been developed, e. g. analgesic-antipyretic drugs, antibiotics, antiarrhythmic drugs, anticonvulsant drugs, antidiarrhoeal drugs, antihistamines, anti – almost everything. New laboratory methods have been introduced (e. g. Coulter counter, enzyme tests, HL-A antigens, radioimmunoassays), new diagnostic methods (e. g. computed tomographic scanner, ultrasound, endoscopy, coronary angiography), and new therapeutic methods (e. g. microsurgery, highly selective vagotomy, dialysis, pacemaker, respirator, insulin pumps, dilatation of coronary arteries). The list could be extended.

Concern about the increase in health care expenditures results from the fact that in the past years health care expenditures have risen faster than gross national products.

Medical Proposals for the Reduction of Health Care Expenditure

What kind of medical solutions can be thought of to avoid a further rise in the fraction of the gross national product spent on health care? (1) Stop medical research. (2) Restrict medical care to the economically active. (3) Increase industrial productivity (how?). These extremes seem unlikely candidates. A fourth solution was originally introduced by Mother Nature: (4) sexual propagation and the birth of new entities seem cheaper than the permanent repair of the old ones (Odum 1971). Does it mean that one should not treat the aged or age-related diseases? Should we restrict the most costly technologies to the youngest? Most people do not like this solution either, but it might be a quite natural one.

Equivalent successive investments in any system lead to diminishing marginal returns. The first dose of fertilizer on a fixed area of land will give a higher yield per ton than the second or third dose. In lectures on economics one is taught how to determine the optimal amount of investment. In lectures on medicine one is taught to take advantage of the smallest return so long as it is positive. A fifth solution is therefore that we should change this type of medical ethic. The following are nine commandments contrary to conventional medical ethics:

Thou shalt learn statistics and medical decision analysis and use them in thy clinical routine

Thou shalt not try everything thou can to treat thy patients and save their lives

Thou shalt not start any therapy – even though it be life-saving – when thy chances of success are lower than 10%
Thou shalt not prolong a man's life were it to mean that he live crippled and lame
Thou shalt not prolong a man's life if it be for less than 6 months
Thou shalt not care about probabilities lower than 1%
People want the physician to reassure, comfort, console, solicit, and take away all their fear, thou shalt not do this
Thou shalt not crave a diagnosis for every patient
Thou shalt have regard for the costs of thy measures and prescriptions

Summary of Workshop Discussion

One special problem in an interdisciplinary workshop is that two very different groups get together, one of which knows a great deal about medicine and the other knows a great deal about economics, but there are only few individuals who are knowledgeable in both areas. There is no hope that an economist will be able to convey the full economic perspective to a clinician in a matter of half an hour, nor can the clinician be expected to transmit clinical knowledge and expertise to an economist in the course of a workshop. These are essential and formidable tasks that can be achieved only through sustained interaction of the kind we had and everybody agreed that this is a worthwhile endavour – indispensable for understanding the way that health care systems work.

The medical practitioner and the economist might take different points of view on certain problems. This was illustrated by the subject of postponement (e.g. of surgical operations). To the physician (and his patient) it is a very important issue to know whether a particular therapy is in some sense permanent or only a temporary postponement of the need for better therapies. To an economist that distinction is far less important, and is mainly a question of "time preference" – appropriate discounting of expected future costs and benefits.

In the eyes of a physician postponement can be viewed as a success (e.g. postponement of hospitalization, postponement of death) or a failure (e.g. postponement of a definitive cure), because he argues at the individual level. To the doctor a medical treatment is not a success if the patient ultimately has to be operated anyway. One reason for using medicine instead of advocating surgery right from the beginning is his speculation that an operation could eventually be avoided.

To the economist this is different, to him postponement is a good thing. If, for instance, there were in the absence of cimetidine 100 surgical interventions required per period, and if the effect of cimetidine were to reduce the surgery rate to 90 interventions in any given year, even though it would never eliminate surgery for any one patient, that would lead to a permanent reduction of ten surgical interventions per year for each and every year. Through a discounting process one could translate that saving into a present value and that would be one part of the benefit in the form of reduced surgical costs and any complications resulting from surgery. Costs are better incurred in the future than now because the resources saved can be put to productive use in the interim.

Things look differently if the case becomes more complicated. If during postponement of treatment the resource costs go up by more than the savings resulting from postponement, then of course the benefit-cost analyst would decide against it. These are questions of optimal timing.

What came out clearly in the floor discussion was that there is no merit in a simple expenditure analysis that looks at the flow of money only. To the economist an expenditure analysis can be profoundly misleading. It is the cost-benefit analysis that is important. To do this with any new intervention, such as cimetidine, the comparison has to be carried out with a realistic alternative. People do not take massive doses of antacids, but studies in Scandinavia have shown that antacids at reasonable doses (50–70 ml/day) can be taken without many side effects. Combined with some anticholinergic drugs, such a treatment apparently gave comparable healing rates to cimetidine in one single study in Oslo. In other studies this combination was no better than placebo, i.e. it has almost never been proven that existing treatment was better than placebo. The assumption that placebo is the same as no treatment is not justified.

The design of a trial and the appropriate specification of the costs and benefits depend crucially on the nature of the question that one is seeking to answer. A placebo is entirely the appropriate comparison when the concern is to identify optimal dosages, duration of treatment, and so on. On the other hand, if the question is about the cost-benefit impact of a new procedure in an existing situation then one has to compare different treatments, different modes of patient management, and outcomes. Absolutely critical in comparing different procedures is the value one puts on human life, e.g. when comparing cimetidine with surgical interventions, there is some additional risk of loss of life associated with surgery (as there is with perforation too!) and the outcome really depends on how much value one puts on that loss. The current developments in the evaluation of life saved are twofold: one is to take the "health status index" or "quality-of-life-years" approach; the other is to leave some of these benefits unmeasured in monetary terms, trying to find better ways of presenting this information to those who have to make decisions.

The methodological point that became evident was to recognize that the appropriate design of a trial as well as the appropriate specification of the benefits and costs depend on the nature of the questions that one tries to answer. From time to time criticism by economists implied that a lot of clinical trials have been misdesigned in some sense or else designed for a purpose other than the purpose that would characteristically interest an economist. On the other hand participants made explicit that one of the purposes of coming together to discuss these topics from a medical point of view is not only to understand the differences in the vantage points but also to think about how in the design of studies there might be ways of introducing elements that would also serve the other purpose. In particular, in the case of cimetidine in addition to the array of controlled trials, which to a very large extent solely reinforce one another at the clinical level, one might begin in a systematic way to collect certain types of evidence that would be pertinent to the economic impact of the agent, for example information on employment and work, about other use of health services among patients etc. Thinking critically about the pertinent aspects of health economics, these should more often be merged with the clinical interest and intent.

19 A Review of the Epidemiological Development of Peptic Ulcers and an Evaluation of Duodenal Ulcers in the Federal Republic of Germany Before and After Cimetidine

B. Horisberger

Interdisciplinary Research Centre for Public Health, St. Gallen

Introduction

In industrialized countries peptic ulcers are one of the "common diseases". It is estimated that 10%–15% of men and 4%–10% of women develop active peptic ulcers at least once in their lifetimes. The majority of patients suffer from recurrent attacks of the disease during a period of 10–15 years. According to information contained in the clinical literature on the subject, in the past between 20% and 30% of sufferers from duodenal ulcer ultimately underwent surgery as a cure for the disease (Fry 1964; Krause 1963; Hafter 1978). Peptic ulcers can occur at any time of life, but 80% of cases occur during the period of active life (between the ages of 25 and 65 years), which brings out the social and economic significance of the disease.

The cost of the disease to the national economy of the United States has been calculated at 3224 million dollars (1977), of Sweden at 480 million krona (1975), and of the Netherlands at 337 million guilders (1975). The cost of duodenal ulcer to the West Germany economy has been estimated for 1980 at 944 million marks (see pp. 232–234 of this report).

Cimetidine

Cimetidine is a member of a new class of histamine antagonists, the so-called H_2-receptor antagonists that inhibit stimulation of acid secretions. Cimetidine, therefore, attenuates an important attacking element in the formation process of peptic ulcers and shifts the balance in favour of the defensive factors. After its introduction in 1976/1977, more and more doctors in every country began to prescribe cimetidine, and its share of all prescriptions for duodenal ulcer now stands at between 30% and 60%, according to country. Generally speaking it was established that patients on cimetidine obtained relief from pain more quickly than those under traditional treatment and that ulcers healed faster with the use of cimetidine.

It was observed in 1978 in the USA, 1 year after the introduction of the new drug, that there had been an unexpectedly sharp decline in the number of surgical operations carried out on ulcers; similar observations were also made elsewhere, e.g. in the United Kingdom, Switzerland, the Netherlands, and France. The wealth of clinical observations led to the assumption that this decline must be connected with the introduction of cimetidine and that the drug may well have altered the picture and course of ulcer disease. These alterations involve both the subjective course of the disease, or the attacks suffered by individual patients, as well as the objective medical findings. This suggests that at the sociomedical and economic levels the benefits produced by cimetidine far outweigh the cost. This assumption is based partly on controlled studies and random sample surveys at the microeconomic level (case studies) and partly on aggregated data at the macroeconomic level (national health statistics, representative hospital panels, surgical statistics, and hospital statistics). Since as a rule such comprehensive data become available after a time lag of 1–2 years, the statistics available on the subject do not go beyond 1980. The short period of observation for cimetidine (1977–1980) is partly made up for by the multiplicity of equivalent observations carried out in different countries. Moreover, to round off the picture, we have added to the present summary from the literature on the subject recent figures from the Federal Republic of Germany, which we have gathered in the course of our own investigations.

This paper is divided into two sections: (1) epidemiological pattern of peptic ulcer, with special reference to duodenal ulcer (1970–1979); (2) pattern of incidence of hospitalization and absenteeism from ulcer disease since the introduction of cimetidine (Tagamet) in the Federal Republic of Germany.

Epidemiology

Epidemiological data are absolutely essential as a basis for calculating the economic cost of ulcer disease and assessing the therapeutic value of particular methods of treatment. Up to and including the first half of this century, autopsies provided the chief source material. They offered some indication as to the spread of peptic ulcer disease among patients dying in hospital, but not among the population as a whole. Unfortunately, on such important issues as the incidence of ulcer disease, hospitali-

Table 19.1. Mortality due to ulcer disease, adjusted per 100000 population and age-groups in various countries

Country	Year	Age-group in years				
		All ages	Under 25	25–54	55–74	Above 75
Austria	1978	9.5	0.1	7.5	41.6	80.8
Belgium	1976	5.1	0.8	3.0	23.8	50.4
Bulgaria	1977	6.0	0.2	6.9	37.8	53.3
Czechoslovakia	1975	6.6	0.1	9.0	40.3	54.0
Denmark	1978	6.6	0.1	2.8	27.2	69.6
Finland	1975	3.5	–	3.4	22.4	39.5
Fed. Rep. Germany	1978	6.2	0.3	6.2	27.6	49.9
German Democ. Rep.	1973	10.0	0.1	11.4	51.2	64.0
Netherlands	1978	3.8	–	2.6	17.9	49.1
Sweden	1978	8.3	0.1	3.5	30.8	76.8
Switzerland	1978	6.1	–	3.6	24.8	66.7
United Kingdom	1978	9.4	–	6.3	44.1	92.1
USA	1977	2.7	0.6	2.8	15.4	29.4
	1977	1.8[a]	–	–	–	–

[a] US National Center for Health Statistics
[b] Source: Vital Statistical and Causes of Death, WHO Annual Statistics

zation, and surgery only isolated figures are available. Hospital statistics tended to indicate the incidence of the disease among the selected inpatients at the hospital concerned, but took no account of cases among outpatients.

Statistics on surgery kept by some leading surgical hospitals were more in the nature of accounts of the operations performed and their outcome at the hospital concerned, and made no reference to the catchment area from which the patients came or to the population factor (i.e. they were not standardized). The same applies to absenteeism as a consequence of ulcer disease. Blumenthal pointed out this deficiency as far back as 1959. The most complete figures were the mortality statistics, but all other statistical data were fragmentary (Bapst and Horisberger 1978). Only in the past few years has there been any improvement in this unsatisfactory situation, though even now the statistics on the subject are often several years old. The following summaries must be interpreted with this in mind.

It is only very recently that the epidemiology of ulcer disease has been analysed in greater depth whereby, in addition to records being kept of incidence and mortality rates, a whole range of other socially and economically significant data are being gathered concerning the incidence of hospitalization and surgery, as well as absence from work through sickness. This form of expanded survey is only the beginning. There is no doubt that the increased interest now being shown is connected with the introduction of new therapeutic drugs, in particular the introduction of cimetidine.

Mortality

Mortality due to peptic ulcers varies in European countries between 3.5 and 10.0 per 100000 population, with a marked increase after the age of 55 years (Table 19.1). In the USA, the mortality fell considerably between 1960 and 1978, a trend that is far less pronounced in Europe (Table 19.2). The number of deaths among the population under 55 years of age as a percentage of total ulcerrelated deaths was, in 1977/1978, 8.2% in the Netherlands, 12.55% in the USA, and 13.4% in the Federal Republic of Germany (Table 19.3).

Table 19.2. Mortality due to ulcer disease, adjusted per 100000 population

Year	USA[a]	Netherlands[b, c]	Federal Republic of Germany[c]
1960	5.2	–	–
1965	4.3	–	–
1970	3.2	4.0	6.7
1971	3.0	4.2	6.8
1972	2.9	4.7	6.6
1973	2.7	4.1	7.0
1974	2.4	4.3	6.9
1975	2.2	4.0	7.1
1976	2.1	3.8	7.2
1977	1.8	3.4	6.7
1978	–	3.8	6.2

[a] Source: National Center for Health Statistics, National Hospital Discharge Survey, Hyattsville, USA
[b] Source: Netherlands Economic Institute (1977)
[c] Source: Vital Statistics and Causes of Death, WHO Annual Statistics

Table 19.3. Absolute numbers of deaths due to peptic ulcer in USA, the Netherlands, and Federal Republic of Germany, 1977/1978

Country	Year	Age-group in Years				
		All ages	Under 25	25–54	55–74	Above 75
USA	1977	5900	50	691	2538	2621
		100%	0.85%	11.7%	43.0%	44.45%
Netherlands	1978	525	1	42	187	295
		100%	0.2%	8.0%	35.6%	56.2%
Federal Republic	1978	3827	15	494	1656	1662
of Germany		100%	0.40%	12.9%	43.3%	43.4%

[a] Source: Vital Statistics and Causes of Death, WHO Annual Statistics

Table 19.4. Mortality due to peptic ulcer in the Federal Republic of Germany, 1970–1978

	1970	1971	1972	1973	1974	1975	1976	1977	1978
Total	4115	4161	4046	4311	4310	4409	4429	4134	3827
Male	2911	2857	2762	2862	2886	2843	2796	2605	2314
Female	1204	1304	1284	1449	1424	1566	1633	1538	1514

[a] Source: Vital Statistics and Causes of Death, WHO Annual Statistics

Table 19.5. Mortality due to peptic ulcer in the Federal Republic of Germany, 1970–1978, per 100000 population

Mortality per 100000 population	1970	1971	1972	1973	1974	1975	1976	1977	1978
Total	6.7	6.8	6.6	7.0	6.9	7.1	7.2	6.7	6.2
Male	10.0	9.8	9.4	9.7	9.7	9.6	9.5	8.9	7.9
Female	3.8	4.1	4.0	4.5	4.4	4.8	5.1	4.8	4.7

[a] Source: Vital Statistics and Causes of Death, WHO Annual Statistics

Table 19.6. Mortality in the Federal Republic of Germany for deaths due to ulcer disease in the male population, age-adjusted per 100000 population

Year	Age-group in years					
	All ages	35–44	45–54	55–64	65–74	Above 75
1976	9.5	3.8	8.4	17.3	43.6	80.4
1978	7.9	2.8	6.4	12.8	33.7	75.1

[a] Source: Vital Statistics and Causes of Death, WHO Annual Statistics

The pattern of mortality due to ulcer disease in the Federal Republic of Germany for the period 1970–1978 (Tables 19.4, 19.5) shows that there was a notable decline between 1976 and 1978, especially among the male population. This applies, as indicated in Table 19.6, to all age-groups.

The decline in mortality may be due to several causes. The simplest explanation would be that there were fewer cases of peptic ulcer. Another might be that more ulcers were less harmful, that there was less recourse to surgery, etc. In the absence of more detailed surveys one can only surmise the answer.

Incidence

By this is meant the rate of occurrence of new cases of acute ulcers (with no previous ulcer history) among the population over a given period of time (1 year, for example). Incidence has changed over the years as has, most notably, the male-female ratio among the population affected. The frequently cited data in Table 19.7 are taken from the literature on the subject.

The incidence of duodenal ulcer (DU) appears to be declining somewhat in the European countries listed in Table 19.7. In the USA, an analysis of patients treated under the Kaiser-Permanente Medical Care Program, Portland, Oregon (220000 members) recorded a decline of over 60% (!) in new cases of ulcer disease and in recurrences between 1967 and 1973 (Vogt and Johnson 1980). The US National Centre for Health Statistics, on the other hand, gives the incidence of ulcer disease in 1968 as 3.0 per 1000 population and in 1975 as 2.9 per 1000 population. In the Federal Republic of Germany we found among a sample of 253 cases of ulcer attack (1979 and 1981) that 43% of the patients had no previous history of the disease and so were new cases (Bapst and Horisberger 1978). In a sample of 3312 cases of DU attacks the proportion of new cases was 44% (Neiss 1981). Of an estimated total of 398000 ulcer patients a year, this would give an estimated number of 172300 new cases. On the basis of a population of 63 million this represents an estimated incidence of 2.73 per 1000 population (1980/1981) (see also Table 19.20).

Table 19.7. Incidence of ulcus duodeni and ulcus ventriculi in selected European countries

Author	Time period	Place	No. of patients	Incidence per 1000	Male: female
I Ulcus duodeni					
Alstedt (1953)	1940	Denmark	141	0.38	4.1 : 1
Alstedt (1953)	1948	Denmark	407	1.00	2.6 : 1
Sponheim (1960)	1950–1952	Norway	458	1.50	4.2 : 1
Pulvertaft (1959)	1952–1957	England	862	1.33	3.5 : 1
Litton and Murdoch (1963)	1957–1959	Scotland	810	2.63	4.2 : 1
Dunlop (1968)	1962	Scotland	259	2.70	3.4 : 1
Bonnevie (1975)	1963–1968	Denmark	1475	1.32	2.2 : 1
II Ulcus ventriculi					
Schanke (1946)	1941–1944	Norway	119	1.14	3.2 : 1
Alstedt (1953)	1948	Denmark	136	0.34	2.1 : 1
Pulvertaft (1959)	1952–1957	England	257	0.40	1.7 : 1
Sponheim (1960)	1950–1952	Norway	139	0.45	1.9 : 1
Litton and Murdoch (1963)	1957–1959	Scotland	134	0.34	1.2 : 1
Dunlop (1968)	1962	Scotland	44	0.44	1.9 : 1
Bonnevie (1975)	1963–1968	Denmark	496	0.44	1.3 : 1

Prevalence

Data on "lifetime" prevalence vary between 5% and 10%, in other words between 5 and 10 of every 100 people develop an ulcer disease of some form at one time or another in their lifetime. Some autopsy statistics put the figure very much higher. But in view of the changes that have been observed in the incidence of the disease over the last 10–20 years, figures on lifetime prevalence are not very conclusive. Prevalence over a shorter period (1 year, for example) is more meaningful in terms of economic calculations and weighting in connection with ulcer disease. The National Center for Health Statistics in the USA has published the figures in Table 19.8. It is interesting to note that this table shows an upward trend in prevalence over the period from 1957 to 1978. A possible explanation is that episodes were more carefully recorded. These figures are in marked contrast to the findings of the survey on patients treated under the Kaiser-Permanenente Medical Care Program (Vogt and Johnson 1980). It was found that among the outpatients of this health maintenance organization (HMO) there was a spectacular decline in ulcer episodes per thousand patients between 1967 and 1973 (Table 19.9). It is conceivable that the discrepancy between the national statistics and those of the Medical Care Program is due to differing demographic structures in the populations surveyed.

For the Federal Republic of Germany, a probable prevalence rate for 1980 of between 14 and 18 per 1000 people can be deduced from the total number of prescrip-

Table 19.8. Morbidity trend for ulcer disease in the USA, 1957–1978

Time period, year	Prevalence (per 1000 per year)	Total persons affected annually
1957–1959	14.4	2440
1959–1961	14.0	2796
1961–1963	17.0	3079
1963–1965	19.0	3500
1968	17.2	3360
1975	18.9	3955
1978	17.7	3778

[a] Source: National Center for Health Statistics, Division of Health Interview Statistics, Hyattsville, MD/USA

Table 19.9. Morbidity trend for ulcer diseases in the patient load of the Kaiser-Permanente Medical Care Program

Year	Ulcer episodes per thousand patients		
	Duodenal ulcer	Gastric ulcer	Total
1967	13.7 ± 2.0	4.6 ± 1.2	18.3
1968	12.6 ± 1.8	2.6 ± 0.8	15.2
1969	10.8 ± 1.6	3.2 ± 0.9	14.0
1970	9.4 ± 1.4	2.5 ± 0.7	11.9
1971	6.3 ± 1.1	2.9 ± 6.7	9.2
1972	5.7 ± 1.0	2.8 ± 0.7	8.5
1973	4.1 ± 0.8	2.2 ± 0.6	6.3

tions for DU, though this figure, as all the other survey statistics on the subject, must of course be treated in itself as being rather uncertain. The most that can be said is that it tallies more or less with the data published by the US National Center for Health Statistics.

Peptic ulcer in the Netherlands occurs far less often. The total number of ulcer attacks in that country fluctuates around 50000 annually, corresponding to an annual morbidity of 3.5 per 1000 (1974). The authors concerned admit, however, that "relatively mild cases" were not covered by the estimates, "the number may be considerable. However, as most of these cases healed without seeing a doctor and without losing productive labour time, they have been ignored" (Netherlands Economic Institute 1977).

The *male-female patient ratio* for both DU and gastric ulcer (GU) has steadily shifted in recent years towards female patients. According to the most recent figures available to us, the ratios in Table 19.10 may be assumed for DU cases.

Hospitalization

Figures for *ulcer patients admitted to hospital* in those countries that keep such statistics indicate a downward trend in the hospitalization rate, especially as regards DU

Table 19.10. Duodenal ulcer according to sex in various countries

Country	Time period	Ratio male: female	
Scotland	1962		3.4 : 1[a]
Denmark	1963–1968		2.2 : 1[a]
Netherlands	1974		2.3 : 1[b]
USA:	1973	Ambulatory cases:	3.6 : 1[c]
Kaiser Permanente, Oregon	1975	Hospitalized cases:	1.8 : 1[c]
Fed. Rep. Germany	1979–1981	Ambulatory cases:	1.9 : 1[d]

[a] Bonnevie (1975)
[b] Netherlands Economic Institute (1977)
[c] Vogt and Johnson (1980)
[d] Bapst und Horisberger (1978)

Table 19.11. Number of US hospital discharges with ulcer disease diagnoses, 1966–1978

Year	No. patients with ulcer as first-listed diagnosis			Discharges per 10000 pop.
	Gastric	Duodenal	Total	
1966	166100	345200	511300	26.4
1970	89200	273500	362700	17.8
1971	94100	251400	345500	16.8
1972	99300	241400	340700	16.4
1973	102900	227100	330000	15.7
1974	101500	239800	341300	16.2
1975	101500	224100	325600	15.3
1976	103400	194000	297400	13.8
1978	105100	166300	271400	12.4

Source: US National Center for Health Statistics

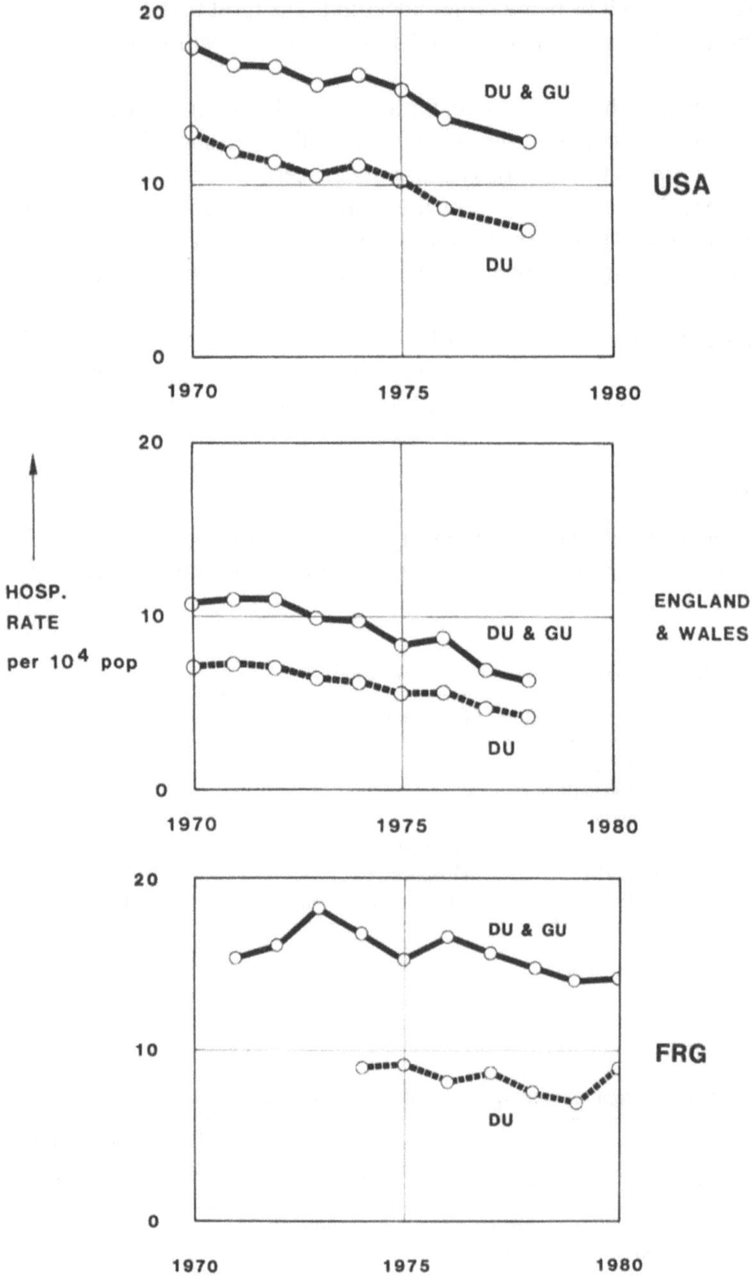

Fig. 19.1. Hospitalization rates for patients with the diagnosis "peptic ulcer" (DU and GU) in USA, England and Wales, and Federal Republic of Germany, 1970–1979. DU, duodenal ulcer, GU, gastric ulcer

patients (Fig. 19.1). The number of patients with "peptic ulcer" as first-listed diagnosis (DU and GU) and discharged from hospital in the USA is shown in Table 19.11.

Table 19.12 shows estimated hospitalization frequencies for the Federal Republik of Germany for 1971–1980 based on our own extrapolation of statistical data provided by the Allgemeine Ortskrankenkassen (AOK), which in 1980 had 16.495 million members (9.795 million of them compulsorily insured). The formula for extrapolation (where GKV = Gesetzliche Krankenversicherung) is:

$$\frac{\text{Compulsory health insurance}}{\text{Total population}} \times \frac{\text{AOK members}}{\text{GKV members}}$$

The DU : GU ratio in the Federal Republic was 1 : 0.7 in 1975 and 1 : 1 in 1980. The hospitalization rates are comparable with those for the USA.

In the Netherlands, surveys carried out by the Netherlands Economic Institute (NEI) in Rotterdam in 1980 produced the statistics in Table 19.13 on annual admis-

Table 19.12. Estimated hospitalization rates for patients with the diagnosis "peptic ulcer", Federal Republic of Germany, 1971–1980

Year	Number of hospitalized patients with peptic ulcer		Hospitalization rates per 10000 population	
	All ulcers	Duodenal ulcer only	All ulcers	Duodenal ulcer only
1971	94700	–	15.5	–
1972	99900	–	16.2	–
1973	113600	–	18.3	–
1974	105100	56000	16.9	9.0
1975	94700	56900	15.3	9.2
1976	102100	56600	16.6	8.2
1977	96800	53300	15.8	8.7
1978	90900	46900	14.8	7.7
1979	87400	44000	14.2	7.0
1980	88000	56900	14.3	9.2

Source: Statistics of the Allgemeine Ortskrankenkasse (AOK), aggregated for the FRG

Table 19.13. Hospitalization rates for patients with the diagnosis "peptic ulcer" in the Netherlands, 1972–1979

Year	Number of hospitalized patients with peptic ulcer disease	Hospitalization rates per 10000 population
1972	13900	10.4
1973	13300	9.9
1974	13650	10.1
1975	12450	9.1
1976	11700	8.5
1977	12300	8.9
1978	10350	7.4
1979	9450	6.8

Source: Bulthuis (1981)

sions of patients with "peptic ulcer" diagnosis (DU and GU). The DU:GU ratio in Holland among hospitalized patients was 2.9 : 1 in 1972, 2.5 : 1 in 1975, and 2.4 : 1 in 1979. Dutch hospitalization rates are far lower than those for the USA and the Federal Republic of Germany. The statistics in Table 19.14 are deducible from the available literature on the position in England and Wales. Figure 19.1 shows the pattern of hospitalization rates for peptic ulcer in the USA, England and Wales, and the FRG. The rough figures are at different levels, but all show a similar downward trend. They are valid for peptic ulcer in general as well as for DU.

Table 19.14. Hospitalization for patients with the diagnosis "peptic ulcer" in England and Wales, 1970–1978

Year	Number of hospital discharges with peptic ulcer diagnosis	
	Absolute	Per 10000 population
1970	51000	10.5
1971	52500	10.8
1972	52000	10.8
1973	49000	10.0
1974	48500	9.9
1975	42500	8.7
1976	44500	9.1
1977	37000	7.6
1978	35000	7.1

Ratio DU:GU, 1970 2.75:1; 1978 2.3:1
Source: Hospital In-patient Enquiry (HIPE), London, HMSO

Table 19.15. Number of operations due to peptic ulcer disease per 100 hospitalized ulcer patients in various countries

Year	No. operations per 100 hospitalized ulcer patients				
	USA[a]	Netherlands[b]	FRG[c]	Switzerland[d]	England[e] and Wales
1970	45	–	–	–	–
1971	–	–	–	–	38
1972	48	45			38
1973	–	45	–	34	37
1974	–	45	–	33	36
1975	44	47	–	32	32
1976	45	47	–	31	32
1977	–	45	–	26	25
1978	33	42	26	23	27
1979	–	42	17	19	–
1980	–	–	20	19	–

[a] US National Center for Health Statistics
[b] Netherlands Economic Institute (1977)
[c] DTI (Diagnose und Therapie Index) statistics, aggregated and adjusted
[d] VESKA (Association of Swiss Hospitals) statistics of hospital diagnoses
[e] Hospital In-patient Enquiry, (HIPE) London, HMSO

Operations

In 1977 there was an unexpectedly sharp decline in the number of operations for peptic ulcer in the USA, the Netherlands, Switzerland, and England and Wales; Table 19.15 shows the ratio of surgical cases to the total number of hospitalized patients. Data concerning the Federal Republic of Germany were obtainable only for the 1978–1981 period but point in the same general direction. In France, studies conducted at 13 hospitals in the Paris region and 12 hospitals in other regions disclosed that between 1977 and 1979 the number of ulcer operations (DU and GU) also declined, viz., by 30%.

As the costs of hospitalization and surgery form one of the prinicpal components of the overall cost of ulcer therapy, the question of whether the recorded decline is significant and may possibly be attributable to the use of cimetidine is of major importance with regard to the benefits to be derived from cimetidine. The figures illustrating the situation in the USA were analysed. It was found that the 1978 ulcer surgery rates did indeed decline significantly more sharply than the drop indicated by the development trend of 1977 (Office of Technology Assessment 1981 b). The figures provided by the US National Center for Health Statistics indicate a decline in the number of gastrectomies and vagotomies (Table 19.16). In the Netherlands especially the number of partial gastrectomies has dropped more rapidly since 1977. There were a total of 1750 surgical interventions of this type in 1977 but only about 900 in 1979, without a corresponding increase in the number of vagotomies. The proportions of patients operated upon for peptic ulcers has declined significantly since 1976, in contrast to the total number of patients hospitalized because of ulcers (cf. Fig. 19.2).

Absenteeism

Sick leave (loss of working hours) because of ulcer diseases varies fairly substantially between one country and another. Apart from the question of the seriousness of complaints, differences in the social security systems of different countries will account for the number of medical certificates issued and the length of sick leave they prescribe. For the Federal Republic of Germany the AOK provides statistics on the overall number of working days lost (Table 19.17). Table 19.17 shows that in 1979, for example, 14.75 of every 1000 compulsory members of the AOK (employees) had lost working time because of ulcer attacks. The average loss of working time per case was 30.7 days making a total of 454 work days per 1000 members. Supposing that the working population of the FRG numbers about 20 million, this is equiva-

Table 19.16. Number of selected surgical procedures due to peptic ulcer disease in the USA

Year	Partial gastrectomy	Vagotomy
1976	54200	48300
1977	51100	45500
1978	39700	29200

Source: US National Center for Health Statistics

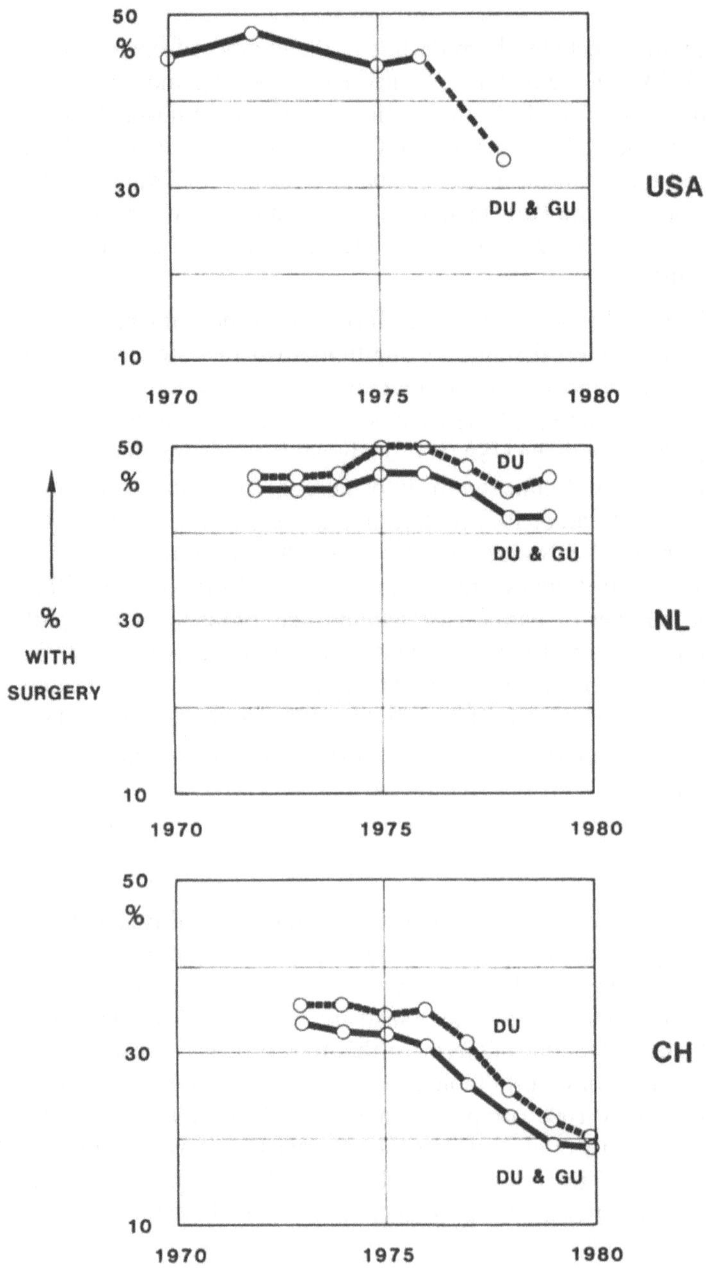

Fig. 19.2. Number of operations due to peptic ulcer disease as a percentage of all hospitalized ulcer patients. DU, duodenal ulcer; GU, gastric ulcer

Table 19.17. Time lost from work by compulsory members of the AOK due to peptic ulcer disease per 1 000 ambulatory and hospitalized cases per year in the Federal Republic of Germany

Year	No. cases per 1 000 members		Time lost from work per 1 000 compulsory members of AOK[a]			
	All ulcers	DU only	Days per 1 000 insured		Days per case	
			All ulcers	DU only	All ulcers	DU only
1971	15.74		529.4		33.6	
1972	16.24		558.6		34.4	
1973	17.10		588.2		34.4	
1974	14.84		538.0		36.2	
1975	13.09	7.7	488.9	269.9	37.4	35.3
1976	14.46	8.8	510.2	294.0	35.3	33.5
1977	14.87	9.3	491.9	294.8	33.1	31.7
1978	14.78	9.3	463.9	283.4	31.4	30.4
1979	14.75	9.3	453.6	278.4	30.7	29.9
1980	14.60	9.4	437.9	270.9	30.0	28.8

[a] AOK, Allgemeine Ortskrankenkassen, 9.8 million compulsory members

Table 19.18. Hospital days for patients with diagnosis "peptic ulcer", 1971 to 1980, per 10 000 population

Year	No. hospital days for peptic ulcer disease per 10 000 population	
	Netherlands[a]	Federal Republic of Germany[b]
1971	–	434
1972	279	449
1973	262	505
1974	259	473
1975	229	414
1976	208	444
1977	210	378
1978	175	344
1979	155	321
1980	–	326

[a] Netherlands Economic Institute (1977)

[b] Estimated value from aggregated statistics of AOK (Allgemeine Ortskrankenkassen) and DTI (Diagnose- und Therapie-Index) data. The DTI is a patterned master sample including data from 300 hospitals on patients suffering from acute diseases, covering 165 000 beds for acute cases (34% of all such beds in the FRG). Out of the total sample, the course of some 6 000 cases a year is completely recorded throughout the hospitalization period (longitudinal studies). The data are compiled by "Infratest Gesundheitsforschung", Munich (Bapst and Horisberger 1981 a)

lent to a total loss of working time caused by ulcers of about 9 million work days in the FRG alone (ambulatory and hospitalized patients). Table 19.18 shows the number of days lost from work through hospitalization.

Summary of Epidemiological Data

A review of major clinical and epidemiological data concerning peptic ulcers shows the following. Peptic ulcers have different causes, but the presence of stomach acid (HCl) and pepsin are prerequisites for their development. Epigastric pains, depending upon food intake, are the key clinical symptom but to confirm the existence of ulcers X-ray pictures or – even better – an endoscopic examination will be necessary. Ulcer diseases are widespread among the population. Millions of inhabitants of industrialized countries fall victim to peptic ulcers in their lifetimes. In the USA and Federal Republic of Germany more than 400000 persons develop new ulcers every year. Males develop duodenal ulcers nearly twice as frequently as females. The death rate due to peptic ulcers ranges from 2 to 10 per 100000 inhabitants and is declining. Nearly half the number of deaths involve patients more than 75 years of age.

In different countries regularly reporting on the subject (e.g. the USA, the Netherlands, FRG) the hospitalization rate of ulcer patients has been retrogressive, particularly since 1977 (e.g. in the USA, the Netherlands, England and Wales, the FRG). The number of hospital days has also dropped to a surprising extent since 1977 (particularly in the Netherlands and the FRG). The number of ulcer operations, especially on DU, has markedly decreased since 1977 in many industrialized countries (e.g. USA, England, the Netherlands, France, Switzerland).

Working hours lost through sick leave due to ulcers showed a decreasing trend in the 1970s and a perceptibly accelerated decline since 1977. The overall decrease in the loss of working time amounted to 10% in the period from 1977 to 1979. The drop in the number of hospital days during the same period was 25% in the Netherlands and 15% in the Federal Republic of Germany.

Epidemiological information comprising aggregate data at the macrolevel has the advantage of being suitable for use as standardized data for comparisons between countries. They are "inert", however, and can demonstrate developments subject only to substantial time lags. The information supplied by national statistics is mostly 1–3 years out of date. In addition, interpreting the causes of a development is often very difficult. To overcome this deficiency and to make possible a causal clarification of changes at the macrolevel, microstudies offer themselves as an effective tool. In the Federal Republic of Germany this tool has been widely used. The results and the corresponding extrapolations are summarized in the following paragraphs.

Studies on Duodenal Ulcers in Federal Republic of Germany Before and After Cimetidine

Cimetidine came onto the West German market in the summer of 1977. The drug was prescribed during 1981 in about 35% of all peptic ulcer cases. The number of quarterly prescriptions issued to ambulatory patients suffering from ulcus duodeni

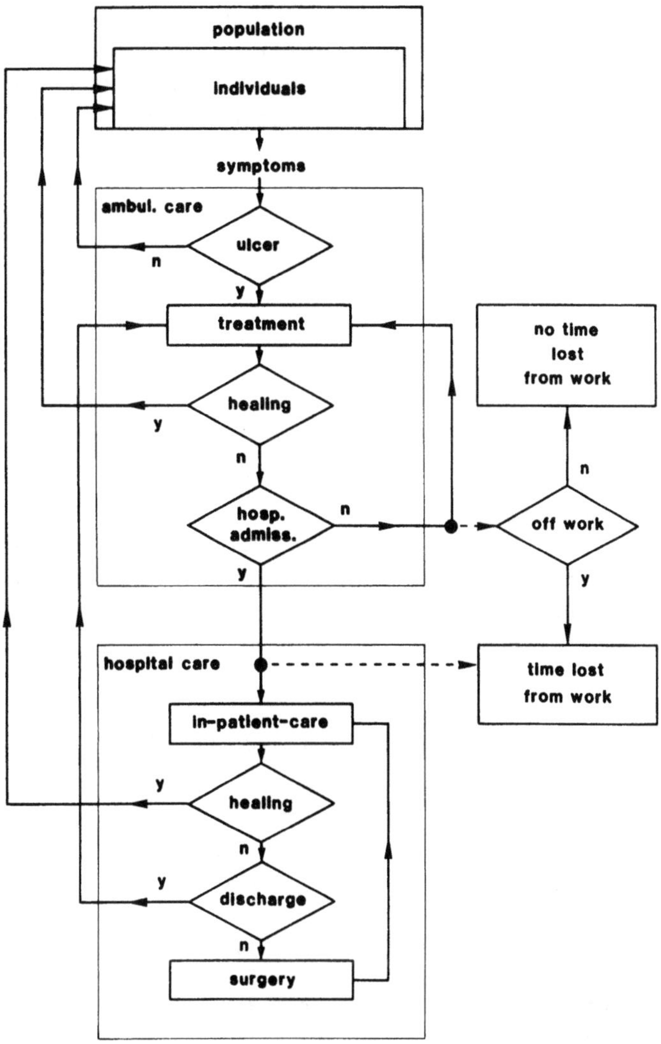

Fig. 19.3. Simplified model for patient management of peptic ulcer disease

attained just under 40% and in ulcus ventriculi cases exceeded 30%. During 1980 a total of 457 000 cimetidine prescriptions were recorded. If cimetidine prescriptions in hospitals are added to this figure, cimetidine is the leading antiulcer drug prescribed today.

Figure 19.3 shows the quantitative and qualitative changes of the factors used in an analysis of the therapeutical effectiveness of cimetidine in the treatment of DU. It is a schematic simplified diagram of the components and decision-making point in the course of an ulcer treatment.

The data presented on pp. 229–236 were obtained from the following *studies*. At the *microlevel* (primary study): (a) one field study each determined the subjective and objective evolution of acute DU attacks in private practice. The first period of field study was autumn 1979 with 103 DU patients; the second period of field study was autumn 1981 with 150 DU patients. The participants in the study were 52 established physicians (33 general practitioners and 19 specialists in internal medicine) (Bapst and Horisberger 1978). (b) Studies were undertaken on the frequency of diagnosis, duration of hospitalization, and modes of therapy of ulcus duodeni (and ulcus ventriculi) in the hospital. Time span of the studies was 1974–1981 (Bapst and Horisberger 1981 a). (c) Interviews were carried out with 101 physicians concerning their assessment of ulcer therapy with cimetidine in private medical practice (Bapst and Horisberger 1981 b). At the *macrolevel* (secondary investigation): processed insurance data supplied by local AOK health insurance branches concerning cases of incapacitation for work, duration of incapacity, and number of hospital cases due to ulcus duodeni and ulcus ventriculi were analysed. Time span of the study was 1971–1979.

Population

The demographic structure is shown in Table 19.19. Of the total population, 43.5% are over 18 years of age.

Concerning the incidence[1] of ulcers (initial occurences per year) in the Federal Republic of Germany we are forced to rely on estimates. A good indication consists of the number of prescriptions for ulcus duodeni recorded in the International Medical Statistics (IMS) data. On the basis of 1327000 prescriptions one is justified

Table 19.19. Demographic structure of the Federal Republic of Germany

	Estimated population according to age and sex			
	1975		1980	
	in 1000	in Percent	in 1000	in Percent
Male				
0–18 years	9130	30.7	9415	30.8
19–40 years	9748	32.8	9745	31.8
41–65 years	7557	25.4	8109	26.5
> 65 years	3309	11.1	3321	10.9
Total	29744	100.0	30590	100.0
Female				
0–18 years	8675	26.9	8945	27.4
19–40 years	8917	27.7	8885	27.2
41–65 years	9366	29.0	9266	28.3
> 65 years	5302	16.4	5607	17.1
Total	32260	100.0	32703	100.0

1 In the Federal Republic of Germany the incidence rate was estimated at three instances. In 1979 and 1981 our institute studied samples of 103 (1979) and 150 (1981) patients with a verified DU in a representative selection of practising physicians in the FRG. The selection of medical practices was done by Infratest Munich. The two groups of patients (age-groups, sex distribution, profession) were almost identical and the proportion of patients without previous ulcer history was 43/100 patients. In 1981 an independent study was performed by Neiss of Munich University; 44% new cases were registered in a sample of 3500 persons.

in estimating the number of ulcer attacks at 625000 (2.12 prescriptions per attack). A survey of 1979 by "Professional Studies (Pharmaceuticals) Ltd.", London, indicates 1.57 attacks per ulcer patient per year in the German Federal Republic. This means 398000 patients undergo treatment per year. According to our own earlier random checks, 43.3% of these have no previous ulcer history, in other words 172000 cases are new occurrences of the disease. On the basis of this figure we arrive at an incidence of 2.73 new cases per 1000 inhabitants (see Table 19.20).

An estimate of the prevalence (total ulcer patients or attacks in relation to total population) is more difficult to establish. On the strength of a representative random sample consisting of 136 patients with ulcer case histories we computed an average number of 5 ± 1 attacks and a mean duration of the disease of 3.2 ± 1.0 years. On the basis of 172300 fresh ulcer cases per year, some 625000–800000 attacks can be estimated for the total population, since it may be assumed that in addition to the treated episodes there occur about 30% cases that are never submitted to treatment at all. This indicates in an estimated subprevalence of 14–18 attacks per 1000 inhabitants older than 18 years, a value of the same order as that in the USA.

Results at Microlevel

A breakdown of ulcer cases into *categories of occupation* of the patients shows the picture in Table 19.21. The *average age* of 253 patients was 44 years (± 12.8 years) whereas the male-female ratio was 1.9 men to 1 woman. *Of the patients 43.3% had no previous ulcer histories* and thus were fresh cases. For the cases having ulcer histo-

Table 19.20. Epidemiological data pertaining to ulcer disease in the Federal Republic of Germany, 1980

Total medication prescriptions for duodenal ulcer	1327000[a]
Total Tagamet prescriptions	457000 (34.4%)[a]
Estimated number ulcer episodes on basis of 1327000 prescriptions	625000
Estimated number ulcer episodes treated with Tagamet	215000
Estimated total of treated patients (1.57 episodes/year)	398000[b]
New cases, no previous ulcer history	172000[c]
Estimated prevalence per 1000 population over 18 years age	14–18
Estimated incidence per 1000 population	2.73

[a] IMS Statistics
[b] Professional Studies (Pharmaceuticals) Ltd. (PSL), London
[c] New cases (no previous ulcer history) in three representative samples (own field studies)

Table 19.21. Ulcer prevalence by occupational category

	1979	1981
Blue-collar workers	30%	33%
White-collar workers	41%	38%
Self-employed	10%	10%
Officials and civil servants	5%	5%
Others	15%	15%
Total	100%	100%

ries an average of 5±1 attacks and a mean duration of the disease of 3.2±1 years were determined. For diagnostic purposes, X-ray examinations were carried out in 73% of cases and 16% were diagnosed endoscopically. In some of the patients ulcers had previously been confirmed, and the examinations were not repeated. In addition, there were 2.9 laboratory studies per attack episode.

Since the symptoms and hence the severity of an ulcer attack may differ from case to case it was necessary, for the purpose of ensuring the comparability of the case evolution (and the degree of therapeutical success), to break down the cases into *categories of severity.* A division of the degrees of severity on the basis of indications supplied by physicians into categories of symptoms according to the four criteria "slight", "moderate", "pronounced", and "severe", shows the distribution in Table 19.22. The proportion of those cases that were submitted to therapy with cimetidine varies according to the degree of severity. In slight or moderate cases, "cimetidine patients" accounted for 33%; in the presence of pronounced or severe discomfort cimetidine was prescribed in 48% of the cases. Of working patients suffering from pronounced symptoms almost half were being treated with cimetidine.

Table 19.22. Distribution of ulcer symptoms

Severity of symptoms	Ambulatory cases	
	Number	Percent
Slight	17	6.7
Moderate	69	27.3
Pronounced	149	58.9
Severe	18	7.1
Total	253	100

Source: own field studies, 1979 and 1981

Table 19.23. Frequency of reported typical ulcer symptoms at different degrees of severity

Type of symptom ($n=253$)	Degree of discomfort	
	Slight to moderate ($n=86$)	Pronounced to severe ($n=167$)
Postprandial pain	76%	67%
Fasting pain (with food relief)	61%	65%
Sleep-disturbing nighttime pains	60%	68%

Table 19.24. Dosages of cimetidine for a 5-week period

	1st week	2nd week	3rd week	4th week	5th week
Dosage no. 200-mg tablets/day	4.31	4.23	4.05	3.88	3.30
Patients	108	107	104	89	70

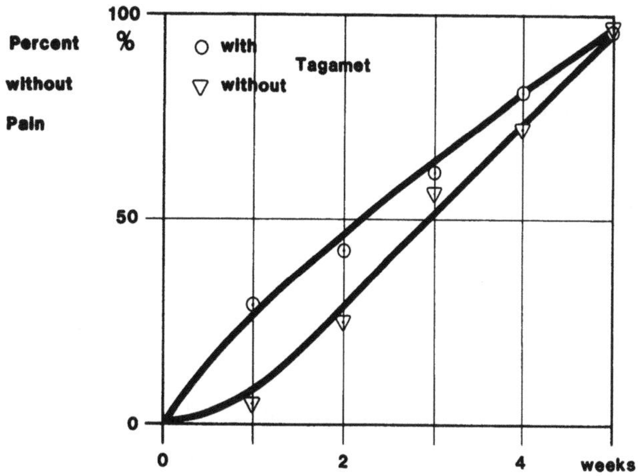

Fig. 19.4. Cumulative distribution of the symptom "postprandial pain" for patients with and without cimetidine. $n = 167$ with severe discomfort. Significant difference after 1 week

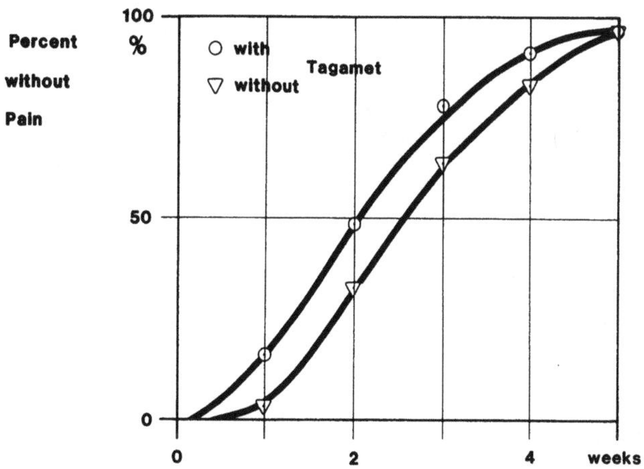

Fig. 19.5. Cumulative distribution of the symptom "night pain" for patients with and without cimetidine. $n = 167$

Typical ulcer symptoms were reported, according to degree of severity, as occurring with the frequencies shown in Table 19.23. The frequency of painful discomfort caused by ulcer attacks is of particular importance in assessing the benefits of any therapy, because freedom from symptoms and pain is considered by physicians to be the primary aim of any therapy (interviews with 101 physicians, 1979). With regard to therapy with cimetidine, the dosages in Table 19.24 were prescribed. In somewhat less than one-third of the cases cimetidine alone was administered: in the remaining cases it was in combination with other drugs. The total number of cases was 253 (108 with and 145 without Tagamet).

On average, treatment comprised an initial examination plus 4.26 subsequent consultations and a final examination. In 40% of the cases complete healing was verified radiologically or endoscopically, in the remaining cases the results were checked out on the basis of clinical findings. Patients suffering from pronounced to severe discomfort treated with cimetidine were rid of their symptoms – depending upon their severity – from 2.8 to 3.5 days earlier than patients not treated with the

Table 19.25. Cost of ambulatory treatment per case

Cost of components	DM million	Percent
Cost of Diagnosis	95.8	43
Cost of therapy	92.4	42
Evaluation of healing process (X-ray or endoscopy)	34.4	15
Total ambulatory costs	222.6	100

Table 19.26. Hospital days of duodenal ulcer patients for 1974–1980 in Federal Republic of Germany

	Hospital days of duodenal ulcer patients		
	Ulcus as primary diagnosis	Ulcus as secondary diagnosis	Total ulcer-related hospital days
1974	1519000	278000	1797000
1975	1346300	325800	1672100
1976	1324200	388800	1713000
1977	1266400	495900	1762300
1978	1123900	NA	NA
1979	1022600	303700	1326300
1980	1134350	323700	1458050

Source: computations based on statistics on types of diseases compiled by AOK and DTI.

Table 19.27. Direct costs of ambulatory and hospital treatment

Cost components	DM million	Percent
Ambulatory costs	222.5	52
Hospital costs	207.0	48
Total direct costs	429.5	100

drug. Per 100 patients this means a gain of 40–50 pain-free weeks for cimetidine patients. The progressive improvement is shown in Fig. 19.4 and 19.5.

The costs of ambulatory treatment amounted to approximately DM 356 per attack or to DM 222.6 million for 625000 episodes. The different cost components were as in Table 19.25.

Results at Macrolevel

Hospitalization

The number of hospital days of patients with ulcus duodeni as the primary diagnosis attained 1134350 in 1980 (Table 19.26). In comparison with 1976 the decrease amounted to about 15%. Average hospital stays for compulsory AOK members were 20.1 days in 1980, as against 26.0 days in 1976. The hospital costs in 1980 amounted, according to AOK, to DM 182.37 a day or to DM 207 million for the 1134350 hospital days. Using these data, the direct costs of ambulatory and hospital treatment for duodenal ulcer were those shown in Table 19.27. Not considered in these computations are surgical interventions. This is because for 1980 no sufficiently reliable surgery statistics are obtainable nor could they be calculated from available data. We would surmise that in 1980 between 18000 and 20000 duodenal ulcer operations were performed. If one assumes a cost of DM 2000 per operation, this would mean an increment in the cost of treatment by a further DM 36–40 million.

Work Days Lost from Duodenal Ulcers

We have used two approaches to obtain figures concerning incapacity to work attributable to duodenal ulcers.

"Bottom-up approach". It has been established, on the basis of microsurveys carried out in 1979 and 1981 that in respect to each 100 attacks 58.5% of the patients were dispensed from working (1979 – 58%; 1981 – 59%). In another sample probe of 3312 attacks (Neiss 1980), 1758 patients were placed on sick leave – i.e. 53%. We have sound reasons to assume that about 55% of all patients suffering severe ulcer attacks are exempted from work. By extrapolation (625000 attack episodes in 1980) we obtain a total of 344000 work exemptions for 1980. It seems reasonable to reduce this figure by 10% because the people involved had no fixed employment, so that a total of about 310000 "genuine" exemptions may be deduced. According to the sample tests we carried out in 1979 and 1981 (149 cases), the mean duration of a sick leave prescribed under ambulatory treatment was 3.43 weeks or 24 days. Related to the total attacks, this means an average incapacity to work of 14.43 days per attack. This is equivalent to an aggregate loss of 7.4 million work days for patients under ambulatory treatment for DU.

Table 19.28. Time lost from work by compulsory members of the AOK due to peptic ulcer disease per 1000 hospitalized cases per year in the Federal Republic of Germany

Year	No. cases per 1000 members		Time lost from work per 1000 compulsory members of the AOK			
			Days per 1000 insured		Days per case	
	Peptic ulcer	DU only	Peptic ulcer	DU only	Peptic ulcer	DU only
1971	3.11		83.8		26.9	
1972	3.32		88.7		26.7	
1973	3.60		95.3		26.5	
1974	3.26		87.6		26.8	
1975	2.94	1.48	77.0	38.6	26.1	26.0
1976	3.18	1.66	82.5	42.4	26.0	25.6
1977	2.92	1.62	65.1	35.8	22.3	22.1
1978	2.64	1.49	56.5	31.9	21.4	21.4
1979	2.46	1.37	50.8	28.0	20.7	20.4
1980	2.34	1.34	47.1	26.7	20.1	19.8

"Top-down Approach". Information supplied by AOK shows that in 1980 those compulsorily insured (9.8 million), i.e. persons able to work, lost 244 work days for each 1000 insured as a result of ulcus duodeni under ambulatory treatment. This implies a total of 2.4 million work days. As the Federal Republic had a total of 26.9 million persons gainfully employed in 1980, the aggregate loss of working time attributable to duodenal ulcers, by extension of this calculation, probably amounts to about 6.6 million work days. Taking the mean figure between the "bottom-up" (7.4 million) and the "top-down" (6.6 million) approaches, we arrive at an estimated working time loss of 7.0 million work days (1980) for DU outpatients.

The AOK figures provide a sound basis for estimates of additional work days lost through hospitalization (Table 19.28). Of the 9.8 million members of the compulsory health insurance scheme, 13200 were hospitalized as a result of diagnosed DU – equivalent to 261000 hospital days. From the cited AOK data a total of 36100 hospitalized patients with the primary diagnosis of DU was calculated for the entire population of the Federal Republic of Germany in 1980. This implies 716100 days of work were lost by hospitalized patients. Accordingly, calculations of indirect costs must take into account 7.7 million ambulatory and hospital patients, which is equivalent to a loss to the national economy of the order of DM 514.0 million (Table 19.29).

On the assumption that cimetidine has exerted a beneficial influence on the capacity to work and that therefore a gain can also be demonstrated in the area of direct costs, we attempted, first, to confirm this qualitatively and, second, to quantify it.

"Bottom-up Approach". In microstudies it was revealed clearly that a reduction in the duration of sick leave of patients suffering from "pronounced to severe" symptoms by an average of 3.7 days was attributable to cimetidine, but it was not possible to show a similar result in patients with "slight to moderate" symptoms. If the gain in work days by patients treated with cimetidine is to be extrapolated on this basis, the following considerations apply. Because of ulcus duodeni, an estimated 310000 persons were ordered on sick leave in 1980. Of these, 66% showed "pronounced to severe" symptoms (cf. Table 19.22), i.e. roughly 204600. Of these, 48% were treated with cimetidine, i.e. 98200 episodes. Now, 98200 times 3.7 is equivalent to a benefit of 363340 days (or DM 24.08 million). This reduction in the number of days lost by ambulatory patients is also confirmed by the development among compulsorily AOK-insured persons.

Table 19.29. Indirect costs of ambulatory and hospital treatment

Components of indirect costs	Days lost from work (in million days)	Equivalent in DM million
Ambulatory care	7.0	466
Hospital care	0.7	48
Total	7.7	514

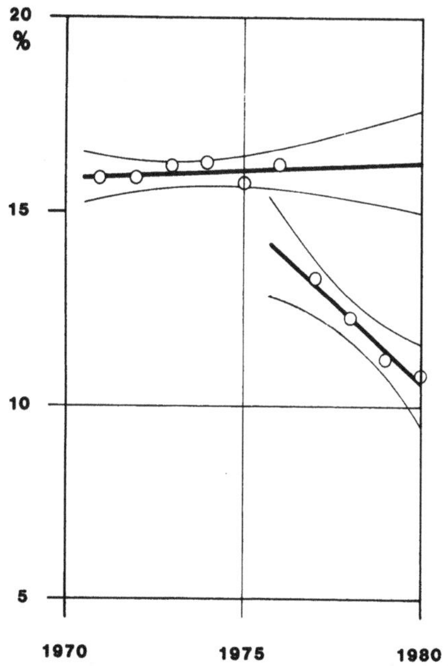

Fig. 19.6

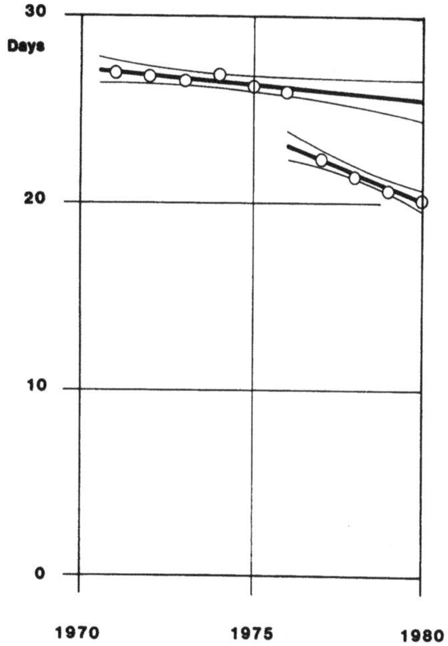

Fig. 19.7

Fig. 19.6. Lost days of work for hospitalized ulcer patients as percentage of total work day loss (100%) due to peptic ulcer disease, computed on the basis of reported data for compulsory members of the AOK. The regression lines with 95% confidence limits are used for comparison with the trend prior to 1977

Fig. 19.7. Lost days of work for hospitalized ulcer patients (number of days per case), computed on the basis of reported data from compulsory members of the AOK. The regression lines with 95% confidence limits are used for comparison with the trend prior to 1977

"Top-down Approach". Figures reported by the AOK make it possible to calculate a significant reduction both in the hospitalization rate (Fig. 19.6) (combined with an increase in the rate of ambulatory care) and in the average duration of hospital stays (Fig. 19.7) (trend differential $p \leq 0.05$). If the resulting smaller number of hospital days and the greater number of ambulatory days of incapacity to work are additionally taken into account, the overall benefit in the area of DU (compared with the development prior to the introduction of cimetidine) can be computed at DM 107.7 million for 1980. The figures in Table 19.17 confirmed at the same time that since 1977, i.e. since cimetidine has become available, a decline from 33.1 days to 30.0 days lost from work per case for compulsory members of the AOK has occurred, so that there is at least some justification in our conservative assumption that the effectiveness of cimetidine is probable. This development is demonstrated even more clearly by the group of hospitalized cases (see Table 19.28). As an analysis of these data shows (Fig. 19.6), there was a significant decline in working days lost after 1977 (trend differential $p < 0.05$).

Finally, the percentage of lost working time due to hospitalization, in terms of overall losses of working time, dropped very significantly after 1977, namely from 16% in 1976 to 10% in 1980. This also proves that the decrease in the hospitalization

Table 19.30. Percentage shares of direct and indirect costs attributable to the duodenal ulcer disease

Cost components	USA[a, b]	Netherlands[a, b]	Italy[a]	Switzerland[a, b]	FRG[c]
Direct cost	53	21	42	24	46
Outpatients	15	3	18	7	24
Inpatients	38	18	24	17	22
Indirect cost	47				
Incapacity to work	47	79	58	76	55
Total	100	100	100	100	100

[a] Bodemar et al. (1979)
[b] Computed as 100, without indirect costs
[c] Own study

rate has not only resulted in a reduction of hospital (and surgery) costs but also has produced an indirect benefit in the form of smaller losses of working time.

From the overall economic point of view the effect of the DU disease in the Federal Republic of Germany, as established on the basis of our analyses in 1980, can be summarized as in Table 19.30. In terms of the national economy we would estimate the direct benefits of cimetidine resulting from the reduction in hospital treatment in 1980 at DM 107.7 million and indirect benefits attributable to the lower incidence of working time losses at DM 24.08 million, which amounts to a sum of DM 131.78 million. If we deduct the amount of DM 43.1 million (retail price in pharmacy, without taxes), which has been spent on treatment of duodenal ulcer with cimetidine, the *resulting net benefit for treatment of duodenal ulcer in the Federal Republic of Germany in 1980 amounts to DM 88.68 million.*

20 Discussion of Paper by Horisberger

B. S. Bloom

University of Pennsylvania

Horisberger's paper highlights many of the health services research problems inherent in attempting to understand the effects of medical care using available epidemiological, economic, and effectiveness data. The difficulties of using data that are collected for nonresearch reasons, such as administration, and are then used to answer specific research questions or hypotheses have been commented upon extensively and are the bane of all health services researchers. It too often leads to making heroic assumptions about the data, to complex, convoluted, and incomplete analyses, and to results couched in the most constrained terms and limited by a variety of *caveats*.

The study undertaken by Horisberger on the effects of cimetidine on peptic ulcer in the Federal Republic of Germany evidently was cognizant of these data shortcomings. It adds to the growing body of evidence dealing with cimetidine efficacy, effectiveness, and cost. It is another piece in the puzzle of the scores of studies improving our understanding of the full range of effects of but one therapy in the armory of medical care.

The researcher's question that must be raised regarding these data problems is: "Why does it require so many various studies, costing so much money, to reach an answer as to the medical and economic consequences of any medical technology?" The answer, quite simply, is that the data bases available have not been developed to provide ready answers to research questions. This is as much the fault of health services researchers as anyone else. It is not that there is a lack of congruence between the needs of decision-makers for good data for programmatic control and the needs of health services researchers for research-oriented data but rather that health services researchers have not been astute in predicting the directions of their research efforts or their data needs; they have instead been responders to the perceived needs of others for answers to research questions. Thus, secondary and tertiary data sources must be relied upon, a multiplicity of studies must be performed, and the partial answers from each one must somehow be integrated to gain some fuller understanding of the effects and costs of medical care technology.

What is the cost-benefit and cost-effectiveness of such a disjointed approach? We are indeed fortunate that cimetidine, a new class of drug for the treatment of a major chronic disease, has been so well accepted by providers, consumers, and policy decision-makers as well as having been so effective and profitable as to allow the corporate manufacturer to fund generously the wide variety of studies that we are utilizing and evaluating at this conference. This is a real phenomenon indeed, for most medical diagnostic aides, therapies, and rehabilitation regimens rarely allow the investment of such large sums of money to the study of disease epidemiology, therapeutic efficacy, cost-effectiveness, and cost-benefit – in essence, providing the full range of information required for rational decision-making.

This rather long and apparently tangential introduction to Horisberger's paper is chosen to remind those of us in health services research that we must be more cognizant of the need for developing well-designed and well-controlled studies of efficacy, effectiveness, cost, risk, and benefit early in the life-cycle of any medical care intervention in order to have an effect on ultimate policy decisions on use, cost, and payment. This requires that we work more closely with decision-makers and policy-makers at all levels of government, with corporate executives, with providers of care, and with our research colleagues to develop jointly the questions to be answered and the data required. There is no necessary incompatibility between the data requirements of government agencies, corporations, providers, consumers, and payers of care and researchers' requirements for specific data. The marginal cost of planning for research data needs and of collecting either specific research data or data in a specific manner need not be great.

We are all aware of the increasingly constrained research budgets in all countries. We must also become aware of the need to work cooperatively with our counterparts in government, industry, and medical care to obtain answers to many of the medical care dilemmas and research questions that have not been addressed or have been dealt with inadequately. As a first problem, most medical care has never been subjected to well-controlled investigation determining efficacy, effectiveness, or cost, let alone cost-effectiveness and cost-benefit.

Objectives of the Study

The main purposes of Horisberger's paper are:

1) To review the epidemiology of peptic ulcer disease, especially duodenal ulcer disease, in different countries and its attendant mortality and morbidity, and to review the changes occurring before and after the introduction and general marketing of cimetidine.
2) To assess whether cimetidine has been responsible for the changing pattern of the incidence and prevalence of treatment in defined populations with peptic ulcer disease.
3) To determine the impact of cimetidine, using data from the Federal Republic of Germany, on hospitalization rates, surgical operations, work loss, and cost in the treatment of persons with peptic ulcer disease.

Critique

There are a number of criticisms that could be raised about this study, most of which are shortcomings in the data base that had to be used. It is unfair to criticize sharply either Horisberger's study or his data sources. It is assumed that the Allgemeine Ortskrankenkassen (AOK) collect statistics for their own administrative or programme control purposes without reference to Horisberger's research requirements. Thus, when he used these available statistics he undoubtedly obtained those that were available. This, unfortunately, can only lead to something less than an ideal study. And so all along, compromises had to be made and many important questions could not be fully answered.

With this major caveat in mind, let me address a few of the study's problems.

Mortality Trends[1]

a) Epidemiological terms are not always specifically defined. For example, in Table 19.1, the rates are adjusted per 100000 population. But does this mean that the rates are age-adjusted to a standard population? This is particularly valuable in age-and-sex-adjusted mortality rates to a standard population. In making international comparisons without age and sex adjustment, variations can easily cause a manifold variation in mortality or disease rates.
b) Standard errors of the rates should have been presented to demonstrate the confidence that could be placed in the data and results. This is particularly important in vital statistics information.
c) Whenever large differences in mortality are observed (Table 19.2), this raises the question "why?" (age and sex adjustment might have explained some of the differences)[2].

Incidence Data

Two peptic ulcer populations were used to estimate the proportion of recurrent and new cases. Little information about the sample was given. Are they representative of the whole population? This is an important point since these results are used as the basis for extrapolation. Standard errors of these rates would also have been of value.

Prevalence

There seems to be some inconsistency in the use of prevalence statistics. At times, prevalence appears to include all persons with the disease at the beginning of the observation period plus all new cases, expressed as a proportion of all persons in the population at the time of observation. At other times, the prevalence data appear to be based upon episodes per person. If the latter occurs, it would mean that there would be more than one occurrence per person and that person would appear more than once in the numerator but only once in the denominator.

---

1 Mortality data are drawn from civil registration systems in each country. The quality of the data, including the completeness of reporting, may vary from country to country. Mortality rates given by age-groups are comparable, e.g. they are age-adjusted. The mortality rates for "all ages" are based on raw data and not on a standard population.

2 Large differences in mortality between countries (Table 19.2) are not due to different age and sex distribution but to a difference in age- and sex-adjusted mortality.

Hospitalization

Why does the rate of operation for peptic ulcer remain constant in Holland whereas it has dramatically declined in Switzerland, the UK, and USA? This decline appears to have begun before the introduction of cimetidine. In fact, duodenal ulcer seems to have been declining, in the US at least, for many years. Is the natural history of the disease changing? Is the severity of the disease changing? What effects has cimetidine had in light of these possible exogenous changes.

Study from the Federal Republic of Germany (AOK)

a) The necessity of using two population samples may confound the study results.
b) If 50% or less of all patients were being treated with cimetidine, would it have been possible to analyze the comparisons between those using cimetidine for more than just symptoms? (For example, demographic variables, work loss, hospitalizations, operations, etc., using a quasi-experimental design with matching, exclusion, stratification, and multiple regression.)

As mentioned earlier, it is important to keep in mind that this critique is directed primarily to the problems of using data that were collected for purposes other than research. Much the same criticism can be directed to a majority of health services research studies. Luckily, most of the studies of cimetidine have not been plagued quite so much with these problems. These studies wisely began very early in the cimetidine life-cycle so that many of the data problems were averted and many of the answers have already been forthcoming.

The study by Horisberger argues, then, most cogently for the need raised earlier, i. e. the cooperative development and implementation of health services research evaluating medical care technologies that include all the stakeholders or parties at interest - government, corporations, providers, consumers, insurers, and research enterprises.

Summary of Workshop Discussion

First, a comment on *international comparison of epidemiological data.* Any epidemiological survey has to take into account that within national boundaries the patterns or trends may be different from those in other countries. It was most instructive to follow the arguments of representatives of a number of European and North American countries based on information that has been generated from a variety of sources and in a variety of national settings. Especially instructive in this respect was a discussion of the methodological difficulty of estimating the *prevalence* of peptic ulcer.

Everyone agreed that the only accurate means of estimating prevalence is by taking a large random sample of the community and subjecting it to endoscopy and perhaps repeated endoscopy. This is the only way to obtain a reliable estimate of the prevalence of the condition. So we must realize at the outset that all other data available are probably inaccurate – assessments of inpatient admissions for peptic ulcer disease, the number of attendances at general practitioners' offices, surgery with dyspepsia, as well as the number of patients dying and having a duodenal ulcer or a gastric ulcer as an incidental finding. All agree that these are inaccurate methods but the best practical way to come to an educated guess. In this respect it is important to study the development of prevalence over time. To this end one has to choose a large population: there is no value in choosing small samples. The population should be studied for a long period of time – several decades because there are variations from year to year. Ideally, there should be a relatively static population. Finally, there should be no overlap of medical services so that if a patient is going to be hospitalized or to have surgery this happens within the region of study.

An interesting report in this respect has been presented from the West of Scotland, where a stable population of just over 2 million people has been studied for almost 50 years (from 1924 to 1973). Some fluctuation in male prevalence was noted with a peak in 1941 (the early years of the war) and the ulcer prevalence in males reached its peak in the early 1950s, since when it has declined fairly steadily. Female prevalence, on the other hand, has increased consistently throughout the 50 years of the survey. It is interesting to note that ulcer prevalence in the last century tended to occur in females rather than in males. With regard to the types of ulcer, duodenal (DU) or gastric (GU), it was shown that in latter years there has been a decline in the ration DU/GU. DU are still far more common, 4:1, but the ratio has declined. Ulcers observed in the last century were mostly GU rather than DU. So perhaps the wheel is turning full circle and we are returning to the nineteenth century pattern of prevalence.

Second, one might try to use *indirect approaches to assess the prevalence* of peptic ulcers both as an alternative and as an indicator for future trends. One way that has been chosen is the incidence of perforation as a measurement of the prevalence of peptic ulcer. The attractiveness of the incidence of perforation is that there is no doubt about the diagnosis. It is confirmed either at operation or postmortem. But the question remains as to whether the incidence of perforation really reflects the prevalence of peptic ulcer, though there are some data which suggest that this is the case.

Third, it is important to make a *distinction between the epidemiological data base and the data needed for economic analysis.* If one is interested in what is happening in the whole population and the total economic effect, then one has to rely on the epidemiological data. Of course, epidemiological data are not as good in quality as clinical data from clinical trials. This, however, is an unfair comparison. One cannot use data from clinical trials because one needs data from populations. In this respect it is important to emphasize that clinical studies and epidemiological studies are not addressing the same kind of questions, and both types of information are needed for projecting consequences. The epidemiological study shows how big the whole problem is. The clinical study shows what is likely to happen in the population that is included in the study. One needs both types of information in order to make assessment of the impact of the agents. But they are not substitutes for one another.

Fourth, in performing *international comparison of results* one can make extensions from clinical studies concerning the medical effects from one country to another because the human body is very similar from one country to another. But in assessing the economic and social effects, the health care systems and social systems in general differ very much in various countries. Economic and social effects cannot be transferred directly, which is why we have to do separate studies in different countries. To illustrate this, consider one point concerning the mortality. There is a striking difference between (for example) Europe and the United States in the mortality trend. In the United States there has been a decline in mortality since the beginning of 1960, but in Sweden and Denmark mortality has remained absolutely unchanged at a higher level, exactly as has happened in the Federal Republic of Germany.

Fifth, in the *macroeconomic studies* the economist would like to take into account direct parameters, for example on ambulatory care, prescription and consumption of drugs, hospitalization, length of stay in hospital, surgical operations, and indirect parameters such as working capacity, sick leave. The last paper (Horisberger) shows that one can use these data for economic analysis and one should improve the data collection with reference to indirect effects of a specific treatment, such as peptic ulcer.

Sixth, the importance of an *early cooperation between physicians, epidemiologists, and economists* was stressed once more. It has already been pointed out there is an abvious need for the economist to come in rather early in the clinical trials. One of the reasons is that it is sometimes impossible to repeat clinical trials and if the economist was not offered the opportunity to collect economic data at that time it could be too late to do it later. The same applies of course for macroeconomic evaluation. Economists should not just take epidemiological data that have been produced for other purposes, they should be involved from the beginning in the design of epidemiological studies.

21 A Review of the Macroeconomic Evaluation of Cimetidine

B. Jönsson

University of Linköping

Introduction

Because of increased interest in the growth of health care costs, a great many questions have been asked about the economic consequences of the introduction of new medical technology. Is the rapid increase in cost due to progress in medical research, progress that has brought about the introduction of new and more expensive diagnostic and treatment methods? Is it possible to reduce the increase in health care costs through systematic investment in the development of new medical technology that is less costly than established therapies? To answer these questions it is necessary to follow the growth of the health care costs of different diagnostic groups and to find methods of calculating how the costs are affected by changes in the therapies used for these diagnoses.

Health economists have frequently pointed out that it is not enough to look at the *direct* costs of preventing, diagnosing, and treating a disease. We also have to measure the *indirect* costs of illness in terms of loss of production due to disability and premature death. In other words, all costs caused by a particular disease, irrespective of whom it affects, should be accounted for in the economic cost estimate. However, intangible costs in terms of pain and suffering are normally not taken into account. The economic cost of a particular disease inform us about the size of the gain that can be realized by reducing the prevalence and consequences of the disease. It also shows how the total cost is divided into different types of cost – direct and indirect. When a new technology is introduced its effects can be seen partly in changes in the total cost and partly in the changes among the shares of different cost categories.

This paper starts with a review of eight different estimates of the economic costs of ulcer disease for 1 year *before* the introduction of cimetidine. These estimates, all from different countries, give the baseline for the evaluation of the impacts of cimetidine. An attempt is made to compare the studies to find out similarities and differences in methods, data, and results. The review will be followed by two sections presenting two different approaches to assessing the impact of cimetidine on the economic costs of ulcer disease. First, there are studies of *expected* changes in the costs after the introduction of cimetidine. These studies represent *ex ante* evaluations. Second, there are estimations of the *actual* effects on the costs of ulcer disease following the introduction of cimetidine. These studies represent *ex post* evaluations. The paper ends with a discussion of the present state of macroeconomic evaluation of health care technologies.

The Economic Costs of Ulcer Disease – a Review of Selected Studies

The first estimate of the economic costs of ulcers was done by Blumenthal (1959)[1]. The purpose of Blumenthal's study was to place the total cost in relation to grants received for research in ulcer disease. The eight international studies included in the present review were published in the late 1970s and were undertaken to provide a basis for analysis of the consequences that the introduction of the drug cimetidine would have for direct and indirect costs of ulcer disease. The results of these studies are summarized in Table 21.1.

We can first conclude that all studies attempt to estimate the economic costs of the *prevalence* of ulcer disease in society for a particular year. None of the studies uses the *incidence* approach[2]. However, there are methodological differences between the studies. One group of studies (von Haunalter and Chandler 1977; Hertzman et al. 1976; Hertzman et al. 1981; Silverberg 1981) included costs that lie outside the market system: loss of production among housewives, for example. The other group of studies (Netherlands Economic Institute 1977; Institute of Studies in Political Economy 1978a; Bureau d'Informations 1978; Schmoranz 1980) aimed at estimating only costs that affect the gross national product; costs outside the market system are not included.

Three studies (von Haunalter and Chandler 1977; Silverberg 1981; Schmoranz 1980) include estimates of loss of production due to premature mortality. The reasons are not explicitly stated but all studies present data about mortality due to peptic ulceration showing that mortality for this disease is low and that 75% of the

Table 21.1. Estimates of the costs of peptic ulcer disease before the introduction of cimetidine

Country	Year	Total costs	Direct costs (percent)	Indirect costs (percent)	
				Morbidity	Mortality
USA (von Haunalter and Chandler 1977)	1977	$ 3224 million	46	41	13
The Netherlands (Netherlands Economic Institute 1977)	1975	fl 337 million	21	79	–
Italy (Institute of Studies in Political Economy 1978a)	1976	L 284 billion	42	58	–
Sweden (Hertzman et al. 1976)	1975	Kr 480 million	22	78	–
Denmark (Hertzman et al. 1981)	1977	Kr 464 million	30	70	–
Norway (Silverberg 1981)	1977	Kr 275 million	27	63	10
France (Bureau d' Informations 1978)	1977	Fr 1740 million	66	34	0
Austria (Schmoranz 1980)	1978	Sch 1477 million	41	41	18

1 An adjustment of Blumenthal's calculation upwards ot the 1963 annual level was published in 1968.

2 See Hartunian et al. (1981) for an analysis of the economic costs of illness applying the incidence approach.

deaths occur in people over 65 years of age. Another reason could be that cimetidine is not expected to have any impact on mortality. One study (Bureau d'Informations 1978) concludes that there are no costs of mortality since the potential loss of production is balanced by an equal reduction in consumption. This study attempts to estimate "economic value of human life" instead of just measuring loss of production. However, the method used has been heavily critizised[3].

From those studies that have estimated the loss of production due to premature mortality for peptic ulcer disease we can conclude that *loss of production due to mortality is much smaller than loss of production due to morbidity.* In three studies (von Haunalter and Chandler 1977; Hertzman et al. 1976; Silverberg 1981) the morbidity costs are divided into two segments: earning losses by those who are normally productive but have lost work days due to ulcer (short-term illness) and those who are disabled by ulcer and unable to work at all (permanent disability). The US study shows that the two types of morbidity have about equal costs in terms of lost production. However, the Swedish estimate reveals that the cost of short-term illness is about four times higher than the cost of permanent disability. The Norwegian estimate, which is done using a "top down approach" based on the results of the Swedish study, also shows that the cost of short-term illness is higher, but only by about 50%.

Most studies point out that decreased productivity while at work should be considered and could be significant for ulcer disease. But they add that there is no way to measure this decrease. Only the French study (Bureau d'Informations 1978) makes such an attempt. The method used is to estimate first the total number of days spent at work by persons suffering actively from ulcer. It is then assumed that their productivity is reduced by 15%[4]. It turns out that this cost is half of the estimated costs of absence from work.

Despite the fact that the French study is the only one that includes loss of productivity at work, this study shows the smallest share for indirect costs of all studies (see Table 21.1). One explanation for this is that the estimate of loss of production is reduced by about 50% to take into account "the present-day economic situation" with, for example 5.3% unemployment. The question about correction of the estimated value of lost production for unemployment is discussed in the Swedish study (Hertzman et al. 1976) but no corrections are made on the following grounds. First, sick leave is usually of short duration and a new person is therefore not hired. Second, it is not certain that an unemployed person can replace a sick one, since the latter's job requires special knowledge and experience. Third, full employment does not mean that there is no existing unemployment; there is always a certain structural and frictional unemployment. Labour market statistics show that job vacancies and unemployment occur at the same time and that the relation between the numbers of both changes with the business cycle. It is hardly relevant to make esti-

3 See Jones-Lee (1976) for a survey of different methods for estimating value of life. The usefulness of a concept like "value of life" could be questioned in macroeconomic evaluation. However, an alternative to estimates of loss of production due to premature mortality could be to multiply the number of life-years lost (or gained) with a common value per life-year. How this should be decided is a delicate matter, but perhaps the most important thing is to use the same value in all studies.

4 The study does not show how this figure was estimated.

mates of the present value of lost production dependent on the present-day economic situation if it cannot be well argued that the present situation will be a fairly permanent one. One conclusion from the estimates of the costs of ulcer disease is that morbidity is probably the most important single cost item. But it is also the cost item for which there are the greatest differences in the methods used to estimate it and where the data are most shaky.

If we look at the distribution of direct costs (Table 21.2) it is obvious that hospital care accounts for the majority of these costs – about 75%. There are differences between countries and it is understandable that countries like Italy and France, where hospital care in general takes a smaller part of health care expenditure than in for example the Scandinavian countries, have the lowest share for hospital care. The share for drugs is about 10%. The very low share for drugs in the estimate from the Netherlands depends mainly on two factors. First that it includes only prescribed drugs and second that it uses a very low mark-up (19%) to convert factory prices to retail prices. The very high share for drugs in the Italian study must not necessarily be wrong, but it is not possible to analyse it further because the source used is not revealed in the study[5].

It is not meaningful to translate the estimates of costs of ulcer disease in different countries into one and the same currency. This is because exchange rates do not

Table 21.2. The distribution of the direct costs of ulcer disease on hospital care, ambulatory care, and drugs

Country[a]	Hospital care (%)	Ambulatory care (%)	Drugs (%)
USA	73	19	8
The Netherlands	85	12	3
Italy	58	17	25
Sweden	68	18	14
Denmark	80	13	7
Norway	78	14	8
France	55	35	10
Austria	82	–	–

[a] Sources are as for Table 21.1

Table 21.3. Share of ulcer disease in total costs of illness in 1975 in the US, Sweden, and Norway

	USA (%)	Sweden (%)	Norway (%)
Direct costs	1.2	0.5	0.5
Indirect costs[a]	1.9	1.3	1.1
Total	1.4	1.0	0.8

[a] Mortality not included

5 However, Table 13, p 24 of the Italian study is headed "Cost of anti-ulcer drugs". If this is a sales figure for all anti-ulcer drugs it should be reduced by some 75% to give an estimate of drug costs for the diagnoses of gastric and duodenal ulcer. If this correction is done we arrive at 8% for drugs and 71% for hospital care.

Table 21.4. Comparison of hospital utilization rates for ulcer disease in different countries

	Denmark	Norway	Sweden	USA	Netherlands	Italy	France	Austria
Share of total number of bed days	1.2%	1.2%	0.5%	1.5%	–	–	–	–
Share of total number of discharges	1.2%	0.9%	0.7%	–	1.0%	–	0.7%	–
Number of bed days per 100000 population								
Peptic ulcer[a]	2229	1647	1650	1797	2374	3740	2177	2752
Gastric ulcer	1061	–	932	–	1011	–	1241	1751
Duodenal ulcer	1115	–	682	–	1363	–	936	1001
Number of discharges per 100000 population								
Peptic ulcer[a]	179	124	119	176	103	187	96	180
Gastric ulcer	84	–	59	48	40	–	55	103
Duodenal ulcer	91	–	57	90	63	–	41	77
Mean length of stay in days	12	13	14	9	25	20	20	15
Gastric ulcer	–[e]	–	–	–	27	21	–	17
Duodenal ulcer	–	–	–	–	24	19	–	13
Number of operations per 100000 population								
Peptic ulcer[a]	65	–	66	44[b]	45	75	38	63
Gastric ulcer	25	–	32	–	17	–	13	36
Duodenal ulcer	39	–	33	–	28	–	25	27
Percentage surgical cases	36	–	55	58[c]	44	40	40[d]	35[d]
Gastric ulcer	–	–	–	–	43	–	–	35
Duodenal ulcer	–	–	–	–	45	–	–	34

[a] Includes cases with gastric, duodenal, and peptic ulcer site unspecified (ICD no. 531, 532, and 533, respectively)
[b] Includes partial gastrectomy and vagotomy, National Center for Health Statistics figures (Fineberg et al. 1981 a, p 43)
[c] Share of bed days for surgical cases, see Note [a]; Fineberg and Peartman (1981 a, p 43) estimates the surgical rate at 25%–29%
[d] Assumed value
[e] Data not available

perfectly reflect how resources are used in the countries but depend solely on the goods and services that are exported and imported. As medical care is not often a part of international trade, it is extremely difficult to judge whether the same relative prices could be used or not. One way to compare the costs of ulcer disease in different countries is to look at the share of ulcer disease in the total costs of illness. To do such a comparison we have to have an estimate of the total costs of all illnesses in the various countries. Such estimates are available only for Sweden, Norway, and the US (Table 21.3). Ulcer's share of the total costs is somewhat higher in the USA than in Sweden and Norway. The biggest difference between the countries is in the share of direct costs. In Sweden and Norway ulcer causes only 0.5% of the total health care costs, while in the USA it causes 1.2% – about 2.5 times as great a share. The numbers indicate that ulcer disease is treated more intensively in the USA than in Sweden and Norway.

One way to circumvent the exchange rate problem in international comparisons is to compare physical units of resources used. Since hospital care is the dominating direct cost it is of special interest to look at the utilization of hospital resources. Such a comparison is shown in Table 21.4. Ulcer disease accounts for about 1% of the total number of hospital discharges. There is a variation from 0.7% (Sweden and France) to 1.2% (Denmark and probably the US). If we look at the number of discharges per 100000 of population we can see that there is a group of countries with high discharge rates (Denmark, US, Italy, and Austria) and a group of countries with discharge rates that are about two-thirds of these values (Norway, Sweden, Netherlands, and France). The variations in average length of stay are considerable, from 9 days in the US to 25 days in the Netherlands. The lowest number of bed days per 100000 of population is found in Sweden and Norway. The variation in the number of operations per 100000 of population is much smaller. The very low number of surgical operations for gastric ulcer in the Netherlands and France should be noted.

The statistics on hospital utilization reveal large differences in the use of medical technology for ulcer disease in the different countries. We also can conclude that the quality of the data used in many cases is not satisfactory. Many numbers used are rather "guesstimates" than estimates. But some interesting interpretations of the direct costs for ulcer disease can be made from the data in Table 21.4: (a) The higher share for hospital cost in the US than in Sweden is mainly explained by a greater number of admissions. The surgical rate is the same[6]. (b) The high share for hospital care in Denmark compared with Sweden is mainly explained by a higher admission rate for medical cases. The number of operations is about the same. (c) The high share for hospital care in the Netherlands is mainly due to long mean length of stay. (d) The low share for hospital costs in France and Italy is not supported by the utilization data. If the estimates are correct the explanation must be found in a low cost per bed day in relation to costs for physician visits and drugs.

Table 21.5 shows a comparison of the mortality in different countries due to ulcer disease. Except for the high mortality in Austria, Denmark, and Sweden compared with other countries, there are no great differences in the pattern of mortality. About two-thirds of the deaths occur in men and in persons aged 65 years or more.

6 If we assume that the high estimate for the US is the correct one.

Table 21.5. Comparison of mortality due to ulcer disease in different countries

Country	Gastric/ duodenal	Total number of deaths	Rate per 100000 population	Percent of deaths in males	Percent of deaths in persons 70 years and older
USA (1977)	1.1	6562	3.1	60	53
Netherlands (1974)	1.6	590	4.3	59	75[b]
Italy (1976)		3653	6.4	76	64[b]
Sweden (1977)	2.1	750	9.5[a]	65	70
Denmark (1975)	1.9	356[a]	7.1[a]	–	70
Norway (1977)		194	4.8	61	67
France (1974)	4.3	2290	4.2	67	61
Austria (1977)	1.4	713	9.5	57	56

[a] Gastric and duodenal ulcer only (1975)
[b] 65 and over

It is of course possible to make a similar comparison of the morbidity data that make up the basis for the estimates of indirect costs due to absenteeism and permanent disability. However, even if we go down to a very detailed level there are a great many limitations for the use of data from cross-national comparisons for macro-evaluation of medical technology. There are so many factors that differ that it is nearly impossible to separate the effects of the specific technology selected for study. More promising is to make a macroeconomic evaluation based on variations within a specific country. Even within a given country different technologies, both new and old, are used at the same time and these variations could be used for practicable evaluations. Such studies could be done in two ways. The first method is to use multiple regression analysis to study, say, how variations in hospitalization between regions are related to variations in the use of cimetidine. If data permit, the relation between the rate of use of a certain technology and the total economic cost of a certain disease could be analysed in this way. However, regional data on health care costs, morbidity, and mortality are usually not available for such analysis. For a study on international and interregional variations in hospital utilization rates for ulcer disease see Jönsson and Silverberg (1981). The second method is to separate the users of the new technology from the users of the old technology. The two groups can be compared in terms of costs of medical care, morbidity, and mortality. It is easier to detect differences in the impact of different technologies this way than by analysing regional variations. However, the problem is to make sure that there is no bias in patient selection for different technologies. We have to make sure that the differences found between the two groups are related to the use of different technologies and not other factors. For studies using this method see Geweke and Weisbrod (1981) and Rhode Island Health Services Research Inc (1981).

Ex Ante Evaluations of the Impact of Cimetidine on the Economic Costs of Ulcer Disease

The economic costs of a particular disease inform us about the size of the gain that can be realized by reducing the incidence and consequences of the disease. It also shows how the total costs are divided into different types of costs – direct and indirect costs. When a new technology is introduced its effects can be seen partly in changes in the total cost and partly in the changes among the shares of different cost categories.

One method of estimating these consequences is to let physicians with a thorough knowledge of the disease make judgements about the expected effects of the new therapy – both about the extent of its usage and about its effects on the patient. Such assessments are naturally very difficult to do and entail great uncertainty. Thus, they are often filled with reservations. They do have the great advantage of being performed *before* the new technology has come into use. Therefore they can be of value to decision-making about the introduction of a new technology. Since we do not know anything about the *actual* effects of the new technology at its moment of introduction, estimates of *expected* costs or cost reductions constitute the only available information. Consequently the value of the information will have to be related to whatever else we know in the decision situation at hand. That calculations of expected effects have a high degree of uncertainty is, consequently, not a sufficient argument for them to be rejected. In cases where the technology was actually introduced there are also possibilities for a control of how good the estimates were. By studying the causes for the difference between an estimated and an actual development, we can probably improve forecasting methods.

The most commonly used method for estimating an expected effect is to start with the actual economic costs of a disease during a previous year, usually the year before introduction of the new technology. This is an acceptable method only if the costs in real terms remain relatively unchanged from year to year. If the cost is rising one obtains an underestimate of gains, and if it is declining one obtains an overestimate. The question to be asked is: what would the economic costs of ulcer disease

Table 21.6. Expected cost changes with the introduction of cimetidine in different studies

Country	Expected percentage cost changes					
	Hospital care	Ambulatory care	Drugs	Morbidity	Mortality	Total
USA[a]	−35	−18	+ 40	−35	−18	−29
The Netherlands[b]	−28	–	+ 90	−21	–	−20
Italy[c]	−66	0	+108	−40	–	−30
France[d]	−15	0	+291	−30	–	± 0
Austria[e]	−63	+12		−64	−25	−54

[a] Robinson Associates (1978)
[b] Netherlands Economic Institute (1977)
[c] Institute of Studies in Political Economy (1978b)
[d] Bureau d'Informations et de Previsions Economiques (1979)
[e] Schmoranz (1980)

have been had we had access to the new technology during that year? That means that we are comparing two "steady states", with or without the new technology. An alternative, and perhaps preferable, approach would have been to make explicit estimates of the expected patterns of direct and indirect costs of the disease for the coming years.

Table 21.6 summarizes the expected change in economic costs due to ulcer disease from the introduction of cimetidine in five different countries. The results from the different studies all point to the same direction but there are differences in magnitude. Costs for hospital care for ulcer patients are expected to be reduced. The low estimate for France is mainly explained by an assumption that a large number of hospitalization cases are "medical-social cases", which do not really warrant the hospital. These cases are not expected to be affected by the introduction of cimetidine. Obviously there are such cases in all hospitals but the number is probably lower in the US and Sweden with higher surgical rates and shorter length of stay. And it is unrealistic to assume that these cases would be unaffected by the new technology. Instead one can argue that these cases will be most affected by a new technology that improves ambulant management of the disease.

The studies for Italy and Austria predict very dramatic reductions in costs for hospital care. These two countries also have the highest number of bed days per 100000 of population (Table 21.4). The savings in hospital costs in the Italian estimate come about equally from a reduction in the *number* of surgical cases (no change in average length of stay) and the *average length of stay* for nonsurgical cases (very small reduction in the number of cases). For Austria the main effect comes from a reduction in the number of hospital admissions, 75% for surgical cases. The distinction between reductions in the number of admissions and average length of stay for reductions in the total number of bed days is important for the estimation of cost consequences. If the reduction in bed days comes from a reduction in the number of patients treated it is acceptable to use average cost per bed day or patient for the estimation of cost savings. But if it is a reduction in average length of stay, the average cost represent on overestimate of reduction in costs (Jönsson and Lindgren 1980). The cost of a marginal bed day is lower than the average cost, probably in the magnitude of 50%. Costs of drugs are assumed to increase in all studies. The estimates vary considerably between studies, from 40% in the US to nearly 300% in France.

The savings that are claimed in all studies come mainly from reductions in loss of production due to morbidity. Since the cost of morbidity is the single most important cost item these savings have a large impact on the total savings. Four of five studies predict considerable reduction in the total costs of ulcer disease as a consequence of the introduction of cimetidine, between 20% and 50%. The only exception is France where the combination of small savings in hospital costs and large increases in drug costs results in constant total costs for ulcer disease.

There are great similarities in both methods and results of all the studies. One reason for this is that they are not done completely independent of each other. The studies from Italy, France, and Austria use assumptions that are derived from the studies from the Netherlands and the US as complements to their own estimates. Divergences between the studies derive mainly from differences in the predicted effects. With the exception of the US study it is not possible to analyse how the different estimates are arrived at. There does not seem to have been any systematic process to derive the expected effects. They are formed on the basis of published clinical studies, opinions of physicians contacted, results from similiar studies in other countries, and informed guesses.

Since the US study was one of the first and has the most clearly described method we can use this study for a discussion of the methodological problems involved in predicting the economic consequences of a new health care technology. The US study is limited to the effects of cimetidine on duodenal ulcer patients while the other studies refer to both gastric and duodenal ulcer. The estimates are based on predictions by physicians experienced in the use of cimetidine. These physicians provided estimates of treatment and response with the use of cimetidine in relation to conventional therapy. We can divide the estimation process into four different steps: (1) selection of physicians; (2) definition of "cases" presented to physicians; (3) predictions of effects on the utilization of health services, morbidity, and mortality; (4) converting changes in utilization, morbidity, and mortality to changes in costs.

To be able to make predictions about the effects of a new health care technology it is necessary to have a good knowledge of the properties of the technology. Those who have this knowledge at an early stage are mainly physicians involved in clinical evaluation of the new technology. But when a new technology is widely used in the health care system these specialists only account for a small fraction of the users – and they may not be representative. There may be differences both in the magnitude of use of the technology and in the effects encountered between experienced physician investigators and the majority of physicians using the technology in the health care system. There is also a risk of bias in the estimates if specialists who were involved in the development and clinical evaluation of the new technology are more enthusiastic over its use and consequences than physicians in general. Therefore it is important to try and select physicians that are representative for the majority of users to predict the effect. The role of specialists should first of all be to assist with relevant information.

The definition of "cases" for which the new technology could be used means dividing the patients into a number of categories that are as homogeneous as possible in terms of severity of the disease and therapeutic effect. This subdivision of patients must be complete, which means that all patient groups together should exhaust the total costs for the disease. For example acute surgical patients are excluded from the study by Robinson Associates (1978)[7].

The prediction of the effects of cimetidine was done in the following way. The physician was first asked to look at the five patient descriptions and to decide what proportion of the current doctor-treated duodenal ulcer population was represented by each[8]. Next, he was asked to estimate how a typical physician would most likely treat each of these patients prior to the introduction of cimetidine and how he

7 For the period 1973–1979 these patients represent one-third of the patients who underwent surgery for duodenal ulcer in Malmöhus county in the south of Sweden. Since the surgical rate was 40% they represent 13% of the total number of patients and their share of costs is probably higher.

8 This information does not necessarily have to be predicted. It is at least in theory possible to investigate this.

would most likely treat them if he were to prescribe cimetidine. This treatment description included all drug regimens plus any dietary changes that he viewed as necessary. The drug information solicited from the physician included the percentage of patients for whom the drug would be prescribed or recommended, the amount prescribed per day, and the duration of the drug therapy. After having established the manner in which each of these patient types would most likely be treated, the physician was next asked to estimate how each of the two programmes would perform in its ability to control the ulcer symptoms and to prevent the progression of the duodenal ulcer condition to a more severe situation. Specifically, for each patient type the physician was asked to estimate: (a) frequency of repeat episodes; (b) frequency of paitent visits to physician; (c) likelihood and frequency of hospitalization; (d) likelihood of surgery; (e) frequency of diagnostic X-rays and endoscopies; (f) amount of missed work; (g) likelihood of death from ulcer complications.

The physician investigators were also requested to estimate for each patient type the likelihood that cimetidine would be prescribed for them after its level of acceptance was stabilized. Although the personal experiences of the physician investigators with cimetidine provided a solid background for their responses, they were asked specifically to estimate how other doctors and specialists in the medical profession would most likely prescribe cimetidine and other drugs.

The predictions from the physicians varied considerably. Therefore there is a problem of aggregating the different answers. Just using the average, as was done in the study, could introduce bias into the estimates. This point is discussed at length in a review of the study by Fineberg and Pearlman (1981 a, b).

The method used in the Robinson Associates study to convert estimated clinical and health system effects into dollar savings were as follows. As a baseline for estimating the cost of duodenal ulcers they used estimates of the costs of peptic ulcer disease in 1977 developed by von Haunalter and Chandler (1977). Within each direct and indirect cost category, the analysts estimated from secondary sources the fraction of peptic ulcer costs attributable to duodenal ulcer disease. The physician's information was then used to compute, on a per-duodenal ulcer patient basis, the percentage increase or decrease that would likely occur between the two alternatives. These percentage changes in per-patient cost were then applied against the national total of duodenal ulcer costs for 1977 to estimate what the costs would have been had cimetidine therapy been used instead of the traditional therapy. However, they were not used directly. The percentage *difference* in cost for the *average* patient was applied to the total cost estimate from the study by von Haunalter and Chandler (1977). Because the total costs estimate and the reduction in costs are computed in different ways there are obvious problems in relating them to each other. Basically the methodology used in the study by Robinson Associates is sound. However, there are elements in it that make it plausible that they overestimate the potential savings from cimetidine. But this will not alter their basic conclusion. Cimetidine does appear to save more resources than it costs. The US $ 305 million savings in direct medical costs from the use of cimetidine are approximately nine times the estimated US $ 34 million increase in drug costs. To this we can add the savings in indirect costs.

There is not much use in speculating about over- or underestimates of potential savings from cimetidine. The proof of the pudding is in the eating. We will after some years be able to estimate the *actual* effects of cimetidine. By comparing *ex ante* estimates with estimates *ex post* we can analyse what was wrong and right in the initial assessment and that will give ideas for further improvements in the methodology.

Ex Post Evaluations of the Impact of Cimetidine on the Economic Costs of Ulcer Disease

As seen from Table 21.7 most studies on what happened to direct and indirect costs of ulcer disease after the introduction of cimetidine have concentrated on the effects on surgery. This is understandable for three reasons. First, hospitalization is the most expensive direct cost and surgery accounts for about half ot this cost. Second, the number of surgical operations is a more accurate measure of the effect of cimetidine than the number of discharges or bed days. Third, clinical studies comparing cimetidine with placebo have shown that patients receiving cimetidine have fewer surgical operations (Bodemar and Walan 1978).

Two studies also investigate the impact of cimetidine on costs for ambulatory care and drugs. Only one study analyses changes in indirect costs. Instead of reviewing the studies one by one we will look at the different costs categories one by one and compare the results from the different studies and with the projections presented in the previous section.

Effects on Surgery and Costs of Surgery

Surgery could be studied either from diagnosis data or surgical data. The first method identifies the number of patients (admissions or discharges) with a certain diagnosis and if the patients have been operated on or not. The second method directly identifies the number of selected surgical procedures. The latter method has several advantages. Surgery data are usually more accurate than diagnosis data and give more detailed information about what is done with the patient. But there are also problems. A certain type of operation could be performed for different diagnoses

Table 21.7. Ex post studies of the effects of cimetidine on peptic ulcer disease

Effects	UK[a]	Netherlands[b]	France[c]	USA[d]	USA[e]
Surgery	×	×	×	×	×
Hospitalization	(×)	×		(×)	×
Ambulatory care		×			×
Drugs		×			×
Work loss					×

[a] Venables (1981) [b] Bulthuis (1980) [c] Lambert (1980) USA: [d] Fineberg and Pearlman (1981 a); [e] Rhode Island Health Services Research, Inc.: The effect of cimetidine on peptic ulcer disease in Rhode Island, July 1980

(×) The main focus of these studies is on surgery but discharge data are also presented. However, no deeper analysis is undertaken for nonsurgical cases and this has to be analysed. It is also common that one patient undergoes several different operations on one occasion[9].

Since estimates of the social cost of a disease usually start from the diagnosis concept it is preferable to estimate the number of patients operated on within a certain diagnosis. More detailed analysis could be made on the kind of operations that are performed. But the most important information is whether the patient has been operated on.

Both methods have been used in the studies of the effect of cimetidine on surgery for peptic ulcer disease. The European studies all start from diagnosis data and estimate the number of operations within the diagnosis "gastric ulcer and duodenal ulcer". The US studies estimate the number of partial gastrectomies and vagotomies, which are the common types of surgeries for ulceration. There is a strong correlation between these operating procedures and the diagnosis "gastric and duodenal ulcer" but it is not a one-to-one correspondence[10]. One disadvantage with us-

Table 21.8. Trends in ulcer surgery 1970–1979 reported in five different studies. Index 1976 = 100

Study / Year	UK[a]	France[c]	Netherlands[d]	USA[e]	Rhode Island[f]
1970	–	–	116	116	–
1971	141	–	115	120	–
1972	137	100	112	120	–
1973	125	100	109	120	124
1974	122	100	113	113	125
1975	94[b]	100	107	104	113
1976	100	100	100	100	100
1977	65	95	102	94	98
1978	66	68	78	67	64
1979	–	70	72	79	58

[a] Operations for gastric and duodenal ulcer in England and Wales (Venables 1981)
[b] Young doctors went on strike this year
[c] Operations for gastric and duodenal ulcer. Data from different sources showed that there was no trend for 1972–1976 (Lambert 1980)
[d] Operations for gastric and duodenal ulcer (Netherlands Economic Institute 1977; and Bulthuis 1980)
[e] Partial gastrectomy and vagotomy (Fineberg and Pearlman 1981 a)
[f] Partial gastrectomy and vagotomy for 12 months ending August 31 each year

9 The number of operation codes registered for ulcer disease (ICD 531–533) in Swedish patient statistics for 1977 exceeded the number of operated persons by 39%.

10 Data from two surgical clinics in Sweden show that partial gastrectomy and vagatomy accounted for 63% of surgical operations for duodenal ulcer for the period 1973–1979:
Number of surgical operations in diagnosis duodenal ulcer at two surgical departments in Sweden 1973–1979

Dept.	Total	440	441	442	443	444	445	446	447	448	449
I	492	2	1	17	1	5	19	137	290	3	17
II	327	5	0	125	0	1	38	43	88	21	6

Legend: 440, gastrotomy; 441, pylorotomy; 442, partial gastrectomy; 443, total gastrectomy; 444, gastrotomy (as single procedure); 445, anastomosis operations; 446, suture of gastric or du-ing surgical data is that we do not obtain a separation of operations for gastric and duodenal ulcer.

Table 21.8 shows the trends in ulcer surgery for 1970–1979 in the five different studies. Table 21.9 summarizes the estimated reductions in surgery and cost of surgery. The estimation of reductions in costs is done by multiplying the reduction in the number of surgical cases with an estimate of average cost per surgical case. The low cost estimate in the Rhode Island study is based on the assumption that there is no reduction in admissions for ulcer, but that only surgery is reduced. The high estimate is based on a reduction in hospital admissions equivalent to the decline in ulcer surgery. The cost estimations in the European studies are based on this latter assumption.

All five studies indicate that there was a 30% reduction in surgery after the introduction of cimetidine for both gastric and duodenal ulcer. The study from the UK shows an even greater reduction – about 50% – but this is mainly explained by the method used. The average number of surgical operations for 1971–1979 is compared with the average number of operations for 1977–1978, not taking into account that there was a downward trend in the period before the introduction of cimetidine. No such trend was evident in France but the analysis of the pre-cimetidine period is insufficient. Only two observations are counted, for 1972 and 1976 and they are based on a very small sample. Regression analysis is used in both studies from the US to predict the number of surgical operations for 1978 and 1979. The prediction is compared with the actual number of operations and the reduction is shown to be significant ($P < 0.05$). The study from Netherlands uses another statistical technique. The number of surgical operations for 1972–1979 is analysed by multiple regression analysis with cimetidine and a trend factor as independent variables. The contribution od these two factors to the reduction in surgical operations over time is estimated[11].

Most studies discuss at length if cimetidine reduces or postpones surgery but of course we need data for more years to answer that question. There is also usually a

Table 21.9. Reductions in surgery and costs of surgery following the introduction of cimetidine

	UK[a]	Netherlands	France[d]	USA[e]	USA[f]
Reduction in number of operations	–	–	–	–30%	–30%
Gastric ulcer	–43%	–20%	–30%		
Duodenal ulcer	–49%	–33%	–30%		
Estimated savings	£9 million[b]	fl 9.9 million	Fr 43 million	–	$ 59–97 million

[a] Venables (1981) [b] Duodenal ulcer only; £ 2.8 million is hospital costs, rest is cost of mortality following surgery [c] Bulthuis (1980) [d] Lambert (1980) USA: [e] Fineberg and Pearlman (1981 a) [f] Rhode Island Health Services Research, Inc.: The effect of cimetidine on peptic ulcer disease in Rhode Island, July 1980

odenal ulcer site; 447, vagotomy; 448, gastroscopy with endoscopic operation; 449, other operations on stomach.

11 The details of the regression analysis are not presented in the study.

comparison of the development of ulcer surgery and other types of abdominal surgery to investigate if some general surgical trends can explain the drop in ulcer surgery for the year after the introduction of cimetidine. This is shown not to be the case.

Hospitalization

No significant changes in hospital discharge rates for gastric and duodenal ulcer can be seen after the introduction of cimetidine. The average length of stay does not exhibit any change either. This is surprising in light of the significant reductions in surgery. Most studies have estimated that between 40% and 50% of hospitalized ulcer patients undergo surgery. However, the ratio between the number of surgical operations (partial gastrectomies and vagotomies) and the total number of patients discharged with the diagnosis "ulcer" was between 0.25 and 0.29 : 1 for the period 1966–1977 and 0.19 : 1 in 1978 in the US.

Since surgical cases are a small part of all hospitalized ulcer patients and in most countries there is a strong downward trend in hospital admissions for ulcer patients (especially nonsurgical duodenal ulcer patients) it is difficult to detect significant changes. We must therefore conclude that all savings in hospital costs come from a reduction in the number of surgical cases. If we compare the estimated reduction in surgical costs with the estimated reduction in hospital costs from ex ante studies we see that these studies heavily overestimate the savings. The US findings show that ex ante estimates are three to five times higher then ex post extimates. For France the ex ante estimate was a saving in hospital costs of 63–94 million francs in 1977 prices. The ex post estimate was a reduction in hospital costs of 43 million francs in 1979 prices. The estimated ex post savings in the Netherlands were fl 9.9 million in 1979 prices. This is approximately fl 6 million in 1975 prices. The ex ante estimate was a saving of fl 15.75 million in 1975 prices, of which fl 4.70 million came from surgical cases. The ex ante studies from France and Netherlands overestimated the savings in hospital costs by a factor of two, mainly because the expected reduction in hospitalization for nonsurgical cases was not confirmed.

Ambulatory Care and Drugs

The development of costs for ambulatory care consultations and diagnostic examinations and drugs has been studied in the Netherlands (Bulthuis 1980). The study found no significant break in the trend of gradually increasing costs for ambulatory care after the introduction of cimetidine. Drug costs increased threefold in current prices after the introduction of cimetidine. We also have to remember that the estimate of drug costs in the Netherlands before the introduction of cimetidine was very low compared with other countries. The data presented in the study permit no deeper analysis.

The costs of ambulatory treatment after the introduction of cimetidine was also studied by Rhode Island Health Services Research Inc (1981). Their estimates were based on a health interview survery done by telephone for a random sample of the Rhode Island population. Persons reporting an ulcer were divided into two groups – cimetidine users and non users. The utilization of health services by the two groups was compared before and after the introduction of cimetidine. The study showed higher (double) costs for medications and physician visits of cimetidine users, but these costs were offset by lower costs for disability days. Total costs, direct plus indirect, were less for cimetidine users. The Rhode Island study is very interesting and presents valuable information about ulcer epidemiology and costs of the disease. However, it does not answer questions about the actual impact of cimetidine on costs for ambulatory care and drugs in the community. Cimetidine users and nonusers were shown to be two very different groups of the ulcer population[12].

Swedish data can be used to discuss further the effects of cimetidine on the costs of drugs for ulcer patients. In 1980 the total costs of drugs for ulcer patients outside hospitals were Kr 113 million. Cimetidine accounted for 18% of these costs[13]. If we make the assumption that there was no substitution of cimetidine for other drugs we can conclude that drug costs for treatment of ulcer disease increased by 18% with the introduction of cimetidine.

Another way to look at drug costs is to concentrate on costs for diagnoses ICD 531–533, gastric and duodenal ulcer and peptic ulcer site unspecified. Drug costs for these diagnoses increased by 40% after the introduction of cimetidine. We have then taken into account that only 25% of the costs of antacids and anticholinergica and 50% of costs of cimetidine relate to these diagnoses. If we compare the total costs of cimetidine with the costs for other drugs prescribed for diagnoses (ICD) 531–33 the cost increase due to cimetidine was about 80%. However, this comparison is only relevant if we could assume that the net effect of cimetidine therapy outside these diagnoses is zero. If this is not the case we have to evaluate the costs and benefits of each separate indication for the technology.

Work Loss

An estimation of days of work loss due to ulcer disease after the introduction of cimetidine was undertaken in Rhode Island in 1981. The study is based on data from the Rhode Island Temporary Disability Insurance (TDI) files, which cover 82% of the employed work force in Rhode Island. In order to receive payments under TDI, a worker must file a claim and be examined by a physician. The TDI programme pays benefit for non-work-connected sickness that results in more than 1 week of consecutive days of lost work and will continue to pay for 26 weeks. Periods of sickness outside this range are not recorded in the study, but any change in work loss due to ulcer disease should be revealed in the TDI data.

The study found a downward trend in work loss for peptic ulcer disease before the introduction of cimetidine (1974–1977). The estimated trend, if extrapolated, results in the expected disappearance of peptic ulcer disease as a reason for work loss by 1985. The observed rate in 1978 was 15.6 days of work lost for ulcer disease per 1 000 covered employees, which was greater than the expected rate of 14.5 days, but

---

12 For a more extensive discussion of the method of comparing cimetidine users and nonusers in the community, see Geweke and Weisbrod (1981). This study is reviewed in the paper by Weisbrod in this symposium.

13 It has been taken into account that 8% is used in hospitals and that 5% of prescriptions are for diagnoses other than ulcer disease.

the difference was not significant. In 1979 the observed rate, 16.3 days, was significantly greater than the expected rate 11.2 days ($P < 0.05$). These results lead to the conclusion that there was no significant acceleration of the trend of declining work loss rates for illness due to peptic ulcer disease after the introduction of cimetidine.

Discussion

The need for macroeconomic evaluation of new health care technologies must be assessed in relation to the shortcomings of controlled clinical trials as a basis for economic evaluation. It is necessary to perform such studies under strict protocols, which differ from ordinary medical practice where subjects are not chosen at random among the disease population. Such trials are usually performed by specialists in university hospital centres. While the controlled conditions are the strength of the trials in determining the efficacy of the technology they are a weakness if we try to extrapolate the results to the general population and the health care system as a whole[14]. This weakness is not avoided even if the clinical trial is extended to include economic and social effects. Therefore there is a need for complementary studies to evaluate system-wide costs and benefits for society.

However, what you gain in generalization when you move from controlled trials to population based studies you lose in precision. It is not possible to measure costs and benefits with the same degree of exactitude in a macrostudy as in a microstudy. Therefore we will only be able to detect the most important changes at the macrolevel, in the same way as the national accounts only give a picture of the overall performance of the economy. If we wish to analyse specific sectors, firms, or products in detail we have to use other data.

Macroeconomic evaluation could be defined as an analysis of the impact of a health care technology on the economic costs of disease in a defined health care system. This points to the important relation between technology and disease. This is not a one-to-one relationship. The same technology could have effects on several diseases and there is usually more then one technology used for each disease. However, the evaluation has to be undertaken as a relation between technology and disease. We see from the reviewed studies that they sometimes refer to all ulcer disease and sometimes to subgroups, such as gastric and/or duodenal ulcer. This makes the matter complicated. Should we evaluate cimetidine in all its uses even outside ulcer disease, or should the analysis be limited to, for example, cimetidine in duodenal ulcer therapy? The definition of the disease determines the borders of the analysis.

The definition of economic or social costs of a disease has been subject to widespread controversy over the years. But in practice, most studies have subscribed to a definition that includes *direct* costs for health care and *indirect* costs from loss of production due to morbidity and premature mortality. Investigators usually regret that they cannot measure the costs of pain and suffering and exclude them from the

---

14 The results from clinical trials can usually be extrapolated from one country to another. This is not the case with wider health system effects. It is necessary to do separate studies of the health system effects in different countries and we should not be surprised that these studies differ in results.

analysis. This may be serious in a microevaluation but not necessarily in a macroeconomic evaluation. Nobody criticizes the national accounts for not measuring the utility derived from different types of consumption or for not including pain and discomfort in the measure of production costs. There are good reasons to exclude these costs in macroeconomic evaluations.

The general methodology in the macroeconomic evaluation of cimetidine has been to start with a study of the economic costs of ulcer disease, continue with an *ex ante* study of the expected effects of cimetidine on these costs, and end with an *ex post* study of the actual effects of the introduction. Basically, this is a sound way to proceed. The cost of disease study provides the baseline for the two other studies and there is a need for both *ex ante* and *ex post* studies at different times in the decision process.

There are three different ways to measure the costs of illness or disease. The *prevalence* approach provides an estimate of the economic burden resulting from prevalence, number of cases, of a certain disease in a year, say 1982. In principle, this measure includes costs of resources used during 1982 for prevention, diagnosis, treatment, rehabilitation, and long-term care, output lost during the year due to short-term illness, and output lost due to permanent disability and deaths in 1982. Because a death or a permanent disability means lost output not only during 1982 but also in future years, the present value of the future production losses is counted. It should be noted that the calculation of future losses would be based on the existence of morbidity in 1982 and not on the onset of a disease in 1982. The underlying cause of a premature death or a permanent disability in 1982 may well be the onset of a certain disease in earlier years.

The incidence approach provides an estimate of the economic burden, discounted to 1982, resulting from the incidence of disease in 1982. Because of an illness starting in 1982 a person may need treatment not only during the same year but for many years ahead; he may lose time from work during these periods of illness; and he may eventually die of the disease that struck him in 1982. In principle, the measure based on the incidence approach includes all present and future costs of health care resources used due to the onset of the disease in 1982. It also includes expected present and future losses of output. So, this measure requires knowledge of the incidence of the disease in 1982 and the expected course of the disease, including sickness, disability, and mortality as well as treatments most likely to be used.

In the third approach, interest centres on the economic burden of disease that is actually borne in 1982. This approach provides a measure that consists of health care costs in 1982, production lost due to morbidity and mortality existing in 1982, and the value of output lost in 1982 because of morbidity and mortality in previous years. Present values of future losses of production due to morbidity and mortality in 1982 are not included in this measure, so no discounting is needed.

The three approaches will give the same estimates of the direct and indirect costs of acute conditions with short duration and no future effects. In the example above the three approaches will assign all costs to the same year. In most cases the three approaches will, however, provide quite different results.

All macroevaluations of cimetidine uses the prevalence approach. The advantage of this approach is that one can compare the direct costs for certain diseases with the total costs of health care known from other sources. It is possible to use a "top-down" approach to estimate the direct costs for a particular disease. This is not possible if the incidence approach is used. This approach needs much more information about the natural history of the disease, with or without different interventions. However, since ulcer disease is a chronic relapsing disease there would be advantages in using an incidence approach, measuring the economic costs of ulcer disease over the life-time for a cohort of patients.

We have seen from the reviewed studies that the main obstacle for macroeconomic evaluations is lack of relevant data about the epidemiological trends in the disease. At the moment the limitations of the data are more serious than the limitations in the methodology employed. The questions asked are relevant and there are methods for giving an accurate answer to them. But this is not possible due to lack of appropriate data. There are wide divergences in the methods applied in the different studies and, as has been pointed out, some are not scientifically acceptable. But there has been progress in the framework and techniques used to estimate the costs of disease. It is not surprising that the standard of practice varies between investigators. There is a long way to go before we have such consistency in the methodology applied that we can with confidence compare studies for different diseases and different countries.

22 Discussion of Paper by Jönsson

H. V. Fineberg

Harvard University

Jönsson's paper reviews a series of national studies on the cost of peptic ulcer disease and the impact of cimetidine on those costs. The paper distinguishes three stages in the macroeconomic evaluation of new medical intervention or technology: (1) Estimates of the cost of the target disease; (2) projections of the *expected* changes anticipated from the introduction of the new technology, called *ex ante* estimates; and (3) assessment of the actual changes produced by the new technology, termed *ex post* estimates. The discussion in the paper is organized into three sections which correspond to these divisions – a review of eight national studies of the cost of ulcer disease, *ex ante* projections of cimetidine's expected impact on costs in five countries, and *ex post* measurements in four countries of some of the consequences of cimetidine.

The paper discusses a number of methodological issues as well as findings from these studies. My brief remarks cannot do justice to the many valuable observations in Jönsson's review. I shall try to summarize here some of the more salient points, make a few observations extending and reinforcing elements in the paper, and raise a number of questions.

Summary

Studies in all eight countries estimate both direct and indirect costs due to ulcer disease. In all but one case, the indirect costs (due to loss of productivity) exceed the direct costs (due to medical expenditures). Indirect loss due to morbidity is probably the largest single cost item for ulcer disease. Jönsson notes that the studies utilize a strikingly varied approach to measuring these morbidity costs, and data to support the estimates in the studies are not very firm. Of the direct cost components in the eight countries, between 55% and 85% are due to hospital care. Ulcer disease accounts for between 0.8% and 1.4% of the total costs of illness in the three countries for which estimates are available.

At the time a new technology appears, it may have two kinds of effect on cost. First, it may change the total cost of disease, and second, it may alter the distribution of costs across different categories. In the case of the introduction of cimetidine, the five *ex ante* national studies project total savings ranging from 0% to 54%. In his discussion of these studies, Jönsson makes a number of nice methodological observations. For example, in estimating the savings due to reduced hospitalizations, the *average* cost per bed day is acceptable if the number of hospital admissions is reduced, but the average overestimates potential savings if reduced bed

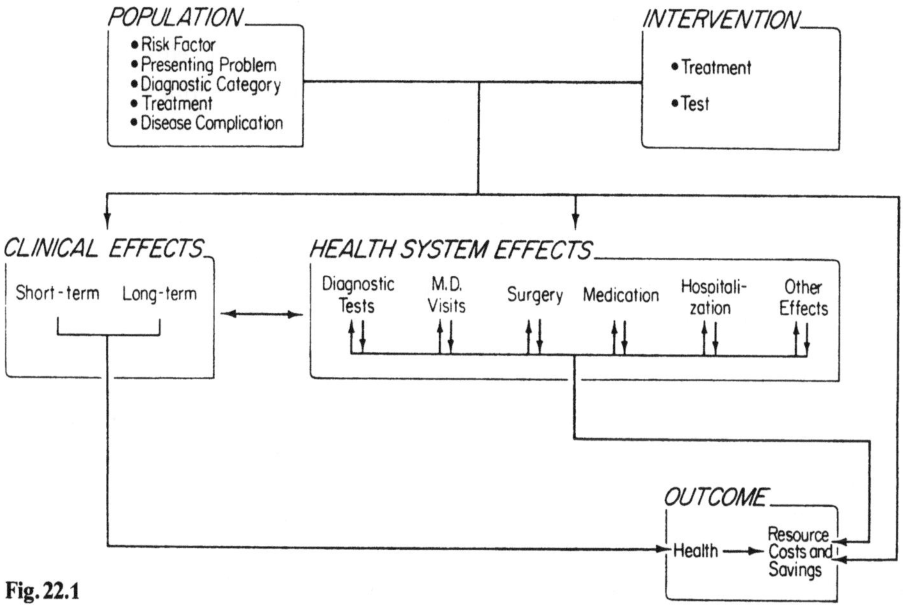

Fig. 22.1

days come in the form of shorter hospital stays. The studies vary in the extent to which they describe the detailed methods for projecting expected savings and in the apparent formality of their estimation methods.

Jönsson sees *ex post* evaluations as useful in their own right and as possibly helpful also for improving future *ex ante* estimates. Five *ex post* studies in four countries examine the trends in surgery before and after the introduction of cimetidine. All show a striking reduction following the introduction of cimetidine; I would like to return to this point later in my remarks. At the same time, overall hospitalization rates and average lengths of stay do not show a correspondingly large decline following the introduction of cimetidine. (Recall that this is all against a background of declining hospitalization rates for ulcer disease in most of these countries.) From this observation, Jönsson concludes that the various *ex ante* studies overestimated the total savings due to hospitalization. Relatively few data from national studies are available on the nonsurgical consequences of cimetidine.

Comments

I would like to organize my comments on some of the issues raised in Jönsson's paper around the elements in an evaluation model to assess the economic and medical consequences of a health intervention. As shown in Fig. 22.1, the evaluation of a new medical technology always entails the assessment of a particular health *intervention* in a particular *population* within a particular health *system* over a particular *time* period. We always have to try to think straight about these four elements (intervention, population, system, and time), in part because data that form the basis of health evaluations typically appear in various combinations of intervention-population-system-time, and not in just the combination that is the object of assessment. For example, in the case of ulcer disease, some pertinent cost and clinical data apply to patients with the diagnosis of peptic ulcer, some to patients with the diagnosis of duodenal ulcer only, some to patients with symptoms of ulcer disease, and some to patients self-reporting the diagnosis of ulcer. Obviously, each population is distinct and estimates based on one apply only partially to the others. In general, a target population may be defined in several ways – according to a risk factor for disease, a presenting clinical problem, a diagnostic category, and so forth. An intervention may be a test, like computed tomography, or a treatment, like renal dialysis or cimetidine. (In this context, preventive or rehabilitative interventions are, like treatment, designed to interdict the development or natural history of disease.)

Changes in any element of the model – the population, intervention, health system, or time-frame – will alter the evaluation. Assessors of new medical technology, like computed tomography (CT), are accustomed to worrying about evolution in the state of technology and the consequences of that evolution for economic and health evaluation. In the case of CT, for example, commercially available technology has progressed over the past decade from a device limited to the head and requiring several minutes to complete a cross-sectional slice to a device that can examine any part of the body in a few seconds per slice.

One lesson from the studies of cimetidine is that evolution in the population with disease can be as important to the assessment as any change in the technology itself. As we have seen in Horisberger's paper, the frequency and severity of ulcer disease has been declining steadily since the 1960s in some, not all, European countries and in the United States. This secular trend needs to be taken into account, both when projecting the expected effects of an intervention like cimetidine (the *ex ante* studies that Jönsson describes) and when attempting to measure its actual effects from regional or national data (the *ex post* studies). As Jönsson points out, some studies fail adequately to consider these trends, comparing for example the average of hospitalization or surgery in the 5 years prior to cimetidine with the rates in the 1st year following its introduction. Even a phantom intervention would appear to be quite effective, granted the advantage of such a calculation.

A key consideration in estimating the costs of a condition is to measure the costs exclusively and completely in the population that is amenable to the particular intervention, i. e., the target population. The key is to match any anticipated proportionate reductions in cost due to the intervention with the actual population subject to that proportionate reduction. Both Jönsson and I would criticize one of the more comprehensive *ex ante* studies of cimetidine because its estimates of percentage change in hospital costs are based on a less than full spectrum of hospitalized ulcer patients and then applied to the hospital costs of all ulcer patients.

The choice between a prevalence and incidence approach in estimating the cost of illness is likewise reduced to the question of gauging the costs in the actual target population of the intervention. The effects of a preventive intervention that has no bearing on the course of established disease should be measured against the costs of incident or newly acquired illness. The effect of a treatment that has no influence on the contraction of disease should be measured against the cost of prevalent illness. To some extent the analyst can choose the population for which to measure costs, but some estimates of the effect of interventions require data collected in economic studies and clinical trials designed for other purposes. The appropriate caution is always to ask whether the population in a study is properly representative of the full target population or if it is more or less inclusive than the target population.

In comparing the economic consequences of a new intervention in different countries, the various health systems are obviously going to be quite varied in organization, in total resources, and in the deployment of resources. In a country like the United States, with a pluralistic health care system, an intervention like cimetidine may have varied economic impact within a single national setting. Hypothetically, for example, suppose physicians in a prepaid group practice have a higher threshold for operating on ulcer patients than do physicians in private practice. Then an intervention like cimetidine could have a proportionally greater or lesser impact on surgery rates in the prepaid group practice depending on the drug's effectiveness in the most severely afflicted patients. The variation in health systems among countries raises questions about the comparability between countries of changes in cost following the introduction of cimetidine, and I will say more about this later in my remarks.

As an evaluation deals with the intersection of a population and an intervention, it is neither a complete assessment of alternative approaches to the population's problem nor of the impact of the intervention. A prominent feature of the use of cimetidine, for example, is the frequency with which it is employed in patients who do not have a diagnosis of ulcer disease (Fineberg and Pearlman 1981 b). The clinical effectiveness, risk, and cost of *all* uses of an intervention contribute to its overall impact. The intended effect of a new technology, properly used (sometimes called its "efficacy") may diverge widely from its actual use and net effects (termed its "effectiveness").

The three subject areas in this volume may be arrayed along several dimensions related to this evaluation model. One of these is the degree of specificity in the target population to which the intervention applies. In this respect, cimetidine rests in the middle, between renal dialysis, which applies exclusively to patients with end-stage renal disease, and CT, which is employed in a wide variety of clinical situations. The task of assessing the overall economic impact of a technology becomes progressively more demanding as the variety of patient types increases.

In terms of net economic consequences, cimetidine is the most likely of the three to produce net savings in resources. Renal dialysis is costly. CT, while an outstanding technological triumph, has the handicap of any diagnostic procedure – to simplify somewhat, its costs apply to all who are examined, and its benefits are restricted to the smaller number who benefit from the treatment that was initiated because of the information gained from the scan. If we believe that economic investments in health are, at root, value judgments about the social benefit of care, then some measure of intangible benefits is most sorely missed in cases where productivity measures fail to show a net economic advantage. In the case of cimetidine employed in patients with peptic ulcer disease, the need is not all that pressing.

Jönsson's paper highlights differences in the methodological approaches used to measure cost consequences in the various studies. He concludes: "There is a long way to go before we have such a consistency in the methodology applied that we can with confidence compare studies for different diseases and different countries" (p. 261).

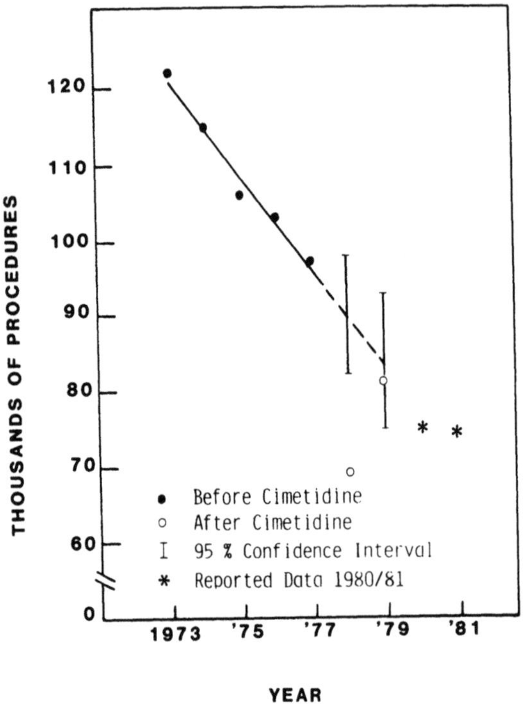

Fig. 22.2. Ulcer surgery in the United States, 1973–1979

For the moment, I would like to stress another observation, the remarkably consistent pattern in surgery in the *ex post* studies in different countries; and I say "remarkably" almost as an understatement. This holds true despite differences in the basis for counting operations noted by Jönsson. (Records in some countries trace the number of surgical procedures, and records in others trace the number of patients in a diagnostic group who undergo surgery.)

Figures 22.2 and 22.3 depict surgery for ulcer disease in the United States for 1972–1978. Figure 22.2 indicates that surgery in 1978, the first full year after the introduction of cimetidine in the United States in mid-1977, declined much more than expected based on the previous 5-year trend. The number of operations rose in 1979, still remaining below the projected level based on the pre-cimetidine trend. The number of operations in 1980, shown on Fig. 22.2, declined again to approximately 75000 procedures and to 74000 in 1981. Figure 22.3 shows the same data normalized to a scale of 100 in the initial year, 1972. Plotted on the same normalized scale are the surgery figures for the Netherlands. Again the introduction of cimetidine in 1977 was accompanied by a marked decline in surgery in the following year.

Cimetidine was introduced in Great Britain in 1976, one year earlier than in the United States or the Netherlands. Figure 22.3 shows the trend in surgery for ulcer disease in Great Britain. The dip in surgery in 1975 reflects a general decline in surgery that year due to a physician's strike. (The total number of *all* operations in Britain decline 0.4 percent between 1971 and 1978. In 1975, there was a 6.1 percent decline compared to the previous year, compensated by a 7.4 percent rise in the following year.) Notice that the striking drop in surgery for ulcer disease in Britain oc-

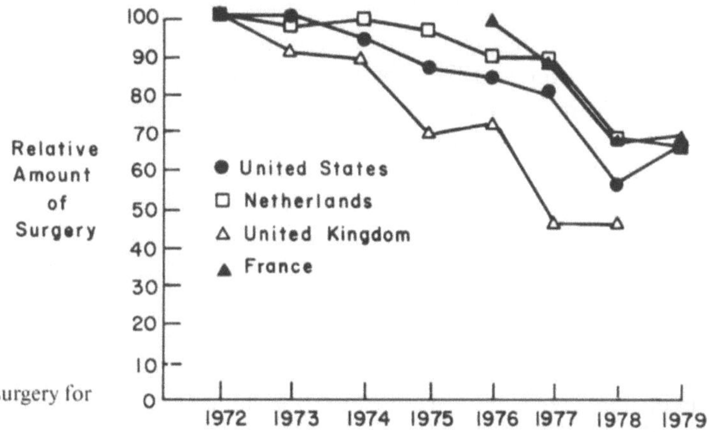

Fig. 22.3. Trends in surgery for ulcer disease

curs in 1977, one year earlier than in the United States or the Netherlands and coinciding with the earlier release of cimetidine in Great Britain (Fig. 22.3).

The data we have from France are incomplete for the years prior to 1976. Here, where cimetidine was also introduced in 1977, the decline is similar to those in the United States and the Netherlands (Fig. 22.3).

Overall in these countries, the average annual decline in surgery for ulcer disease was 4% during the five years prior to the introduction of cimetidine. In the year following the introduction of cimetidine, the average decline was 24%, and this figure is remarkably consistent in all four countries. Nature tends to proceed in a continuous fashion, and it is difficult to imagine any sudden epidemiologic aberration that would create the parallel discontinuities in the rates of surgery that we see in each case in the year after cimetidine's introduction. Credibility strains to the breaking point if we postulate a natural force that appears by chance a year earlier in Great Britain than in the United States, France or the Netherlands.

Based on the projection of earlier surgical trends and the actual rates observed, I would estimate conservatively that in the first two years following the introduction of cimetidine in these four countries, there are savings of more than 60,000 operations for ulcer disease. In a few countries there is evidence for a rebound in surgery in the second year following the introduction of cimetidine, but still not to levels that exceed the projection based on earlier trends. Translating the reductions in surgery into relative economic savings depends on the particular mix of resources required for surgery in each country relative to other expenditures for ulcer disease, relative to all health expenditures, and relative to the total resources available in the economy.

Queries

Reflecting on Dr. Jönsson's review, I would like to raise several questions for more general consideration.

Who is the audience for macro-economic evaluations of new technology? In his paper in this volume, Weisbrod points out that expenditure analysis, as distinct from resource analysis, may be the most pertinent form of assessment for decision makers who supervise fixed budgets for the reimbursement of medical services. Who are the decision makers who should be attending to macro-economic evaluation? In particular, are cross-national comparisons of results, as distinct from a single national study, of special interest to any policy makers?

In its review of systematic resource studies in health, the U.S. Congressional Office of Technology Assessment concluded that cost-effectiveness analysis and cost-benefit analysis can helpfully array the consequences of medical interventions, but they are not in general sufficiently reliable and consistent to serve as a trusted basis for policy making. Do you agree? Based on the review of these macro-economic studies or on other experience, do you believe the quality and consistency of studies can be improved? To what extent are variations in studies due to differences in the objectives or values of the analysts; to inadequacies in the clinical, epidemiological and health system data bases; to knowledgable disagreements about methodological approaches; to methodological errors and misjudgments; and to other factors?

Throughout Jönsson's review, I detect a quiet yearning for comparability across the national, macro-economic studies. Is such comparability attainable? We are all familiar with the reasons why traditional market forces do not apply to pricing in the health system. Different countries vary in almost every important element that makes up macro-economic assessment of a medical intervention: the total wealth of the country; the resources devoted to health (absolutely and relative to the total); the epidemiological patterns of disease; the prominence of any one disease relative to others; the measured units of health services and the mix of resources that comprise each unit; patterns of diffusion and utilization of new technology; and cultural patterns of work, family life and response to illness. In the face of all this variation, what can we conclude from comparative figures about, say, the proportion of total costs of ulcer disease due to indirect losses? Country A may have a lower proportion of indirect costs compared to Country B. Yet if the total cost of the disease is sufficiently higher in Country A, the per capita indirect costs of the disease relative to all disease costs may be higher in Country A than B. Depending on the total burden of illness and the Gross Domestic Product (GDP) in the two countries, the comparative indirect cost relative to GDP may flip in the opposite direction. I despair of making sense out of comparative changes in proportions where the numerators and denominators are each subject to so many fluctuations and interpretations. I tend to think that data on disease epidemiology (deaths, incidence rates, prevalence) and on units of health service (physician visits, hospital days, operations) are more readily comparable than are the resources assigned to different components of the cost of illness in different countries.

Jönsson and others have suggested that clinical trials may be more extensively utilized for the purposes of gathering socio-economic data pertinent to the economic analysis of a new technology. He alludes in his paper to area-based comparisons intended to ascertain the effects of a new technology.

Weisbrod has likewise described a detailed study in a defined population. The principal theoretical limitation in relying on controlled clinical trials is the frequently inappropriate comparison group (placebo rather than alternative therapy) and a major limitation of area-wide studies is the possibility of selection bias. To what extent can these and other drawbacks be overcome for each type of study?

Finally, Jonsson makes the intriguing observation that by comparing studies with our previous *ex ante* projections, we might learn something about how to adjust future *ex ante* estimates for new technology. I would caution that this is likely to be a long learning process because each *ex ante* – *ex post* pair represents a single observation, and we can only learn by discerning patterns and causal connections in a series of observations. The nature and possible causes of mismatch in the *ex ante* – *ex post* estimates of economic consequences are innumerable. Perhaps some systematic mis-estimates in a component of cost would emerge after a few examples, but there is no assurance of that result, especially when one considers the potential variety in technologies that may be subject to *ex ante* and *ex post* analysis. Are there other, more ready ways in which we can learn from comparing *ex post* to *ex ante* studies?

Summary of Workshop Discussion

The discussion that followed Fineberg's comments and his synthesis of results obtained in various countries after the introduction of cimetidine (ex post) concentrated on the following points.

1. *International comparison:* everybody was struck by the similarity of trends in the different countries. This is especially astonishing since there are no two countries that define their hospitals, length of stay, and so on in the same way; there are many factors that differ, yet one obtains similar results in all health service system. The only factor that is the same in all countries is the technology, e. g. a drug or a medical device. Thus at the macroscopic level the new device produces perfectly comparable effects although there exist many limitations in the use of data for cross-national comparison. Therefore, in future, systems evaluation should focus on such problems as to why cimetidine, used by two different groups of physicians in the same country, is less effective in one group. We do not know the cause but most probably some physicians are more proficient than others. Such studies would enable us to define patient management better.
2. *The overall systems effect* can be observed only if the new drug or device is widely accepted by physicians and patients alike. Attractivenes to the physician may be due to effectiveness, while convenience is the main factor to the patient. In the case of cimetidine there was general agreement that it is the remarkable convenience, together with the subjective pain relief, in contrast to the inconvenience and side effects associated with larger doses of antacids. These factors in turn will result in a better diffusion of the new technology through the health services at the individual, clinical level. The generalized systems effect then is the result of a myriad of individual clinicians' decisions to prescribe cimetidine and of their patients' compliance in taking them.
3. In the *assessment and evaluation* of a new drug or device, performing a cost-effectiveness or cost-benefit analysis is only one tool. It should, however, not be the only tool upon which to base public decisions, especially macrodecisions. But along with other kinds of information, by providing another perspective, by rounding out the full answers to a medical technology utilization questions, it can help to decine whether in fact use of the new technology should be expanded or not. Cost-benefit and cost-effectiveness analyses are not such that they provide a cookbook recipe so that anybody, whatever his training, can, by just following the recipe, proceed with such analyses. But there is another aspect. By doing such analyses economists and physicians become interested in the process of assessing. With all the shortcomings of existing methods, what is the alternative? It was the general belief that up to now the economist had no better procedures than to use cost-benefit and cost-effectiveness analyses. Everybody agreed on the limitations of these techniques but the limitations of the data (in both quantity and quality) were seen as more serious than the limitations of the methodology itself.
4. There is a *need to train* economists, epidemiologists, and medical doctors in the application of these decision technologies. Decision-makers in senior positions trying to deal with their daily problems of social control may be alerted by studies

which they cannot appreciate in detail. Existence of these studies will eventually exert an impact on their behaviour, reasoning, and decision-making. However, one must keep in mind that such analyses should take into consideration the various aspects of medicine and society. A bias is introduced if cost-benefit analyses serve as relevant values or rationing devices and if benefits, in the eyes of the individual consumer, are evaluated on an inappropriate scale. This means that "system rationality" may differ from "individual rationality" or preference.

Part IV

Computerized Tomography of the Head

23 Critical Questions Regarding a New Diagnostic Technology: A Case Study Using Computerized Tomography of the Head

B. J. McNeil and J. A. Hanley

Harvard and McGill

Controversy among neurologists, radiologists, public health planners, hospital administrators, and politicians has marked the use of computerized tomography (CT) since its inception in 1973. At one extreme, some have pointed to its high costs and unproven efficacy and say we should be concerned about its rapid diffusion and potential overuse (Office of Technology Assessment 1978b). At the other extreme are those who have pointed to its safety, its freedom from discomfort for the patient, and its unique ability to image soft tissues as reasons for encouraging its rapid diffusion and availability to larger segments of the population (Baker 1975). Both extremes have highlighted three key questions that must be asked of any new technology;

(1) Is it more efficacious than existing alternatives? (In this case the existing alternative is radionuclide imaging). How much so?
(2) Can we direct it towards those who need it the most? (Or, keep it away from those who need it least?) What tradeoffs would be involved if we were to try to be more selective in its use?
(3) How much does it cost?

This paper will address briefly the first two questions using data from several studies conducted in the United States.

Calculation of Its Effectiveness

In evaluating the amount of diagnostic information available from a new imaging technology (e.g., CT) relative to that available from an existing one [e.g., radionuclide (RN) imaging] it has become apparent that the receiver operating characteristic (ROC) curve is the best approach (Swets 1979). It requires the development of a series of true-positive (TP) and false-positive (FP) ratios representing different levels of confidence associated with separating normal from abnormal cases. The advantages of the ROC approach over single TP/FP pairs are twofold: (1) It eliminates the ambiguity associated with observer bias – a tendency to overcall or undercall lesions. It does this with little extra effort on the part of the readers participating in the study; specifically, instead of merely calling an examination normal or abnormal they grade (usually on a four- or five-point scale) the chance that it is abnormal. (2) From the above series of TP/FP ratios a curve can be drawn so that one can project for a given TP ratio the corresponding FP ratio, and conversely for any FP ratio, the TP ratio.

Three years ago Swets and his colleagues used this approach to compare CT

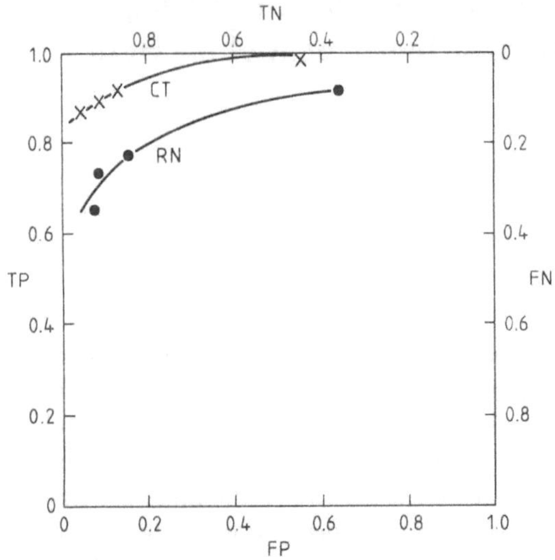

Fig. 23.1. ROC curves for CT and RN scanning of the head. The data for CT are on an ROC curve everywhere above the curve for RN imaging, thus indicating the superiority of the former technique. For example, at a TP ratio of 85%, the FP ratio of CT is only about 4% whereas that for RN scanning is about 35%. Source: McNeil (1982). (Clinical Decisions and Laboratory Use, p. 195, 1982. University of Minnesota Press)

and RN imaging of the brain (Swets et al. 1979). The authors compared the abilities of each modality to identify mass lesions in the brain, to localize these lesions, and to classify them into one of several disease categories. For simply *detecting* lesions and with an FP ratio of 10%, the TP ratio or sensitivity of CT was about 92% and that of RN scanning 72% (Fig. 23.1). By this index CT appears superior to RN. One other index can be used to document this; it is the area under each curve. The closer the area is to 1.0 (i.e., 1.0 times 1.0) the better the performance. The area under the CT curve in Fig. 23.1 is 0.97 and that under the RN curve is 0.87.

Swets carried the comparison of CT with RN one step further and demonstrated that in more specialized tasks, e.g., detection *and* something else, CT was also superior to RN (Fig. 23.2, right panels). For example, in combining detection and disease classification and with an FP ratio of 10%, the sensitivity proved to be 70% for CT and 55% for RN scanning.

The data displayed in Figs. 23.1 and 23.2 convincingly indicate that CT is superior to RN at all levels of diagnostic information. Two related questions remain: (1) what effort or experimental design is required to obtain this type of information; (2) if the differences in area were not so dramatic, how would we approach the statistical analysis?

Apart from instrument-related issues, four requirements must be met. First, if two competing modalities are being tested, examinations must be conducted independently of one another such that the results of one cannot dictate the technique employed in the other. Second, the study must be prospective (otherwise, we could never be sure requirement 1 was met) and all images graded on a four- or five-point scale to allow the drawing of ROC curves. Third, there must be independent proof

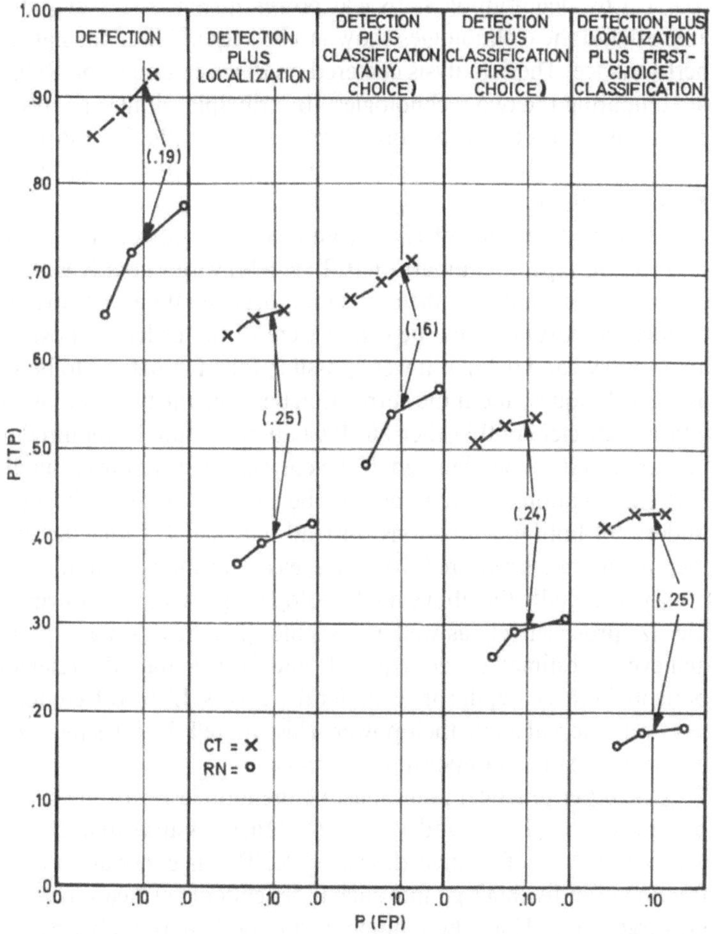

Fig. 23.2. ROC curves for CT and RN scanning for five tasks. On the *ordinate* is the TP ratio, *P(TP)*, and on the *abscissa* is the FP ratio, *P(FP)*. The *ordinate* runs from *0* to *1.00*, while the *abscissa* goes only from *0* to approximately *0.15* for each of the five tasks. These tasks range from pure detection to detection plus localization plus disease classification on the *far right*. The data indicate that for each of the five tasks, the ROC curves for CT were above those for RN scanning. For all tasks involving detection plus something else (panels two to five), the ROC curves are depressed relative to those for detection alone. This phenomenon occurs because these combined tasks are a subset of the detection tasks alone. (Swets et al. 1979).

of the final disease status for those patients included in the ROC curves. Fourth, the sample size must be sufficient to ensure that the statistical power is high if differences in performance appear small.

The first three of these requirements are relatively straightforward and have been discussed elsewhere (McNeil 1979); the fourth is more complex. Recent studies by Hanley and McNeil (1982a, b) have addressed this issue in two ways: (1) by showing *before* the study begins how to calculate sample size using real differences in the performance of the two competing techniques that would be important to detect; (2) by determining statistical power *after* a series of patients has been examined and the technologies shown to be "equal" (i.e. not statistically different) in performance. Their analysis centered on the area under the ROC curve as a means of comparing the two technologies. [In principle, similar analyses should be possible for other indices of performance, e.g., a sample TP/FP point along the curve, but these are only just now being developed (Hanley and McNeil 1983; Metz and Kronman 1980)].

In brief, the results of Hanley and McNeil showed that the sample size necessary for this type of comparison (CT vs. RN) varies greatly with the accuracy of the two modalities and with the correlation between them. For example, if the real differences important in the detection were of the order of those finally shown (i.e., areas of 0.97 and 0.87), if it were possible for each patient to be studied by *both* imaging techniques, and if the correlation between the two areas were high (e.g., correlation coefficient of 0.5), then 80–100 patients would be required for statistically significant results to be obtained. If the correlation were lower but all patients still had *both* examinations, the required numbers would rise. Finally, if none of the patients underwent both examinations (instead half had CT and the other half had RN), then the numbers required would increase enormously, in this case to 300 or 400.

Operationally the above methodology suggests the following: (1) estimate sample size prospectively as well as possible; (2) study as many patients as possible to achieve the estimated size required; and (3) calculate the relevant indices of comparison, in this case, the areas under the curves. If the differences in the indices are not dramatic, calculate their power. This will tell the investigator the chance that he or she is missing an important difference.

One other practical point must be mentioned regarding sample size. The numbers present in Hanley and McNeil (1982a, b) assume that the patients have *all* had independent proof of their disease state. This is generally not true because only a fraction of individuals go into such independent verification via angiography, biopsy, surgery, etc. Thus, these numbers are too low, probably by several fold at least. Our experience at the Brigham and Women's Hospital in Boston suggests that two institutions and 1½–2 years of study are generally minimum requirements for obtaining adequate numbers of patients for studies of this sort.

Can We Be Selective in the Use of CT?

Determining who benefits the most from a CT examination of the head is a difficult, if not impossible, task. Determination of who should be examined first, were CT resources to be limited, can be conceptualized somewhat more easily. For example, we might examine those with the highest probability of having disease detected by CT, those with the highest probability of having treatable disease identified, those with the highest probability of having potentially curable disease identified, or those most problematic diagnostically. Different types of methodological approaches would exist for each of these alternatives. This review will mention only the first – in other words, can we identify individuals with a very high or very low chance of having an abnormal CT? If this separation cannot be fully achieved what would be the consequences?

Table 23.1. Evaluative characteristics in patients having CT of the head (Roberts et al. 1981)

Findings	Frequency of occurrence in entire population (%)	Likelihood ratio
Aphasia	9.4	2.5[a]
Papilledema	2.2	2.02[a]
Gait disturbance, noncerebellar	11.8	1.68
Dementia or altered behavior	27.5	1.62[a]
Depressed consciousness	17.1	1.59[a]
Motor weakness	32.4	1.50[a]
Head trauma	8.8	1.48[a]
Fever or infection	5.4	1.39
Sensory alteration	19.1	1.25[a]
Altered vision	12.8	1.24
Posterior fossa sign, cerebellar ataxia	13.3	1.05
Nausea, vomiting	7.5	0.96
Altered hearing	3.2	0.91
Endocrine dysfunction	2.6	0.82
Seizure	16.4	0.82
Headache	24.0	0.78
Dizziness or vertigo	9.8	0.58

[a] Significantly different from 1.0 by χ^2 test.

One approach to this problem was taken by the Departments of Radiology and Neurology at the Brigham and Women's Hospital in Boston and the Baystate Medical Center in Springfield (McNeil et al. 1981). More than 2500 patients with new neurological problems at each institution were studied and their clinical characteristics correlated with CT head results. Two techniques were used to analyze these data. In the first technique, a disjunctive analysis was performed. It indicated that if only those patients with one or more significant findings (Table 23.1) were examined by CT, then the total number of computed tomograms performed at the Brigham and Women's Hospital would have decreased to 74%, but at the same time only 82% of the CT-detectable abnormalities would have been found. At the Bay State Medical Center, examination of only patients with significant findings would have led to a decrease in the total number of examinations to 68% and to the discovery thereby of 82% of patients with abnormal CT results.

In the second technique, a more detailed linear logistic analysis was performed in order to quantify further the probabilities. With it, however, most of the predicted probabilities were in the middle range (0.2–0.7) such that these predictions did not clearly separate between those who had abnormal results and those who had normal results. In other words, there was a nearly linear relationship between the percentage of patients with identified disease and the percentage of the original population that might have been examined using different probability cutoffs in the logistic expression (Fig. 23.3). Thus, using either the disjunctive or logistic approach for classifying patients was also associated with a sizable reduction in sensitivity, i.e., in the percentage of the population with positive CT studies thereby identified.

It could be argued that neither of the above methodological approaches in complete enough, and that, for example, a more sophisticated system of sorting might

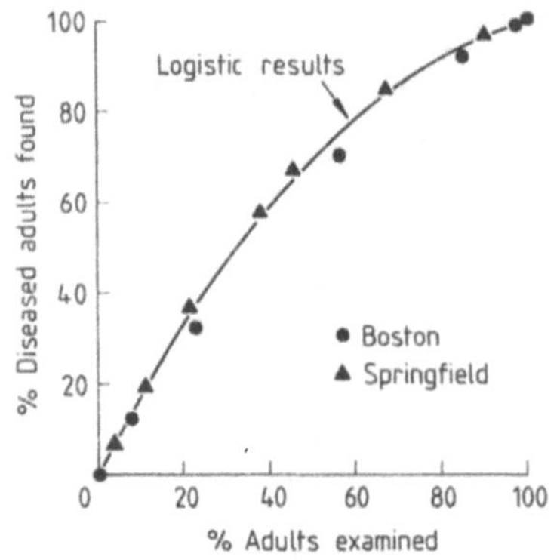

Fig. 23.3

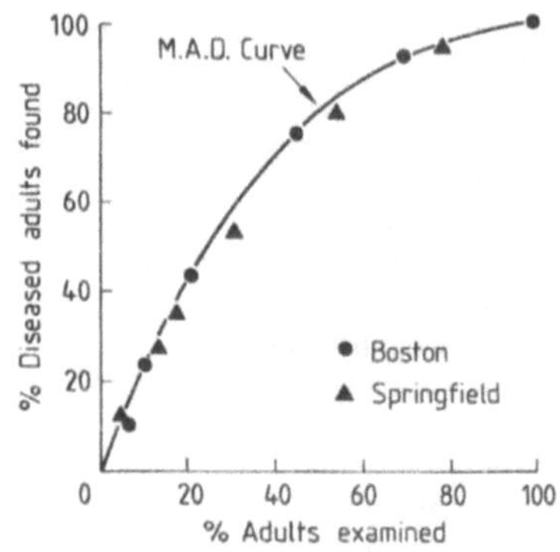

Fig. 23.4

Fig. 23.3. Discrimination results for CT examinations of the head. The *abscissa* represents the percentages of nearly 2500 patients that might be examined, ranging from a small portion to almost all; the *ordinate* shows what percentage of the total of all diseased patients would be found by CT if examinations were limited to the percentage shown on the *abscissa*. The *curve* shows the results of the logistic regression analysis described in the text. There is a close relationship between the percentage of diseased patients found and the percentage of total patients examined. For example, the analysis indicates that examining 60% of the total population would lead to detection of about 74% of diseased patients

Fig. 23.4. Maximum attainable discrimination (M.A.D.) curve for CT of the head. The *ordinate* and *abscissa* are as labeled in Fig. 23.3. However, the *curve* describes the *theoretical* limit of detectability using 20 pieces of data on each patient. The *curve* is only slightly convex *upward* and is only slightly better in performance than the logistic expression shown in Fig. 23.3

have led to better separation of normal patients from diseased ones. To address this problem we now present an approach that proves that such "negative" results are real. The approach rests on the concept of the *theoretically* or intrinsic maximum attainable discrimination available between patients with disease and those without disease (Hanley and McNeil 1982). It uses all available clinical data and requires that the patients be placed into unique sets, where all patients within a single set have exactly the same symptoms and are thus indistinguishable from one another but are different (by at least one symptom) from patients in any other set; the subsets so formed are the finest partition possible on the basis of available data. These subsets can be used to generate a performance curve whereby the percentage of patients with a relevant endpoint correctly identified is plotted against the percentage of the original population studied. This curve differs from the curve plotted in Fig. 23.3 in that the latter is an empirical one created on the basis of a *simple* logistic model. The former is the *theoretically* best one and may, in fact, not be approached by any simple linear logistic empirical model.

Figure 23.4 plots such a curve from the data base on patients having CT of the head. It shows that under the *best* of circumstances if CT examinations were performed on only 80% of the population about 8%–10% of diseased patients would be missed. This is an improvement over that found with a simple linear logistic model where 13%–15% would be missed (Fig. 23.3) and thus provides a *minimum* percentage of patients missed. Under these circumstances 63 patients (3% of all diseased patients) with intracranial masses, hemorrhage infection, or hematoma would not have been examined; another 101 patients with infarction, ventricular enlargement, or changes in their gray or white matter would similarly not have been examined. These results indicate that if an investigator were to try to improve separability by making the results of any numerical scoring or priority system approach those of the theoretical or best model minimum of 8%–10% of diseased patients would not be identified and their diseases would be as just indicated.

Summary

From a general point of view this review has discussed two of the three major problems associated with the application of new diagnostic or therapeutic technologies. For CT of the head we recognize that the debate over its usefulness is probably over – at least the recent National Institutes of Health consensus conference would suggest so. We believe, however, that the debate might have been over years ago had systematic studies relating to the questions posed in this paper been completed earlier. Such studies obviously require the timely availability of research funding, and the need for assuring this is great.

From a more specific methodological point of view, this paper has emphasized two areas. First, ROC analyses are becoming more useful as their statistical properties become better known; this phenomenon should increase the quality of analyses on effectiveness. Second, the maximum attainable discrimination concept allows investigators for the first time to say that their failure to achieve separation was a function of the patients' characteristics, not their analyses. The availability of this approach to validating "negative" results suggests that similar analyses might be useful on other previously published studies which, like ours, failed to achieve separation.

24 Discussion of Paper by McNeil and Hanley

A. H. W. Wahba and B. C. Visinescu

World Health Organization

We would like to underline the emphasis on evaluation research as it is prescribed in McNeil and Hanley's paper. Both the growing complexity of the diagnostic, therapeutic, and rehabilitative potential at the disposal of the physician and the increased cost from the excessive use of technologies of not necessarily proven efficacy and utility call on the responsibility of the medical and health professions to amplify their efforts to provide evaluation studies of high quality. It is quite true that one impediment to not having more evaluation studies done might be the scarcity of research funds directed to this area. Nevertheless one should try to stimulate a change in mentality in health care professionals as to the *status* of evaluation studies, which are often considered second rate from a scientific point of view.

McNeil and Hanley's paper shows well that highly scientific and intellectual reasoning is necessary for evaluation studies. The paper presents clinical work to test the usefulness of two new methods that should be considered important contributions to the methodology of evaluating diagnostic techniques: (1) The receiver operative characteristics (ROC) method, which we would describe as a method of measuring the combined sensitivity and specificity of the technology taking into account the variation that might result from subjective interpretation of the results; (2) the concept of maximum attainable discrimination (MAD), which can be used to analyze whether a reduction in the number of patients to be examined by a specific diagnostic method can be achieved without undue loss of its analytic power and vital clinical information. We will comment briefly on both methodologies but first we would like to take a somewhat broader approach to the methodology of evaluating new medical technologies in general.

The activities of the World Health Organization (WHO) Regional Office for Europe's unit for Appropriate Technology for Health are concentrating on the development of a health technology assessment network. In this network several institutes with different disciplinary backgrounds from different countries will engage to embark jointly in the area of evaluation. In the preparatory activity for this network we have found that it is fundamental to have a multidisciplinary approach. Also, we found that with the present state of affairs it is very difficult, though not impossible, to organize this multidisciplinary collaboration successfully. It appears that as a first approach it is necessary to consider evaluation in a rather broad sense combining in a systematic way all existing evidence on efficacy, technical quality, safety, cost-effectiveness, and patient and social acceptability of medical technologies.

Although it is very tempting to try and develop some sort of overall index of utility of a technology to compare with the financial resources that are spent in providing the respective service, for various reasons, especially with the case of diagnostic technologies, this has been difficult to achieve and so we are left with a weak methodology assessing the relation between effectiveness and technical quality of a technology and its expected impact on health outcome. The ROC method presented is a very elegant method of establishing the relative accuracy of a diagnostic technique, relative to any other (standard) technology. Swets et al. (1979) have already indicated in their paper on the ROC method that this method should be considered as a basis for further evaluation of the utility of a diagnostic technology. It would also include elements of medical efficacy, risk associated with a use of a particular technology, and cost evaluation. This type of evaluation, sometimes described as formal clinical decision analysis, involves the use of probability of responses from the use of diagnostic and therapeutic technologies in terms of health outcome.

The ROC method provides a good basis for determining the probability distribution in formal clinical decision analysis. An estimate of the cost involved may be compared with a net benefit in terms of health outcome. Alternatively it is feasible to try and estimate the extent to which an improved diagnostic technique would improve therapeutic management or make a rough prognosis of health outcome. Goitein (1980) used this type of estimation to provide indications of the cost-effectiveness of computed tomography (CT) in cancer radiation therapy by comparing the increment in benefit in terms of health outcome due to CT with the cost of diagnosis and therapy. CT was found to be cost-effective by a factor of 5.5 over traditional methods. Other studies have concluded that CT is cost-effective over traditional diagnostic methods used in the diagnoses of brain diseases (Jonsson et al. 1976; Barral 1980).

Cost analysis in these cases also deals with cost savings that might be achieved because CT would replace other more expensive technologies involving hospitalization and a much higher risk to the patient. These methods are pneumoencephalography and cerebral angiography in the case of brain scanning. This leads us to a point that very often proves crucial in the discussion of policy implications of imaging technologies like CT scanning. Although CT scanning in itself might be more cost-effective than other diagnostic technologies, savings will be achieved only when suitable organizational changes of improvements can take place, *redistributing the* available *capacity* of competing techniques that might also to some degree be considered as complementary. Availability of more than one technique seems to be correlated with the defensive use of more overlapping information than is strictly necessary.

So the answer to an appropriate use of imaging technologies would seem to be a proper planning system – possibly on a regional basis – assuring collaboration between several diagnostic centres that would concentrate on one or two technologies and provide services to those patient categories that have been demonstrated, in terms of health outcome, to benefit from the technology. This would enable: (1) maximum accessibility to all facilities of patients in need of a specific technology (assuming that not all the institutions would be able to purchase all diagnostic technologies); (2) sufficient work load for each unit can be obtained to justify experienced staff in a centre and provide high quality health care; (3) sufficient work load assures optimum economic utilization of a unit. The reasoning behind this is that although a technology might be both effective and cost-effective in itself, savings at the community level will be achieved only if organizational measures are taken to observe *cost-productivity* as well. Also, it is necessary to avoid using complex diagnostic technology in these areas where it cannot be expected to influence (in a positive way) the therapeutic process and thereby to have a positive contribution to health outcome. The MAD concept presented in McNeil and Hanley's paper appears to be an excellent analytical tool for the researcher and clinician but not for the health economist and health planner. We would advocate the combination of this concept with some index indicating the ability to influence therapeutic management of care of *specific groups* of patients affected by particular diseases. Both for reasons of quality of care, to avoid unnecessary discomfort to the patient, and economic reasons, it appears necessary to direct more effort to define these groups of patients from the epidemiological point of view.

A changing responsibility pattern is imposed upon the medical profession. Although its main *responsibility* should remain with the *individual* patient, an economy of scarce resources imposes on the profession the nescessity of providing the basic elements for the assessment of realistic needs for technological health care at the community level. The clinical elements of efficacy and safety should be combined with economic data and systematic assessment of other data such as patient and social acceptability of technology to provide guidance to policy-makers. Limited resources impose a choice at the community level between *rationalization* and *rationing* of health services. For both processes an adequate input of medical data is necessary for two reasons: (1) if rational choices cannot be made at the community level, groups probably most in need of medical care, such as the chronically ill and the elderly, are most likely to suffer from the nonavailability of health care resources for basic health care; (2) if it proves impossible to provide valid clinical reasons to guide rationalization or even rationing of health care services, scarce resources will enforce the necessity of choices to be made on another basis like budget restrictions based on financial criteria alone.

The example of the CT scanning is very illustrative in this respect. Because of the high cost of investment and exploitation related to its use, efforts were undertaken in many countries to restrict the diffusion of this technology. Very often nonhealth reasons were used as a basis for planning and this was due mainly to the lack of comprehensive evaluation studies on safety, effectiveness, and cost-effectiveness. Several authors (Banta 1980; Office of Technology Assessment 1981 a; Sterman et al. 1980) have shown that this sometimes leads to the installation of this costly technology in inappropriate places and to lack of capacity where it is really needed. An example of where comprehensive guidelines for appropriate use are provided on a national basis is to be found in Canada (Health Services and Protection Branch 1980). Guidelines were also developed in some European countries but generally not adhered to.

As already indicated more health services research is needed to demonstrate for which patient groups, in terms of health outcome and cost-effectiveness use, CT scanning is most indicated. Husband et al. (1982) recently reviewed the best indications for a CT whole-body scanner. It would appear helpful to implement this type of clinical retrospective study with prospective studies to quantify the relative benefit that specific indications can have from CT scanning.

Computed tomography is indisputably a powerful diagnostic tool especially in the area of cranial scanning and cancer treatment planning. In summary, the following conclusions seem to emerge:

(1) ROC, as a measure of accuracy of diagnosis, should be further developed as a tool to measure benefit to groups of patients in terms of health outcome
(2) Systematic multidisciplinary assessment of efficacy, as well as safety and cost-effectiveness, can and should provide data for policy-makers. These data refer to a system where all conditions are optimal. The inclusion of social and ethical points as well is desirable in such assessment
(3) The addition of utilization studies and epidemiological studies providing estimates of performance under average conditions can provide the basis for the planning of resources necessary to achieve savings at the national level
(4) Further research efforts into evaluation methodology would seem necessary
(5) The identification of those patient groups that positively benefit from CT in terms of health outcome would in particular need further clarification.

Summary of Workshop Discussion

The results of the workshop on evaluation of the effectiveness and efficiency of the computed tomographic (CT) scanner may be classed into: (1) those relating to the goals and purposes of the evaluation, (2) those pertaining to methodologies, and (3) those delineating basic limitations of all assessment studies. The following overview, however, does not follow this schema strictly so as to give an impression of the interaction between the participants.

Evaluation of *effectiveness* of technologies, using the very powerful receiver operative characteristics (ROC) and maximum attainable discrimination (MAD) techniques, should be symptom-centred or centred on specific diseases, the natural histories of which are known. In addition, benefits should be specified in relation to the population. *Population-based evaluation* is clearly necessary for the definition of effectiveness as well as for economic assessment and for planning health services. Thus, assessment requires weighing benefits against costs at the level of the patient and the population, as well as at the level of the health care institution and the health system.

Assessment studies of future medical technologies (the efficacy of which may not be demonstrated as clearly as in the case of CT scanning in certain, select diseases) should therefore include not only their impact on treatment and outcomes in certain well-defined cases, but also bring these results into relation with the size, age, and morbidity of the population cared for. The population-based analysis of changing strategies in care used in the case of doudenal ulcer and cimetidine might serve as an example.

Secondly, it is equally important to characterize the *institutional* framework in which a technology is used and evaluated, both with respect to its relation to the environment (referring practitioners, catchment area and demographic characteristics, access, etc.) and with respect to its structure (number and kind of specialities and special services with access, within the hospital, to the technology), Moreover, information on the organization of the health and financing systems (including some of the prevailing control mechanisms) may be needed for the characterization of the institutional framework.

Belgian experience has shown that it is preferable to assess a new technology under "controlled conditions", in pilot studies, in a few centres to obtain information on utilization (of the new and existing technologies), effects, outcomes, and costs. Only such a comprehensive evaluation allows for the development of criteria for planning, for authoritative negotiation about reimbursement rates, etc.

In many countries it seems that new technologies are often overutilized, a process favoured by a fee-for-service system. One form of (goal-oriented) rationing is attained by restricting (within a hospital) access to the (new) technology. In the case of CT scanners, utilization may be limited to neurosurgeons, neurologists, certain internists, and otorhinolaryngologists (Finnish experience). Flexible fee-for-service systems, as applied in Belgium, can have stronger effects on utilization. Once medical effectiveness is evident, reimbursement rates are continuously adjusted to volume (of utilization). Another, additional approach to influencing or curbing utilization is exemplified by the American Radiologists Association, which published guidelines, i.e. compilations of indications for CT scanning. Depending on the agency issuing the guidelines for utilization these may or may not describe optimal usage. In any case, *systems effects* of another type should be taken into account. If access (by physicians) to certain technologies has been established, or if the capacity of departments using certain technologies has reached a particular level, the difficulties in controlling and changing utilization are greater. Technology by itself establishes indications for its use; nobody is rewarded for not using a technology. This is why marginal benefits have to be looked into very thoroughly. It is also the reason why conventional medical technologies (not requiring very large investments, such as clinical chemistry and ultrasound) should also be evaluated.

25 Economic Evaluation of CT Scanning of the Head: A Review

E. Jonsson and P. M. Jonsson

Swedish Planning and Rationalization Institute of the Health Services and the University of Stockholm

Economic evaluation of medical technology implies, in brief, calculation of the costs of resource inputs in relation to what can be achieved by them. In theory the approach essentially is to identify, quantify, and assess all relevant inputs and relate these to their outcomes. However, this may be difficult in practice.

The problems in calculating costs are clearly minor compared with the difficulties in determining and measuring valid end-points in an economic evaluation of diagnostic technology. The benefits or measures of effectiveness of a diagnostic technology may in principle be sought in its (a) pure technical merits, (b) diagnostic implications, (c) impact on therapeutic processes, and/or (d) influence on patient health outcome. Technical merits refer to equipment safety, operational aspects, less complicated machinery etc. The diagnostic implications of a technology – disregarding therapeutics and treatment outcome – could be addressed according to its ability to: (a) produce accurate information (including both true-negative and true-positive findings) measured in sensitivity, specificity, and predictive values; (b) produce intermediate outcomes such as reduction of risk, relief of pain, anxiety, and discomfort from testing, measured as number of patients affected and in terms of actual consequences of physical and psychological risk; (c) directly and indirectly replace other diagnostic procedures, measured in volume and cost (i. e. directly to replace entirely an alternative method or indirectly to eliminate the need of further testing due to findings in the process of the diagnostic work-up).

Impact on therapeutic processes could focus on measurable aspects (expected versus actual measures) of a technology's ability to: (a) provide more precise guidance for planned therapeutic procedures; (b) provide information that actually changes physicians' treatment plans, for example away from an "unnecessary" intervention; (c) provide guidance in choosing between several therapeutic alternatives, for example between surgical intervention and palliative therapy.

The ultimate endpoint would be to measure patient health outcome in terms of changes in mortality, morbidity, and quality of life. In certain cases it should be possible to arrive at a common manifestation of the diagnostic and therapeutic values in changes in treatment outcome. This would be the case if a diagnostic technology provided an opportunity for: (a) detecting a preventable or curable disease at an earlier stage; (b) defining the location and extent of a disease more precisely, therefore improving its prognosis.

The great majority of studies published on economic evaluation of computed tomographic (CT) scanning of the head have focused on diagnostic implications mainly measured in the technology's ability to replace other, sometimes less effective and more costly, diagnostic procedures. In most, or all, of these studies CT scanning is more or less implicitly assessed by its ability to produce positive findings. Little or no systematic effort has been directed at the economic implications of the technology's ability to diagnose nondisease, i.e. to establish the positive value of negative findings.

Some General Methodological Concerns

An evaluation of any technology must relate to the objective or objectives for which it is used. In the health context the objective is generally assumed to be optimal health outcome (Weinstein 1979). However, a diagnostic technology may not itself directly relate to the health outcome of patients – except for more immediate outcomes in terms of mortality and morbidity related to the risk of a diagnostic procedure. Therefore, a more complex definition of the effectiveness of CT scanning of the head will be needed.

Several suggestions have been made as to how effectiveness of CT scanning could be determined. Fineberg et al. (1977 a) have identified a hierarchy of five levels representing the routes by which CT scanning could influence outcome. These are: *technical capability* – does the device perform reliably and deliver accurate information? *diagnostic accuracy* – does use of the device permit accurate diagnoses to be made? *diagnostic impact* – does use of the device replace other diagnostic procedures? *therapeutic impact* – do results obtained from the device affect planning and delivery of therapy? *patient outcome* – does use of the device contribute to improved health of the patient (Office of Technology Assessment 1978 b). Fineberg notes that since CT scanning of the head is employed in the diagnosis of serious neurological conditions where even the best available therapy may not affect longevity, "studies of the effectiveness of CCT for such patients must be sought in treatment changes that affect morbidity and quality of life".

Abrams and McNeil (1978 b) also state that although health outcome as the criterion of effectiveness is „a general one and clearly the best one" such a measure when applied to diagnostic technology has both theoretical and practical limitations. Health outcome may not be altered because of the nature of the disease. And even if it does, this takes a long time to measure and "adequate studies cannot usually be performed before decisions regarding regulation and diffusion must be made". Abrams and McNeil suggest that valuable measures of effectiveness can be found in whether new diagnostic information is actually received. This can be measured in three different ways: 1) accuracy, 2) short-term morbidity/mortality from diagnostic testing, and 3) effect on therapy planning.

Many other authors have brought up methodological issues and in particular discussed the limitations in assessing CT scanning with respect to health outcome (Wortzman et al. 1975; Carrera et al. 1977; Evens and Jost 1977; Knaus and Davis 1978; Swartz and Des Harnais 1977). Among the arguments put forward are: CT scanning is a single test among many whose individual effect on health outcome would be almost impossible to distinguish (Evens et al. 1977), and measures of health outcome do not reflect the value of reassurance (Larsson et al. 1980) or the value of negative findings (Zimmermann et al. 1978). Although many such limitations could be reasonably dealt with in an economic analysis it seems as though the effectiveness of CT scanning of the head has to be sought in a less definitive context until treatment alternatives for many of the neurological conditions have emerged or more valid indices for measuring changes in morbidity and quality of life are developed.

A technique that would at least explicitly illuminate – array – all relevant factors and should be taken into account in an assessment of medical technology, has been proposed for policy-making purpose (Office of Technology Assessment 1980). One such study has been performed on CT scanning of the head (Jonsson 1980). In this study a number of potential consequences of the introduction of CT scanning were listed. Some of these – replaceable pneumoencephalographies and cerebral angiographies – were quantified and assessed in monetary terms and also weighed against the costs of introducing CT scanning. The resultant "net" monetary value was put against all nonquantified remaining factors and the final judgement was left to the individual policy-maker.

Costs and Utilization of CT Scanning of the Head

The cost of CT scanning of the head includes of course not only the purchase price of a scanner (now ranging from $ 0.2 to 0.5 million) (Jonsson and Marké 1981) but also operational costs. These are, in essence, costs of personnel, costs of equipment maintencance, costs of supplies, and indirect costs jointly shared by several departments such as costs of administration, transportation, heating, electricity, cleaning, laundry. A number of studies have examined capital and operational costs of CT scanning in relation to utilization, patient volume etc., revealing varying agreement in costs and cost relationships (Lille and McCullough 1977; Office of Technology Assessment 1978b; Gempel et al. 1977; Jacobsen et al. 1975; Banta and McNeil 1978; Winter 1978).

In a model study on the economic implications of CT scanning (Evens 1981) it was estimated that the largest single cost item – 33% of total costs – were overheads (close to 80% of these being cost of administration, education, and fringe benefits). Salaries accounted for 24% and depreciation for 20% of total costs. The costs of supplies were estimated at 7% and equipment maintenance at 16% of total costs. A similar study on the cost of CT scanning in Sweden, covering all hospitals in the country with experience of the technology (Jonsson and Marké 1981), shows the main cost item being costs of personnel (29%), followed by cost of depreciation (25%), and cost of equipment maintenance (16%). Cost of overheads – differently defined from above – was calculated at 13%.

Studies of CT scanning at three hospitals in the US (Enlow et al. 1979) showed that utilization of a particular scanner is a function of patient demand, scan time, ratio of head to body procedures, and medical practice. Factors affecting the number of procedures performed were idle time, scheduling delays, and scanning speed. A survey of all operating CT installations in the United States in 1976 emphasized that costs vary due to factors such as depreciation method, maintencance requirements, number of personnel, geographical area, utilization, and overheads allocation (Evens and Jost 1976). Patient volume – average 55 per week – was thought to have a minimal effect on total costs since only the variable costs and some indirect costs were said to be affected by increased volumes. On the other hand increased patient volume has a significant effect on the cost per patient. In a follow-up study, (Evens and Jost 1979) it was found that average patient volume per week had risen from 55 to 63 and the total cost had increased by almost 5%. This increase in total cost may partly be due to an 8% increase in the use of contrast studies. It was also found that the majority of the institutions surveyed in this study (49 of 67) were meeting the US national guidelines on utilization – 2500 patient procedures per year.

Impact on Other Diagnostic Procedures

Computed tomographic scanning of the head has had an impact on several other diagnostic procedures, notably pneumoencephalography, cerebral angiography, radionuclide brain scanning, echoencephalography, electroencephalography, skull X-ray, and exploratory surgical procedures. Many of the early studies on the impact of CT scanning on the utilization of other neurodiagnostic tests were somewhat speculative in their approach. Some were based on interviews with physicians and others were retrospective studies of records, whereby it was either estimated how many different examinations *would* have been necessary in the absence of CT scanning (Wortzman and Holgate 1979) or how many could be replaced *if* CT scanning would have been available (Ekbom and Marké 1975; Broman and Pedersen 1975). However, weak though the data base for these projections has been, the estimates have proved to be fairly correct. The ability of CT scanning to replace a number of other diagnostic procedures is now well documented (in addition to references already stated, see Hillier and Baker 1976; Ambrose et al. 1980; Winston 1978). For example, the number of pneumoencephalographic examinations has been reported as having declined by up to 84%, cerebral angiography by up to 35%, radionuclide brain scanning by up to 90%, skull X-ray by up to 24%, and exploratory surgery by up to 58% as a result of the availability of CT scanning.

An examination with CT scanning of the head does in principle not require hospitalization as is usually the case in examinations with pneumoencephalography and cerebral angiography. Thus there should be a concomitant reduction in the number of patients admitted for inpatient care as these kinds of examinations can to a certain extent be replaced by CT scanning. An analysis of neurological and neurosurgical admissions at a major US hospital prior to and after the introduction of a CT head scanner revealed a decreased length of stay of 7 days for patients with extracerebral collections after the introduction of the scanner. Patients with tumours had a reduction of 8 days. A subgroup of patients matched by age, diagnosis, and physician showed a shortened length of stay of 3 days per hospitalization (Bahr and Hodges 1978). From another study, conducted at a major hospital in the UK, it was found that the average length of stay for patients undergoing neurosurgery was reduced from 18 days in 1970 to 13 days in 1976, although CT scanning was only one factor in this overall reduction. The waiting list for neurosurgical admissions was completely eliminated and the patient volume at the unit increased by 10%.

Estimated cost-savings of replaced neurodiagnostic procedures with CT-scanning rest very much on shortened hospital stays in many studies (in addition to previous references, see Thomson 1977; Bartlett et al. 1978). In one of these (Jonsson and Marké 1981) a fairly detailed statistical analysis was undertaken to demonstrate the cause and effect relationship in reduced hospital stays at neurology and neurosurgery departments and the introduction of CT scanning. The results indicated a valid relationship. However, there is a frequent need for continued hospitalization among patients with neurological diseases regardless of diagnostic procedures undertaken (Fineberg et al. 1977; Abrams and McNeil 1978b). Cost-savings obtainable from anticipated reduction in hospital stay may therefore be overestimated.

In an early Canadian evaluation of the diagnostic impact of CT scanning of the head substantial savings in costs were anticipated from replaced examinations and averted hospital stays (Wortzman et al. 1975). However, in a reappraisal 4 years later it was concluded that the health care system had induced increased costs in all areas where savings had been anticipated (Wortzman and Holgate 1979). Savings in hospital beds were not truly realized because the total number of beds required to handle the patient care load within the entire community did not decrease. Length of hospital stay remained unchanged since more complicated cases were admitted. The costs per neuroradiological diagnostic procedure, which could not be replaced by CT scanning, were calculated as having increased substantially since fixed costs were deemed to have remained as high as before.

The evidence of cost-savings obtainable from the trade-off between CT scanning and other neurodiagnostic procedures is somewhat contradictory and shows a complicated pattern of underlying assumptions. Evens and Jost (1977) concluded that CT scanning is cost-beneficial in comparison with radionuclide brain scanning in spite of the fact that the latter procedure is less costly. An analysis of the the clinical efficacy (measured in sensitivity, specificity, and accuracy) of the two procedures showed that CT scanning would increase accuracy at a marginal cost of US $ 70. However, clinical experience demonstrates that a negative radionuclide brain scan will be followed by CT scanning at a joint cost of US $ 181. As this may happen frequently the authors conclude that a cost-benefit approach is to establish CT scanning as the first procedure of these two options.

A substantial reduction, 94%, in craniotomies for head trauma was found as a result of the advent of CT scanning in a study by Ambrose et al. (1976). This should produce considerable savings by reducing exploratory surgical procedures. Such savings will, however, only be fully realized when the number of operating room personnel, supplies, and overheads are reduced. Otherwise, the general effect of fewer procedures is an increase in unit cost (Abrams and McNeil 1978b).

It has been shown that for certain subgroups of patients undergoing neurosurgery and neurological treatment there are cost decreases (Winston 1978; Bahr and Hodges 1978) for example for intracranial tumours, as well as cost increases (Bahr and Hodges 1978), for example for cerebrovascular disease, in the total costs for neurodiagnostic work-up after the introduction of CT scanning. There are also studies claiming overal cost increases in the diagnostic work-up of patients referred to neuroradiological examinations due to a substantial increase in the number of patients examined by CT scanning (Knaus and Davis 1978; Abrams and McNeil 1978b). A study of two hospitals in the US demonstrated a marked increase in the total number of neurodiagnostic procedures since the introduction of CT scanning with no parallel increase in the number of in patients in neurology and neurosurgery departments nor of outpatient neurological examinations (Abrams and

McNeil 1978b). It seems quite likely that a "noninvasive" procedure such as CT scanning would be applied with much less strict indications for use than other invasive neurodiagnostic examinations and additional costs may be generated when many more CT scanning procedures are carried out than the total number of examinations replaced, as shown in some studies (Knaus and Davis 1978; Bahr and Hodges 1978). However, other studies show that such an increase in the total number of diagnostic procedures does not necessarily lead to total increases in costs, at least not when savings of bed days are included. In studies from the he UK (Thomson 1977) and Sweden (Jonsson 1980; Jonsson and Marké 1981), it was found that total estimated savings, including bed days, outweighed the total costs of CT scanning despite the fact that substantially more CT examinations were carried out than the number of procedures estimated to have been replaced. However, in the Swedish study it was concluded that predicted savings could quickly be offset by a rapid diffusion of the technology. The study was based on the prevailing circumstances up uptil the 1980s in Sweden when CT scanning was available mainly at regional hospitals. These have a large catchment area and the subsequent ability to utilize fully the capacity of the CT scanning technology for patients with strict indications for referral for this kind of investigation. As was pointed out: "... even if there is technical and personnel capacity to investigate many more patients ... it is possible that too broad indications for examinations may also create indirect economic consequences which will not correspond to the economic benefits put in prospect".

The accessibility of a fairly uncomplicated diagnostic procedure carrying almost no patient risk at all may challenge any limiting indication for use. An expanding number of patients "eligible" for CT scanning will certainly also have cost implications. For example, in a follow-up study of patients with a chief complaint of headache the cost for obtaining a positive result increased nine fold (from US $ 500 to $ 4363 in 1977) from patients with headache *and* abnormal neurological findings present to patients with headache only (Carrera et al. 1977). In another prospective analysis of more than 3000 scans performed during 1 year it was shown that the cost per case found also increased ninefold (from US $ 411 to $ 3500 in 1978) from patients in coma to patients with headache as their only indication for CT scanning (Office of Technology Assessment 1980). In a third study from 1980 it was demonstrated that the cost of finding a case of brain tumour in nuclear diagnostic medicine including CT scanning was US $ 1265 for patients with headache *and* abnormal findings on neurological examination. This cost increased nine fold to $ 11901 for patients with headache as the only finding on neurological examination (Larsson et al. 1980).

It was suggested that these findings should encourage physicians "to reduce their reliance on this diagnostic procedure where possible in favour of clinical judgement" (Larsson et al. 1980). However, it was also noted that as the costs relate only to abnormal findings they do not consider the value of reassurance in patients with neurological signs or symptoms. Physicians, patients, and the medical system as a whole are not willing at present to carry the consequences of underdiagnosis, no matter how small, but willing to pay the marginal costs, no matter how high.

Therapeutic Planning and Patient Outcome

Improved patient outcome from adequate therapeutic measures may be the yield of a diagnostic technology through its ability to detect early a curable disease or injury by giving precise information on location and extent of disease or symptom and by differentiating between conditions for which there are quite opposite therapeutic alternatives. There are a few studies published that systematically aim at demonstrating the impact of CT scanning of the head on therapeutic processes and/or the concurrent patient outcome. The impact of CT scanning on the treatment of patients with a broad range of (cancer) disease sites, for which radiotherapy was indicated, has been assessed in a number of studies (Goitein et al. 1979; Hobday et al. 1979; Ragan and Perez 1978) revealing changes for 38%–52% of all tumour patients studied. However, no clinical study of the impact of CT scanning on tratment outcome has been reported in this area (Goitein 1979, 1980).

The effect of CT scanning on physicians' diagnostic and therapeutic plans was also demonstrated in a prospective study by Fineberg et al. (1977). The study was based on perceived need of diagnostic work-up and treatment plans compared with actual measures taken in these respects. Therapy was altered in 19% of 194 patients scanned consecutively. There were four types of changes in therapy among these patients as a result of findings from CT scanning: new treatment was started, previously planned treatment became more precise, anticipated treatment as abandoned or found unnecessary. The authors maintain that the fraction of patients for whom therapy was altered represents an upper limit in this study since it is possible that factors other than CT scanning may have contributed to the decisions to change therapy. In commenting on their study the authors called attention to the fact that changes in treatment plans do not necessarily benefit the patients in terms of longevity. Attempts to assess the effects of altered therapy on outcome for patients with serious neurological diseases have to include measures of morbidity and quality of life along with figures of mortality.

In a study by Zimmerman et al. (1978) the aim was to establish possible prognostic values of CT scanning in patients with acute head trauma. In three subgroups of patients with life-threatening haematomas (extra- und intracerebral) diagnosed by CT scanning the postoperative survival rates "compared favourably" with the equivalent rates from the pre-CT era. The explanations for this were suggested to be the circumventing of delays and risks encountered with the traditional diagnostic procedure (arteriography) and the more rapid and accurate identification of lesions made possible by CT scanning.

In a similar study of patients with head trauma no difference was found in the overall mortality rates between patients seen before and after the advent of CT scanning (Ambrose et al. 1976). In another assessment, of 10 years' experience with radionuclide brain scanning for patients with brain tumour no significant difference in 2 year survival after surgery was found (George and Wagner 1975). This was in spite of a tenfold increase in the number of radionuclide brain scans, a shortening of the time interval from onset of symptoms to performance of surgery by 75%, and a decrease in postoperative mortality.

Summary and Conclusions

Few, if any, diagnostic technologies have been the target for such an extensive interest of economic analysis as CT scanning. Nevertheless, to date no single study demonstrates a thorough investigation of all the pros and cons of CT scanning of the head from an economic perspective.

The calculation of costs, whether of CT scanning or of other neurodiagnostic procedures, poses fewer difficulties than the identification and measurement of all direct and indirect consequences relevant to an economic evaluation of CT scanning of the head. There seems to be a fairly widespread agreement that patient outcome – in terms of mortality, morbidity, and quality of life – should remain the ultimate validator in assessments of medical technology including CT scanning of the head. However, there are many problems in this respect. A diagnostic technology is subordinated to important factors such as efficacy of treatment, which in turn is subordinated to the natural history of the disease. The potential quantitative impact on quality of life of CT scanning must await the development of methodology to conceptualize and measure these aspects.

The majority of economic evaluative studies published to date of CT scanning of the head have focused on costs versus cost savings of other, replaced, diagnostic procedures. Some of these are based on rather thin data and are somewhat anecdotal. Others are meticulously performed studies based on empirical facts, however, in many instances they make questionable assumptions. Most analysis demonstrate that CT scanning of the head is cost-effective despite the fact that only a minority of variables have been taken into account.

There are many pitfalls and biases to be aware of in the design of future scientific economic evaluations of CT scanning of the head. A prominent methodological problem will be to include the dynamics of all medical technology; the expanding indications for use as a technology become diffuse and the technology becomes more generally accessible. Another much neglected aspect of CT scanning of the head, which should deserve more attention in future economic evaluations, is the value of negative findings. The present approach suggests that all costs are to be set against the positive findings. This implies that a diagnostic technology producing almost only negative findings is vastly cost-ineffective however accurate these findings may be and whatever impact this may have in making other diagnostic procedures more cost-effective.

26 Discussion of Paper by Jonsson and Jonsson

U. Wiggli

University of Basel

Evaluation of patients' health outcomes is extremely difficult for the following reasons: it does not reflect the value of negative computed tomographic (CT) findings (– negative CT findings predominate); CT is only one factor influencing outcome – its influence in different diseases is not of equal importance; health outcome may not be altered because of the nature of the disease; definition of health outcome is relative – from individual to individual, from culture to culture, maybe even from health care system to health care system. This kind of evaluation (evaluation of health outcome) will take much too long to affect physicians in their choice of diagnostic and therapeutic measures.

There should be a mid-term or even short-term solution to integrate not economic *evaluations* but economic *thinking* into medical practice. Physicians have a well-developed sense of responsibility for their patients (to give the best treatment) and for themselves (to make the correct diagnosis) but there is only a moderate degree of responsibility for costs imposed on the health care system. By responsibility for the latter I mean giving due consideration to those instances where cost may outweigh benefit (where it is possible that cost is higher than benefit or where there is only cost and no benefit).

In most papers only cognitive aspects of diagnosis and treatment have been discussed. But there exist also social aspects, for example, the ways physicians see, think, and feel under everyday stresses and strains, the way each physician decides, what each one considers to be important, what each one considers ought to be done.

Decision-making is a complex mixture of actual expectation of yield from the procedure, personal approaches of the individual physician, and pressures in the decision-making environment. Here are some of the reasons for requesting an investigation: to prove or eliminate a diagnostic hypothesis; to document the clinical impression of normality; to do it for the record; for the physician to protect himself from legal consequences; to do it out of uncertainty; to obtain social and professional reward for the discovery of a new pathological condition; to do it routinely because of clinical inexperience. In addition, there are pressures from the patient, from relatives, or even from the referring physician.

To make a short-term solution possible for the evaluation of economic aspects of CT, the CT section (which is a multispeciality section) must know from year to year how valid its services have been in regard to patients' outcome – factors such as the final diagnosis, cause of death, and treatment obtained must be known. True-positive, true-negative, false-positive, and false-negative CT diagnoses may be extracted easily from the patient files. This makes necessary a good information flow within a hospital with all its affiliated services with the help of computer facilities. This greater information capacity should lead to increased diagnostic accuracy and more effective treatment.

Summary of Workshop Discussion

The salient results of the workshop on economic evaluation of the CT scanner may be summarized as follows. *The calculation of costs* of resource inputs should first consider specific, frequently occurring disease entities. It is known, for example, that costs for treatment of brain tumours have decreased with CT, whereas costs of treatment of cerebrovascular diseases have increased with CT. Secondly, evaluation needs to take into account the fact (1) that many negative results are obtained, and (2) that CT also produces unexpected findings. *Negative findings,* i.e. information on the nonexistence of a disease, may have reassurance value. Symptoms or quality of life, however, cannot always be expected to improve by the certainty that a suspected disease does not exist. More importantly, out-of-pocket as well as genuine opportunity costs are also incurred by tests with negative results. The values of the consequences of negative results may be estimated if the negative answer obviates other tests and procedures (which may themselves be risky). Health economists will have to develop techniques to value reassurance of the patient. The literature on insurance and the value of reducing uncertainty and on standard gambles should be consulted as to appropriate methods.

Any economic assessment of medical technologies comprises *technical evaluation.* Very few studies are available comparing machines from the engineering viewpoint related to economy. Price – performance ratios certainly should and can be established. Technical performance depends on the design and quality of the technology embodied in a machine. Too often prototype-like machines find their way into hospitals. First-generation machines all too often do not perform as expected, thus prohibiting an acceptable level of clinical effectiveness. Moreover, high running costs are incurred due to excessive maintenance and repair. The WHO Regional Office for Europe is now setting up a network of collaborating institutes for technology assessment. It will be coordinated by a body that will allocate resources, ensure rationality, divide the tasks (technical, clinical, economic), ensure quality, deter duplication, and collate and distribute results. Results of technical assessment of quality, performance, limitations, human engineering, maintenance needs, and need for personnel training in relation to purchase prices should also be available to financing agencies (e.g. hospitals).

Results of *educational programmes* aimed at physicians on the one hand and the public on the other to improve awareness about the costs of medical technology have not always been positive. Successful programmes, however, have been reported from Iceland. Medical students were told the prices of the procedures they prescribed. In addition, special clinical conferences were organized for all physicians in order to raise cost-consciousness and newsletters were circulated discussing clinical cases in connection with cost analysis. Apparently, the effects of these programmes in the relatively small Icelandic medical community were positive. Results with similar programmes using the news media may be achieved. It seems important that press releases are used to explain what should be done in specific cases and how benefits relate to costs in these cases. The WHO Regional Office for Europe reported two seminars for medical correspondents of the main European newspapers and networks with the titles "Alarm or Education?" and "Sensation or Sense?"

27 The Evaluation of Computerized Tomography: A Review of Research Methods

I. Russell

University of Newcastle upon Tyne

Introduction

The word "evaluation" spans a very wide spectrum of meaning – ranging from the ill-defined usage of the popular press through the careful but nontechnical explanations of the Oxford English Dictionary to the rigorous definition used by economists. This paper therefore begins by summarizing what the author, a health care researcher, understands by "health care evaluation". This phrase will be used to describe the process of choosing between alternative health care policies (in the widest sense, i.e. including alternative diagnostic technologies) by estimating the net value of each. It is helpful to break this process down into three main components:

1. The identification and measurement of the inputs consumed and the outputs generated by each policy. These inputs and outputs (which it is convenient to group together under the generic heading of "effects") may be subdivided into tangible effects and intangible effects. Tangible (or economic) effects are those, such as staff time, upon which is *relatively* easy to place a monetary value. Intangible effects, more difficult to value in monetary terms, may be further divided into clinical effects, such as a change in prognosis, and social effects, such as a change in patients' leisure activities. In the author's view, the major role in the identification and measurement of tangible effects should be taken by economists, of clinical effects by clinicians, and of social effects by behavioural scientists.
2. The valuation of the inputs and outputs thus measured. Although the author believes that the major responsibility for this task should be given to economists, there are other disciplines that would lay claim to it!
3. The estimation of the "technology matrix", i.e. the numerical relationships between the measures of input and the measures of output. To the author, it seems appropriate for epidemiologists and statisticians to play a major part in this activity.

Thus health care evaluation is both a complex process and one which requires close collaboration between a wide range of disciplines for its success.

This paper has two main aims. First, the main body of the paper discusses the potential contribution of epidemiological methods to the evaluation of computerized tomography (CT), in particular its technology matrix. Secondly, appendices A, B, and C present critiques of some of the epidemiological methods used in the literature to estimate this technology matrix. However, this paper is not intended to be comprehensive, for two reasons: first, if evaluation requires interdisciplinary collaboration, as argued above, then so does any comprehensive review; secondly, there have already been many excellent reviews (American Hospital Association

1977; Institute of Medicine 1977; Abrams and McNeil 1978a, b; Office of Technology Assessment 1978b, 1981b; Stocking and Morrison 1978).

Evaluation of Diagnostic Technology

Many authors, including Banta and McNeil (1978), McNeil (1979), and Wagner (1981), have stressed the particular difficulties of evaluating diagnostic technology. The estimation of the technology matrix as defined an p. 298 is even more difficult than in the evaluation of therapy. Not only is there a wide range of clinical conditions to be considered, but the chain of events by which any improvement in technical capability might improve patient outcome is long and complex.

Fineberg et al. (1977a) therefore suggested that the evaluation of diagnostic technology should be considered at four separate levels, subsequently extended by the Institute of Medicine (1977) to five (illustrated here by specific questions about CT): (a) technical capability – does CT provide better pictures than other diagnostic procedures? (b) diagnostic accuracy – does CT increase the proportion of correct diagnoses? (c) diagnostic impact – does CT replace other diagnostic procedures? (d) therapeutic impact – does CT lead physicians to change therapy? (e) patient outcome – does CT generate improvements in patients' clinical prognosis (e.g. as measured by longer survival)?

It has been suggested, for example by Ragan and Perez (1978), that this specific taxonomy for the evaluation of diagnostic technology is analogous to the general taxonomy for health care evaluation proposed by Donabedian in 1966 and elaborated by him in 1980 (also illustrated here by specific questions about CT): *structure* – does the institution (or physician) to be evaluated possess (or have access to) a CT scanner? what is the technical capability of this scanner? is it appropriately located, equipped, and staffed? *process* – does the institution (or physician) make "appropriate use" of the scanner? *outcome* – does the scanner improve patients' general health status?

At first sight, the analogy between Fineberg's specific taxonomy and Donabedian's general taxonomy appears useful. The evaluation of technical capability is contained within that of structure; the evaluation of patient outcome is contained within that of outcome. Nevertheless, it would be wrong to deduce that the evaluation of diagnostic accuracy, diagnostic impact, and therapeutic impact can all be regarded as evaluations of process. To evaluate diagnostic accuracy, diagnostic impact, or therapeutic impact is to apply objective criteria to assess the result of using CT a posteriori; to evaluate process is to apply normative criteria to assess the appropriateness of using CT a priori.

Although normative criteria for evaluating process can, and sometimes do, incorporate rigorous scientific findings, they are more often based on the pooled experience of groups of expert physicians. Norms for the "appropriate use" of CT have been widely developed in the United States, notably by the National Professional Standards Review Council and the Institute of Medicine (Office of Technology Assessment 1981a). An example of the application of such criteria to assess the use of CT is provided by Mehta et al. (1981). They inspected the medical records of patients who had been scanned by CT to check whether their scans met normative criteria developed by the hospital's utilization review committee.

In contrast, diagnostic accuracy, diagnostic impact, and therapeutic impact can all be measured objectively and do not require that normative criteria be developed before they can be assessed. By placing them between technical capability and clinical outcome, Fineberg et al. (1977a) are merely arguing that although positive changes in these variables may lead to an improvement in clinical outcome, such an improvement is not guaranteed. As argued on p. 299 however, Donabedian's (1980) concept of outcome is broader than that implied by Fineberg's taxonomy. More importantly, the concept of output adopted on p. 298 is even broader still, consisting as it does of all the identifiable effects of health care, whether clinical, social, or economic.

Hence diagnostic accuracy, diagnostic impact, and therapeutic impact should all be regarded as outcomes in Donabedian's terms, and outputs in the terms of p. 298. This argument may be supported by four examples. First, the diagnostic accuracy of CT confers benefits on patients anxious about the nature of their illness. Second, the therapeutic impact of CT confers benefits on patients spared unnecessary operations. Third, CT confers benefits on patients spared invasive diagnostic procedures. Finally, and in contrast, CT places patients who would not otherwise have been subjected to radiation at a very slightly increased risk of contracting cancer.

As well as supporting the argument that diagnostic impacts should be regarded as outcomes in the widest sense, these last two examples also serve to illustrate both the general difficulty of evaluating diagnostic technology and the specific difficulty of estimating such outcomes. First, to assess the expected benefit from fewer invasive procedures, one needs to estimate both the global proportion of patients spared such procedures and the expected benefit to each. Appendices B and C provide few grounds for confidence in the various estimates of the global proportion; furthermore, Harvey (1981) has shown that many of the papers which claim to estimate the risks of invasive procedures are methodologically unsound. Second, to assess the expected cost of increased radiation, one needs to estimate three parameters: the net change in the frequency of radiological procedures (the methodological problems of which are discussed by Kendall et al. 1980), the dose of radiation from each scan (Wall et al. 1980; Darby et al. 1980), and the relationship between dose and risk of cancer (International Commission on Radiological Protection 1977; Darby and Reissland 1981; Webster 1981).

It was argued on p. 298 that health care evaluation is concerned, in principle, only with inputs and outputs. Three conclusions for the evaluation of CT now follow. First, investigation of the process of CT scanning is not fundamental to the task of evaluation. However, this does not imply that this task can be entirely divorced from any consideration of process. Indeed, Brook et al. (1977) – strong proponents of the study of outcome – propose that outcome studies should also measure process with a view to identifying *how* improved outcomes are achieved. Second, since diagnostic accuracy, diagnostic impact, and therapeutic impact may all be regarded as outcomes in the widest sense, all three are relevant to the evaluation of CT, at least in theory. In practice, however, few (if any) attempts have been made to estimate the direct benefit of, for example, reduction in patient anxiety. Therefore, diagnostic accuracy receives relatively little attention in this paper. Finally, it is clear that the methodological problems of estimating the outcomes of CT scanning are profound. Although this conclusion stems from the apparently superficial discussion of two examples, it is reinforced by the case-studies reviewed in appendices A, B, and C. In the face of these problems, the remainder of the paper proper is devoted to a general discussion of the methods of health care evaluation as they relate to CT. Appendices A, B, and C add flesh to this theoretical skeleton by discussing a wide range of case-studies, four of them in detail.

Methods of Health Care Evaluation

There are essentially three approaches to the general problem of estimating a technology matrix:

1. Observational studies. This approach may be adopted only when the various health care policies to be compared can all be observed without intervention.
2. Quasi-experimental studies. This approach may be adopted whenever a decision-maker replaces one of the policies to be evaluated with another such policy; the evaluator may then compare these two policies *as if* the resulting data had arisen from a scientific experiment. Thus the typical quasi-experimental study is opportunistic. However the evaluator can adopt this approach deliberately, for example when there are practical or ethical objections to conducting a genuine experiment.
3. Experimental studies. This approach requires, not only that there should be an intervention in the status quo for the sole purpose of evaluating alternative policies, but also that the resulting comparison should exhibit all the essential attributes of a scientific experiment, in particular random allocation.

In theory at least, all three approaches suffer from three basis types of methodological problem. First, there are economic problems of comparability – problems that fall outside the scope of this paper – for example, what is the trade-off between survival and quality of life for cancer patients? (That this and many of the following examples relate to cancer does not imply that CT is more effective in the care of cancer than in the care of other conditions; it merely reflects the fact, illustrated in appendix C, that the *evaluation* of CT in the care of cancer is more advanced than in the care of other conditions). Second, there are statistical problems of measurability:

1. Validity – for example, is "local tumour control" a valid proxy for outcome in cancer patients?
2. Reliability – for example, do assessments of the quality of life vary between and within observers?
3. Accuracy, which requires both bias (i. e. systematic error) and random error to be minimized – for example, to estimate the 1-year survival rate from a given form of cancer with an acceptably low standard error would require a very large and unbiased sample.
4. Timeliness – for example, to estimate the 5-year survival rate from the same form of cancer would take at least 5 years.
5. Accessibility – for example, it is more difficult to measure outcome in patients who improve sufficiently to justify their discharge from hospital.

6. Feasibility – for example, quality of life indices are much more expensive to measure than survival.

Third, there are epidemiological problems of attributability. If the statistical problems of measurability can be overcome, the evaluater is likely to be faced with the question of whether statistically significant differences in outcome can be attributed to differences between the policies being evaluated rather than, for example, to differences in other prognostic variables such as severity and age. The fundamental objection to observational and quasi-experimental studies lies in the fact that such differences can only rarely be attributed with confidence to the policies themselves rather than to concomitant variation in any other factor that affects those outcomes.

In observational studies, problems of attributability usually arise from one of three basic sources: (a) underspecification, which occurs when one or more prognostic variables affecting patient outcome are unknown to, or ignored by, the evaluater; (b) multicollinearity, which occurs when one or more prognostic variables, either known or unknown to the evaluater, are naturally correlated with some other variable beyond the control of the evaluater; (c) selection bias, which occurs, for example, when patients are selected for CT on the basis of prognostic variables. These causes can be ameliorated, but never eliminated, by the skilful application of epidemiological techniques such as matching and standardization, and statistical techniques such as analysis of covariance. Unfortunately, the evidence of appendix C is that very few observational studies that claim to evaluate CT make any attempt to control for bias in these and other ways and thus reduce the problems of attributability.

Although quasi-experiments take many forms (Cook and Campbell 1979), health care evaluaters have rarely looked beyond the before-and-after study. In such a study, the experimental treatment is given, either to all patients (uncontrolled study) or to all patients in a predetermined subpopulation (controlled study) provided that they are treated after a particular time; in both designs, all the patients treated before that time are given the control treatment. The uncontrolled before-and-after study gives little more protection against underspecification, multicollinearity, and selection bias than an uncontrolled observational study.

One way of emphasizing the weakness of the uncontrolled before-and-after study is by listing some of the potential biases to which the demonstrably more powerful controlled before-and-after study is at risk:

1. Biased or haphazard choice of controls.
2. Secular trends in outcome or prognostic variables.
3. Seasonal trends in outcome or prognostic variables.
4. Discrete changes in prognostic or other variables.
5. Regression towards the mean. If the decision to introduce the new policy is triggered by poor outcomes over a relatively short period of time, there will be a natural tendency for outcomes to improve whatever the new policy (Davis 1976).
6. The learning process implicit in the introduction of a new policy.
7. Problems in statistical analysis arising from the temporal nature of the data, in particular autocorrelation (Box and Tiao 1965).
8. The Hawthorne effect, i.e. the tendency for data to be biased by study participants' awareness that they are being observed (Moser and Kalton 1971).
9. Secular trends in measurement errors.

Although appendix B identifies a considerable number of before-and-after studies claiming to evaluate CT, none took the precaution of recruiting a genuine control population. This is particularly disappointing since many of the papers in this field acknowledge the theoretical superiority of the randomized, and therefore controlled, trial. Even if, as these papers argue, randomization would be unethical under the particular circumstances of the study, this should be regarded as strengthening the case for a controlled study rather than undermining it completely as these papers seem to imply.

Apparently, only one randomized trial of CT has been published; although two randomized trials of diagnostic technology are discussed in appendix A, the second is not directly concerned with CT, though relevant to it. Hence the quality of the epidemiological evidence for the effectiveness of CT scanning depends almost exclusively on the quality of observational and quasi-experimental studies. Furthermore, the observational studies reviewed in appendix C and the quasi-experimental studies reviewed in appendix B are generally superior in quality to those studies not so reviewed; in particular, appendix C does not include any observational studies that were entirely uncontrolled. Unfortunately, as already mentioned, the combined evidence of appendices B and C is that very few studies of CT can be regarded as rigorous evaluations. Thus the evidence that CT scanning is effective in improving patient outcome is very weak. However, as argued on p. 298 and as the proceedings of this symposium demonstrate more cogently, a complete evaluation of CT scanners needs the full contribution of many other disciplines.

Although appendix A suggests that only one randomized trial of CT scanning has ever been published, there are three reasons for examining the methodology of such trials in some detail. First, the prospect of more trials being successfully completed is good, at least in Britain. Second, it is important to establish that randomized trials are far more effective in combatting the problems of attributability than either observational or quasi-experimental studies. Third, it is also important to discuss some of the problems that randomized trials generate and thus to try and dispel the widely held view that once the ethical hurdle has been surmounted randomized trials are simple.

Randomized Trials

Page 302 lists many of the biases inherent in judgmental methods of allocating patients to "treatments" for the purpose of evaluation. Many authorities, including Cochrane (1972) and Hill (1977), assert that randomization is essential to remove these biases. However, Fisher (1966) argues that there is an even stronger justification for randomization – that of providing a probabilistic basis for statistical inference.

The ethical basis of randomization, as laid down by both the World Medical Assembly and the British Medical Research Council, is that the rights of the individual patient are paramount (Hill 1977). Two principles follow from this. First, the only patients who may be randomized are those for whom we are ignorant of the relative value of the "treatments"; if we are *not* ignorant, if there is good evidence that one "treatment" is better than the other (either on average or for the patient in question), then the better cannot be withheld. Second, the patient must give his informed consent to take part in the trial (except in exceptional circumstances when patient psychology indicates otherwise). Once these two principles of *individual ethics* have safeguarded the interests of individual patients, the principles of *collective ethics* come into effect. Ex hypothesi, we are ignorant of the relative value of the "treatments". Hence a randomized trial is justified or, as some would argue, required as being in the best interests of the commonwealth of patients. Those patients included in the trial receive one of two "treatments" which are equivalent (a priori if not a posteriori), while those to whom the results are applied receive the "treatment" that performed better in the trial.

Although these principles have been published and widely accepted for 20 years, the debate over their interpretation is becoming fiercer as more and more trials are carried out. Two particular problems of interpretation have emerged – the meaning of equivalent treatments and the nature of informed consent.

At least in theory, more and more evidence as to the better treatment is accumulated as the trial proceeds. This raises the question of whether a trial the size of which has been carefully calculated in advance (not all trials come into this category!) should be stopped prematurely if the accumulating evidence heavily favours one treatment or the other. The most widely publicized example of such a decision occurred in the University Group Diabetes Program Study (Meier 1975). This trial was designed to compare the effectiveness of Tolbutamide, an oral hypoglycaemic agent, in treating diabetes with that of standard treatments such as insulin. Although cardiovascular mortality was not among the outcome variables as originally defined, the trial was eventually stopped when cardiovascular mortality in the Tolbutamide group exceeded that in other groups, nominally at the 5% significance level.

Two major proposals have been made to ameliorate the general problem of accumulating evidence – sequential trials (Armitage 1975) and adaptive allocation. Sequential trials have only their maximum sizes calculated in advance. If the difference between treatments achieves statistical significance at any time before the final patient is recruited, the trial is stopped. In adaptive allocation, the allocation probabilities are determined by the accumulated data. The simplest method of doing this is the "play the winner" rule (Zelen 1969). According to this rule, each success (however defined) on a given treatment generates a future allocation of that treatment to a new patient; conversely, each failure generates a future allocation of the other treatment.

For the present at least, the interpretation of informed consent is much more of a problem in the United States than in Britain. This led Zelen (1979) to suggest a fundamental change in the conventional design (Fig. 27.1). He proposed that the giving of information and the seeking of consent should come after randomization and be restricted to those patients randomized to the experimental therapy (Fig. 27.2). This provides an attractive solution to the immediate ethical problem of consent: the control patients are in the same position as they would have been without a trial while the "experimental" patients have to decide whether to accept the experimental therapy, arguably a more meaningful decision than whether to consent to randomization.

Once these ethical problems have been resolved, the investigator has to decide whether the objective of his randomized trial is to draw scientific conclusions (an

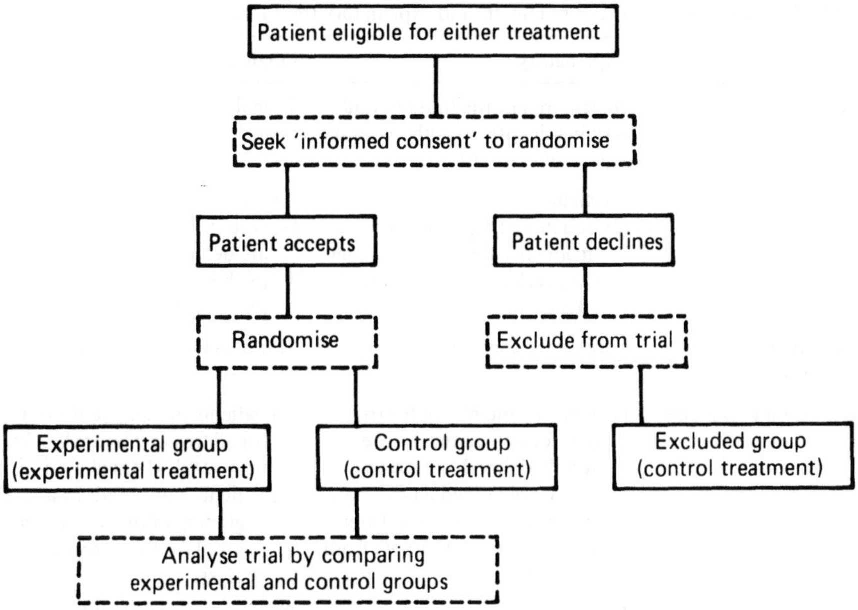

Fig. 27.1. Conventional design for randomized trial

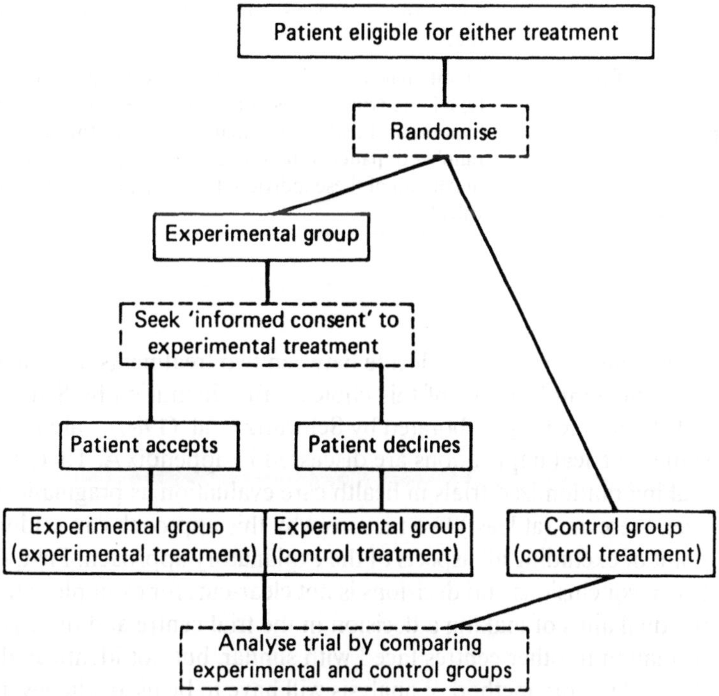

Fig. 27.2. Zelen's design for randomized trial (Zelen 1979)

Table 27.1. Differences between pragmatic and explanatory trials (Schwartz and Lellouch 1967)

	Explanatory	Pragmatic
Objective	To acquire information relevant to certain scientific hypotheses and thus to draw *conclusions*	To make a *decision* between two treatments
Definition of treatment	(1) Rigid (2) Equalized (in particular, treatments are defined so that the psychosomatic or placebo effect is the same for each)	(1) Flexible (2) Optimal (in particular, treatments are defined so that each makes the best of any psychosomatic or placebo effect)
Experimental conditions	Laboratory conditions	Normal clinical practice
Definition of patients	(1) Patients suitable for the trial (i.e. for all treatments) are strictly defined a priori and may be redefined a posteriori (2) Patients who withdraw from a treatment are withdrawn from the trial	(1) Patients suitable for the trial (i.e. for all treatments) are flexibly but irrevocably defined a priori (2) Patients who withdraw after the beginning of treatment remain in the trial for the purpose of analysis
Nature of criteria	Single or multiple	Single criterion only. Multiple criteria must be weighted (with weights based on practical considerations so as to form a single decision function
Method of analysis	Traditional significance test for each hypothesis (but no formal relationship between significance tests)	Select treatment which gives the best weighted decision function (no formal significance test)
Number of patients	Traditional calculation, based on type 1 and type 2 errors, for each hypothesis. Ideally, the actual number of patients should be the maximum of these individual calculations	Calculation based on the weighted decision criterion and on type 3 error (the probability of concluding that treatment A is superior to treatment B when the reverse in true)

"explanatory" trial) or to decide between two treatments (a "pragmatic" trial). The theoretical implications of this choice – first identified by Schwartz and Lellouch (1967) and recently elaborated by Schwartz et al. (1980) – are set out in Table 27.1; some practical implications are discussed in appendix A. There is a strong case for making randomized trials in health care evaluation as pragmatic as possible. However, there are (at least) two reasons why this approach can seldom be taken to the point of excluding all aspects of the explanatory approach. First, the distinction between conclusions and decisions is not clear-cut; for example, a trial will often have the dual aims of making a decision in the trial centre and of providing relevant information to other centres faced with similar, but not identical, decisions. Second, the explanatory method of analysis will have to be used whenever we are unable to assign weights to the individual criteria (Table 27.1).

Conclusions

In the evaluation of alternative health care policies, the estimation of the technology matrix, i. e. the relationships between inputs and outputs, is crucial. Evaluative studies that use observational or quasi-experimental methods are likely to generate biased estimates of this technology matrix, even if properly controlled. Bias is even more likely in uncontrolled studies. Unfortunately, very few evaluations of CT have been controlled. Nevertheless, it is argued in appendix B that the diagnostic impact of CT is so marked that it can be regarded as established despite these methodological shortcomings. In contrast, the evidence that CT is effective in improving patient outcome is very weak.

Since the diffusion of CT scanning is already widespread, especially in the United States, these conclusions are arguably less relevant to CT scanning than to the latest innovation in diagnostic technology – nuclear magnetic resonance (NMR) (Doyle et al. 1981; Hoult 1981; Young et al. 1981; Karstaedt and Maynard 1982; Moseley 1982). Since NMR will compete directly with CT, sound research methods will be needed to compare their diagnostic accuracies, let alone their effects on therapy and patient outcome.

Randomized trials are much less prone to bias than observational and quasi-experimental methods, even when these methods are applied more rigorously than they generally have been in evaluating CT. Hence randomized trials should be the method of choice for evaluating NMR. Nevertheless, in undertaking randomized trials there are many obstacles to be overcome, both ethical and practical. For example, randomized trials of CT are generally regarded as unethical in the United States; even in Great Britain, apparently only one randomized trial of CT has been published. It is to be hoped that these obstacles to rigorous evaluation will be tackled more effectively in the case of NMR than they have been in the case of CT scanning.

Appendix A – Selected Randomized Trials

A1. St. Bartholomew's Hospital, London

Reference: Dixon et al. (1981).

Summary of Method
Type of scanner: EMI 5005
Condition studied: palpable abdominal mass
Study population: 60 consecutive adults referred with new mass
Experimental group: 28 patients given CT as first imaging investigation and further imaging techniques as required
Control group: 25 patients given other imaging techniques
Excluded patients (all after randomization): two control patients given immediate laparotomy; one experimental patient found to have been partially investigated at another hospital; four patients lost to follow-up

Summary of Findings

Diagnostic accuracy (not statistically significant):

1. Experimental group, 27 "correct"/28
Control group, 22 "correct"/25 } not all histologically proven

Diagnostic impact:

2. Total time "needed" to reach diagnosis (statistically significant at 1% level) – experimental group, 2 days (median); control group, 12 days (median)
3. "Need" for inpatient investigation (not significant) – experimental group, 15/28; control group, 19/25
4. Time as inpatient "needed" to reach diagnosis (1% level) – experimental group, 3 days (median among 15 inpatients); control group, 9 days (median among 19 inpatients)

5a. Number of imaging investigations (1% level)
Experimental group, 1.14 (mean)
Control group, 2.08 (mean) } after excluding "review" investigations, since clinicians still learning about CT

5b. Number of potentially hazardous investigations (not significant) – experimental group, 0.32 (mean); control group, 0.48 (mean)

6. Financial cost per patient including inpatient stay (5% level) – experimental group, £ 266 (median); control group, £ 1122 (median)
7. "Need" for laparotomy (not significant) – experimental group, 11/28; control group, 8/25

Commentary

General:

a) On the basis of their literature search, Banta and McNeil (1978) were confident that no randomized trial of CT scanning had been published by that time. Dixon et al. (1981) was the only randomized trial of CT uncovered by the present author's literature search, undertaken through the British Library Automated Information Service (BLAISE); this is based on MEDLINE, the information retrieval system of the US National Library of Medicine. Although one cannot be certain that Dixon and his colleagues published the first trial in this field, they are certainly to be congratulated on a pioneering study. The comments that follow are intended to guide the design of future trials, not to belittle the contribution of the team from St. Bartholomew's Hospital.

Statistical:

b) The effective sample size of 53 was large enough to demonstrate that four of the findings (numbers 2, 4, 5a, and 6) were statistically significant. However, it is arguably too small to yield statistical tests of the other four findings (numbers 1, 3, 5b, and 7) that are sufficiently powerful to identify as statistically significant all differences which may be relevant to clinical practice. When there are many hypotheses to be tested, the sample size should ideally be chosen so as to yield an adequate test of all such hypotheses (Table 27.1).

c) In the report of any randomized trial, it is desirable to quote confidence intervals for all recorded differences between experimental and control groups. This is especially important when, as in this trial, the sample size is too small to yield adequate statistical tests of all such differences. Otherwise, the reader may be misled into thinking that differences which have no statistical significance also have no clinical relevance. For example, the proportion of patients undergoing potentially hazardous investigations was 16% lower (in absolute terms) in the experimental group than in the control group (finding 5b). (In the absence of any statement to the contrary in the published paper, I have made the simplifying assumption that no patient received more than one such investigation.) However, the standard error of this difference is 13%. Hence the confidence interval for the "true" difference lies between −10% (i.e. 10% more patients receiving such investigations after CT than after its absence) and +42%. In other words, this trial does not exclude the possibility that CT reduces the proportion of patients undergoing potentially hazardous investigations by 40% – a reduction that clinicians would regard as very important.

Epidemiological:

d) It is very desirable that future randomized trials of CT should incorporate measurements of patient outcome and, to a lesser extent, of therapeutic impact. In principle, there is a strong case for mounting large trials and collecting relatively few items of data on each patient; in particular, such trials would measure outcome by survival and other simple variables. However, if the number of patients available to be randomized is small (presumably true for this trial), the critical issue of patient outcome can be effectively pursued only by adopting more sensitive, and therefore more expensive, variables. Such variables fall predominantly into two categories – psychological scales to measure such concepts as quality of life, suffering, and anxiety, and empirical variables to assess the effect of the abdominal mass on employment, leisure, and daily life.

Methodological:

e) The published paper suggests that participating clinicians were allowed considerable freedom in their choice of investigations, subject to the requirements that experimental patients should first be given CT and that control patients should not be given CT. This degree of flexibility in the definition of "treatments" is one of the hallmarks of a "pragmatic" trial (Table 27.1) and therefore welcome. In contrast, if Dixon and colleagues had opted for a strictly "explanatory" trial, they would have had to draw up a rigorous protocol to determine the choice of diagnostic procedure at each stage of the investigation. Although the designers of any future "pragmatic" trial should therefore avoid the use of diagnostic protocols, they could profitably collect more data on the diagnostic "process" than Dixon and colleagues appear to have done. For example, participating clinicians could be asked to give a differential diagnosis (i.e. to list possible diagnoses and to estimate the subjective probability of each) along the lines adopted by Wittenberg et al. (1978) in case-study C1.

f) Although this trial is "pragmatic" to the extent that the alternative diagnostic regimes are relatively flexible, it exhibits a number of features typical of explanatory trials (Table 27.1):
   1. Objectives. Although not stated explicitly, these seem to be concerned more with scientific conclusions than with pragmatic decisions.

2. Definition of "treatments". Although relatively flexible, the control treatment was not so flexible as to permit immediate laparotomy.
3. Definition of patients. Seven patients who "withdrew from a treatment" after randomization were all withdrawn from the trial. In particular, it seems unlikely that the four patients lost to follow-up had nothing to contribute to the analysis.
4. Nature of criteria. The seven findings are presented more or less independently without any serious attempt to combine them into a single decision criterion.
5. Method of analysis. Each of the seven findings is subjected to a traditional significance test.

Economic:

g) Although the author's brief is epidemiological rather than economic, it is questionable whether Dixon's apparent use of the published average cost of hospital stay represents the true opportunity cost of an inpatient (see, for example, Russell et al. 1977).

A2. Nottingham City and General Hospitals, England

Reference: Dronfield et al. (1977).

Summary of Method

Type of technology: Olympus GIF-K endoscope (end view)
Olympus JFB-2 endoscope (side view)

Condition studied: acute upper-gastrointestinal-tract bleeding (definite or probable)

Study population: 318 consecutive patients referred with bleeding to Nottingham City Hospital and 99 consecutive patients referred with bleeding to Nottingham General Hospital.

Experimental group: 162 patients given endoscopy as first investigation

Control group: 160 patients given radiology as first investigation

Excluded patients (all before randomization):

32 with trivial bleeding not needing investigation
17 for whom radiology was inappropriate
7 for whom endoscopy was inappropriate
4 refusals
26 for other reasons
95

Summary of Findings

1. Diagnostic "yield" (statistically significant at 5% level): experimental group, 108 lesions (considered to be site of blood loss) detected/162; control group, 88 lesions detected/160
2. Therapeutic impact (not statistically significant): experimental group, 37 operations/162; control group, 42 operations/160
3. Patient outcome (not significant): experimental group, 18 deaths/162 (11%); control group, 13 deaths/160 (8%)

Commentary

General:

a) Since Dixon et al. (1981) was the only randomized trial of CT scanning uncovered by the author's literature search, Dronfield et al. (1977) has been taken as the second case-study of a randomized trial. It too is concerned with the evaluation of diagnostic technology and has implications for the future evaluation of CT. Like Dixon et al. (1981), it is to be welcomed as a pioneering study; again, these comments are intended, not to belittle its contribution, but to guide the design of future trials of CT.

Statistical:

b) The authors report significance tests only implicitly and confidence intervals not at all. (The significance level quoted above for finding (1) was calculated from Table 2 of the published paper.)
c) The effective sample size of 318 was large enough to demonstrate a significant difference in diagnostic yield. Although it is six times larger than the effective sample size used by Dixon et al. (1981), it is nevertheless inadequate to detect any plausible difference in intrinsic mortality between the two technologies. Although the observed mortality of 11% in the experimental group was 3% higher than that of 8% in the control group the standard error of this difference is also 3%. For the trial to have had a worthwhile chance of detecting a plausible difference it would have needed a total sample of at least 2000, i.e. 1000 experimental patients and 1000 controls.

Epidemiological:

d) It follows from comment (c) that randomized trials of diagnostic technology can only hope to identify differences in mortality if they are carried out in many hospitals simultaneously. Conversely, trials restricted to one or two hospitals, such as this one, should concentrate on more sensitive measures of outcome, as suggested in comment (d) on case-study A1.

Methodological:

e) The authors are to be congratulated on conducting an essentially pragmatic trial, as demonstrated by the following features (Table 27.1):
   1. Objectives. Although these are not stated explicitly, the final sentence of the paper "we therefore believe that an early endoscopic diagnostic service is not essential where there is an adequate radiological service" is the epitome of pragmatism.
   2. Definition of "treatments". Subject to the requirements that experimental patients should first be given endoscopy and that control patients should first be given radiology, participating clinicians were free to choose subsequent investigation and therapy.
   3. Definition of patients. All randomized patients were analysed as such.
   4. Nature of criteria. The authors' main conclusion is that since "endoscopy is not accompanied by any discernible benefit to the patient, these findings cast doubt on the need to provide emergency endoscopic facilities where radiological services are already adequate". These statements seem to imply a commit-

ment to a single decision criterion (or, in economic terms, to some form of cost-effectiveness analysis?)

5. Method of analysis. Table 27.1 stipulates that pragmatic trials should be analysed by selecting the "treatment" that gives the best decision function, without recourse to any formal significance test. (Statistical considerations play their part, not in significance testing, but in the choice of sample size and in the estimation of the decision function). Can the absence of significance levels and confidence levels from the published paper now be seen as further evidence of the authors' commitment to a single decision criterion?

f) Both Dronfield et al. (1977) and Dixon et al. (1981) provide evidence that diagnostic technology can be evaluated by randomized trials, in particular pragmatic trials. Although that of Dixon et al. (1981) possessed few pragmatic features, the participating clinicians were allowed considerable freedom in their choice of investigations; no rigorous protocol was imposed. Moreover, in the trial now under discussion, much more pragmatic than Dixon et al. (1981), the participating clinicians were free to choose both subsequent investigation *and* therapy; again, no rigorous protocol was imposed. As the authors seem to hint in their discussion, this double freedom can give rise to an inferential problem: suppose diagnostic technology A is more often followed by therapy C and technology B is more often followed by therapy D; can any valid conclusion be drawn about the relative value of technologies A and B?

In one sense, all pragmatic trials face an analogous problem, since each compares two pragmatic policies rather than two rigidly defined treatments. Nevertheless, the problem is demonstrably more severe in the evaluation of diagnostic technology, since therapy is so much less tied to diagnosis than, for example, postoperative care to choice of surgical procedure. The solution to the problem seems to depend on the extent of agreement among participating clinicians about the relative value of therapies C and D. If there is a clear preference for one therapy over the other, there is a case for introducing a therapeutic protocol that incorporates this preference. If there is no such preference, serious consideration should be given to randomizing both diagnostic technology and therapy, for example by adopting a 2×2 factorial design (Cochran and Cox 1957).

Appendix B – Selected Quasi-experimental Studies

B1. Atkinson Morley's Hospital, London

Reference: Ambrose et al. (1976).

Summary of Method

Type of scanner: EMI 1010

Condition studied: head injury

Research design: uncontrolled before-and-after study

"Before" group: last 100 consecutive patients transferred from general hospitals to regional neurosurgical unit for further management of head injury before introduction of CT scanning

Intermediate group: first 100 consecutive such patients after introduction of CT scanning
"After" group: 100 consecutive such patients 4 years later, i.e. after the learning process was complete

Summary of Findings
Diagnostic impact:
1. Number of technetium scans (statistically significant at 1% level) – "before" group, 22; "after" group, 8
2. Number of arteriograms and pneumoencephalograms, i.e. invasive and potentially hazardous procedures (0.1% level) – "before" group, 39; "after" group, 8
3. Number of exploratory operations (0.1% level) – "before" group, 33; "after" group, 2
4. Therapeutic impact (not statistically significant): "before" group, 14 definitive operations; "after" group, 13 definitive operations
5. Patient outcome (not statistically significant): "before" group, 23 deaths; "after" group, 23 deaths

Commentary
a) This study is uncontrolled in two fundamental respects. First, it provides no information on the trends in diagnostic procedures, therapeutic procedures, and patient outcome that would have been expected in the absence of a CT scanner; the usual method of seeking such information is by persuading one or more (preferably at least three) regional neurosurgical units in which no CT scanner was expected, to provide strictly analogous control patients over the entire period of study. Second, the study provides little information on changes in the pattern of transfer of patients with head injuries to the neurosurgical unit under study as a direct result of CT scanning; such innovations can be expected to generate additional transfers whose diagnoses and prognoses may differ substantially from those of the "before" group. Even if this study had been controlled in both these respects, it would have been at risk to the many potential biases listed on p. 302. In the absence of such controls, Cook and Campbell (1979) categorize the before-and-after study as a design that "does not permit reasonable causal inferences". Nevertheless the diagnostic impact of the CT scanner in this study is so dramatic that it cannot be entirely undermined by this criticism. However, it would be very risky to try to draw firm conclusions about therapeutic impact or patient outcome.
b) Many of the comments on case-studies A1 and A2 are also relevant to this study. However, it seems prudent not to repeat them here lest that be taken to imply that the absence of controls is anything less than a barrier to rigorous evaluation.

B2. Other Quasi-experimental Studies

The literature on CT contains many examples of quasi-experimental studies similar to that of Ambrose et al. (1976). Presumably, most of the investigators, if not all, took the view that CT was demonstrably superior to the alternatives in technical capability and diagnostic performance, if not in patient outcome. Arguing that randomization was therefore unethical, they adopted quasi-experimental designs as the best alternative to experimental designs. Unfortunately, the author's literature search has not uncovered any such studies which took the additional, but essential, precaution of recruiting a genuine control population.

Nevertheless, the apparent diagnostic impact of the CT scanner in these studies is so marked that it can be regarded as established beyond reasonable doubt, even in the absence of controls. By the same token, economic evaluations, in particular cost-effectiveness analyses, based on the resulting estimates of diagnostic impact are probably robust, at least in an epidemiological sense. Thus, the following studies, together with that of Ambrose et al. (1976), do make a positive contribution to the evaluation of CT scanning, but only up to the level of diagnostic impact:

1. Five before-and-after studies reported from the University of Washington, Seattle, USA, each covering a separate topic: cerebral angiograms (Larsson et al. 1977); suspected brain tumour (Larsson and Omenn, 1977); cerebrovascular disease (Larsson et al. 1978 a); suspected hydrocephalus (Larsson et al. 1978 b); headache (Larsson et al. 1980). All but the fourth of these adopted the same basic design as Ambrose et al. (1976), using an intermediate group as well as a "before" group and an "after" group. However, none of the groups contained more than 60 patients.
2. Three before-and-after studies at Johns Hopkins Hospital, Baltimore, USA, concerned with extracerebral fluid, intracranial neoplasms, and transient ischaemic attacks or known cerebrovascular accidents, respectively (Barr and Hodges 1978). These authors also made a valiant attempt to strengthen their research design by creating pairs of patients matched for age, diagnosis, and physician, one patient of each pair being taken from the "before" phase, the other from the "after" phase. Unfortunately, only nine such pairs could be found.
3. Four studies based, at least in part, on "interrupted time-series", i.e. a continuous series of patients spanning an extended period on either side of the introduction of CT scanning (Baker 1975; Knaus et al. 1977; Thomson 1977, 1979; Robbins et al. 1978). Although this research design is potentially more powerful than the less flexible before-and-after study, this potential can only be exploited by the use of sophisticated statistical analysis (Box and Tiao 1965; Campbell and Ross 1968). The study reported by Knaus and his colleagues from George Washington University Hospital, Washington DC, USA has two other noteworthy features. First, it provides a striking illustration of the vulnerability of uncontrolled quasi-experimental designs to changes in the pattern of referral: a "before" group of 124 patients with cerebrovascular disease had a mean age of 63 years while the corresponding "after" group of 100 patients had a mean age of 47 years. Second, in an attempt to correct this bias, the authors restricted comparison to within each of 16 diagnoses – nine cerebrovascular diagnoses and seven categories of brain tumour. However, although this stratification ameliorated the problem of differential referral patterns somewhat, it conflicts with du Boulay and Radue's (1978) plea that evaluative studies should select patients according to their presenting problem rather than their final diagnosis. In the terms of Table 27.1 stratification by diagnosis converted a pragmatic, but biased, study into an explanatory study with slightly less bias.

Appendix C – Selected Observational Studies

C1. Massachusetts General Hospital, Boston, USA

References (a) Fineberg et al. (1977a), (b) Wittenberg et al. (1978), and (c) Wittenberg et al. (1980).

Summary of Method

Type of scanner: (a) EMI head scanner; (b, c) EMI 5000

Study population: (a) 241 consecutive patients referred for CT head scan over a period of 17 days; (b, c) 1398 consecutive patients referred for CT body scan over period of 19 months

Conditions studied: (a) all; (b, c) those falling within one of ten protocols – mediastinum, retroperitoneum, bone or soft tissue mass, jaundice, pancreas, lung, liver, lymphoma, pelvis, urology

Excluded patients: (a) 34 with incomplete data, 13 second or third scans during study period; (b, c) 509 ineligible for all 10 protocols, 266 with incomplete data or technically unsatisfactory

Research design: observational study controlled by questionnaire completed by referring physician before and after scan, specifying:

1. Differential diagnosis (i.e. a list of possible diagnoses together with the subjectively estimated probability of each)
2. Proposed diagnostic plan in the absence of CT scan
3. Proposed therapeutic plan in the absence of CT scan

Summary of Findings

1. Diagnostic "understanding": (b, c) "improved" in 52% of patients
2. Diagnostic impact: number of angiograms – (a) reduced by 52%; (b, c) reduced by 83%

Therapeutic impact:

3. Choice of therapy – (a) "improved" in 14%; (b, c) "improved" in 14%
4. Precision of therapy – (a) "improved" in 10%; (b, c) "improved" in 23%

Commentary

a) This thoughtful design requires referring physicians to specify their differential diagnosis and therapeutic plan both before and after the CT scan, thus reducing bias in the estimation of the change brought about by the scan. Unfortunately, the question whether this change represents an improvement or a deterioration can often be judged only by the physician himself. Thus the estimates of percentage "improved" are basically subjective.

b) The original research design for the study of CT body scans (Wittenberg et al. 1978) proposed to match patients in whom planned surgery was abandoned with historical controls from a computerized research index. A patient discomfort questionnaire was also administered to 100 consecutive patients. However, the authors accord little weight to the resulting findings, thus acknowledging the difficulty of drawing unbiased conclusions about patient outcome from observational studies, however carefully controlled.

c) CT scanning is now so common in the United States that randomized trials are generally regarded as unethical and well-designed quasi-experiments are probably impossible. Under these circumstances, controlled observational studies such as those conducted at the Massachusetts General Hospital provide one of the few robust means of estimating the therapeutic impact of CT scanning. Furthermore, the relationship between therapeutic impact and patient outcome can be investigated independently of CT scanning. The next section suggests how these two approaches might be combined to estimate, if somewhat unreliably, some of the effects of CT scanning on patient outcome.

C2. Other Observational Studies

Although the studies by Baker and Way (1978) and by Bartlett and Neil-Dwyer (1978) are both superficially similar to those of Wittenberg et al. (1978, 1980), both estimated the diagnostic impact of CT scanning retrospectively rather than prospectively. However, conscious of the danger of bias, both pairs of authors sought to justify their subjective estimates. Bartlett and Neil-Dwyer backed theirs up with historical data, while Baker and Way verified each other's independent estimates.

The study by Baker and Way is also noteworthy for their attempt to estimate the effect of each CT scan on an arbitrary 18-point scale. This can be criticized on two grounds: first, although the scale has only one dimension, it is used simultaneously to measure diagnostic impact, therapeutic impact, and patient outcome; second, although the scale is defined as ordinal, it is later converted into a cardinal scale for the purpose of a "cost-effectiveness analysis".

In contrast, the controlled observational approach adopted by Wittenberg et al. (1978, 1980) has been more faithfully applied in studies of the effect of CT scanning on the precision of radiation therapy for cancer (e.g. Emami et al. 1978; Goitein et al. 1979; Prasad et al. 1981). Since the CT scanner can specify the location of known tumours with some accuracy, therapeutic plans drawn up before and after the CT scan can be compared more or less objectively. As a result, such studies can estimate the extent to which CT scanning can improve the effectiveness of radiation therapy, as measured, for example, by the dose deficit and the percentage tumour volume outside the field of radiation.

While acknowledging the theoretical superiority of experimental methods, Goitein (1979, 1980) shows how such estimates can be combined with existing observational data to estimate the effect of CT scanning on patient outcome. Using a statistical technique known as probit analysis to model the relationship between the effectiveness of therapy and the probability of tumour control, he estimates that CT scanning can improve the probability of 5-year survival by more than 3%. Nevertheless, the elegance of Goitein's mathematics and his careful use of sensitivity analysis should not be allowed to obscure the fact that his conclusion relies heavily on uncontrolled observational data and is therefore suspect. The same reservation applies, a fortiori, to three other papers that have combined data from two or even more uncontrolled observational studies in imaginative attempts to estimate the effect of CT scanning on patient survival (McNeil et al. 1977; Zimmerman et al. 1978; Knaus et al. 1980).

28 Discussion of Paper by Russell

A. Williams

University of York

The paper has two main aims: the main body of the paper discusses the potential contribution of epidemiological methods to the evaluation of CT and in particular its technological matrix. I will come back to that in a moment. Secondly, the appendices present epidemiological critiques of some of the research methods used in the literature to estimate such technology matrices. I do not propose to say anything about the appendices since I think they represent a review of the material to back up the general statements made in the main part of the paper. So I am simply going to comment upon the main part of the paper.

The main part of the paper is concerned with the technology matrix and I should first explain what the author means by that. He says that the process of evaluation can be broken down into three stages: the identification and measurement of the inputs consumed and the outputs generated; the estimation of the medical relationship between the measures of input and the measures of output, whatever they are; and the valuation of the inputs and outputs. He leaves valuation questions on one side as being the economist's problem and says that he sees the epidemiological contribution as being what goes on within a "black box", which has inputs going in on one side and outputs coming out of the other side. This leaves open the question of the appropriate way to measure inputs and outputs. The "black box" is the technology matrix.

He then goes on to discuss Fineberg's classification already presented in earlier papers, so I will not go through that again. He then comes to an important point, which is to pick up Donabedian's distinction between evaluation concerned with *structure,* evaluation concerned with *process,* and evaluation concerned with *outcome*. The natural assumption to make is that the black box is about process rather than about outcome. He then goes on, however, to say that in his view it would be wrong to deduce that the evaluation of diagnostic accuracy, diagnostic impact, and therapeutic impact can all be regarded as evaluations of process. The basic principle of process evaluation is that appropriate use is judged against normative criteria and, although such criteria can and sometimes do incorporate rigorous scientific findings, they are usually based on the pooled experience of groups of practitioners. In contrast, diagnostic accuracy, diagnostic impact, and therapeutic impact are all essentially objective and do not require normative criteria to be developed before they can be assessed. He then interprets Fineberg's classification, in which diagnostic categories are placed between technical capability and clinical outcome, as meaning that although these phenomena *may* lead to an improvement in clinical outcome, they do not *guarantee* such an improvement. Hence diagnostic accuracy, diagnostic impact, and therapeutic impact should all be regarded as outcomes in Donabedian's terms.

He then says that this view could be supported by three examples: first, the diagnostic accuracy of CT confers benefits on patients anxious for reassurance about the nature of their illness. Second, the therapeutic impact of CT confers benefit on patients spared unnecessary operations. Third, CT confers benefits on patients who would not otherwise have been subjected to radiation at a very slightly increased risk of contracting cancer. So as well as supporting the argument that diagnostic impact should be regarded as an outcome in the widest sense, his last two examples also serve to illustrate both the general difficulty of evaluating diagnostic technology and the specific difficulty of estimating such outcomes. First, to assess the expected benefit from fewer invasive procedures, one needs to estimate both the global proportion of patients spared such procedures and the expected benefit to each. Second, to assess the expected cost of increased radiation one needs to estimate three parameters – the change in frequency of radiological procedures, the dose of radiation from each scan, and the relationship between dose and risk of cancer.

Since it has earlier been argued that health care evaluation is concerned in principle only with inputs and outputs, and that the main contribution of epidemiology lies in estimating the relationship between them, three conclusions for the evaluation of CT now follow.

1. Investigation of the process of CT scanning is not fundamental to the task of evaluation. However, this does not imply that the task can be entirely divorced from any consideration of process. Indeed, strong proponents of outcome measurement might advocate that all outcome studies should also measure the process with a view to identifying how improved outcomes are achieved.
2. Since diagnostic accuracy, diagnostic impact, and therapeutic impact may all be regarded as outcomes in the widest sense, all three are relevant to the epidemiological evaluation of CT – at least in theory.
3. Finally, it is clear that the methodological problems of estimating the outcomes of CT scanning are quite profound.

I shall be more brief about aspects of the rest of the paper. There is a section on methods of health care evaluation going through material that I shall leave undiscussed since it is not particularly controversial. He compares observational studies, quasi-experimental studies, and experimental studies as alternative ways of deriving evidence and considers the criteria by which one might judge between them and the advantages and disadvantages of each technique. There is a section about randomized trials and the interesting Fig. 27.2, which suggests that one way of overcoming some of the problems with randomized trials may be to introduce randomization and the seeking of informed consent in a slightly different way from the way it has been done hitherto – a point I will not dwell on here.

The conclusions of the paper are set out in three concluding paragraphs on p. 307. These relate to the evaluation of alternative health care policies and the estimation of the technology matrix (that is the relationship between inputs and outputs). Evaluation studies that use observational or quasi-experimental methods are likely to generate biased estimates of the technology matrix, even if properly controlled. Bias is even more likely in uncontrolled studies. Unfortunately, very few evaluations of CT have been controlled. The use of randomized trials to evaluate health care technology is intrinsically much less prone to bias. However, it is fraught with difficulties both ethical and practical. In particular, randomized trials of CT are generally regarded as unethical in the United States and as a result apparently only one randomized trial of CT has been published. (That is not to say only one randomized trial of CT has been done.) It is to be hoped that the fundamental obstacle to the effective epidemiological evaluation of CT can still be overcome.

That is the optimistic conclusion of the paper. I am no epidemiologist and I have limited my role as a discussant to raising four rather general issues that arise from my reading of the paper. They are as follows:

1. What is the minimum information needed to generate a useful technology matrix (or, as economists would call it, a production function)?
2. How in principle is it best generated and what are the main obstacles to conducting such an investigation?
3. What is the closest we are likely to be able to come to this ideal in practice?
4. What is the proper relationship, that is, what is the appropriate division of responsibilities between the epidemiologists, the clinicians, the economists, and anyone else you care to think of, engineers, physicists, etc.?

Summary of Workshop Discussion

Undoubtedly more systematic studies are needed to demonstrate to what extent and at what cost improved diagnostic accuracy is converted into "diagnostic impact". Russell's paper provides an excellent overview of the methods of choice. However, several additional points need to be taken into account, both at the level of clinical decision-making and at the level of the health care system.

First, extremely careful experimental planning and appropriate methods are necessary since the influence of the observer in interpreting X-ray or other images is large and, as McNeil points out, must be eliminated. Unfortunately, little information is available so far on inter- and intra-observer variations in interpretation of images other than X-ray, e.g. only recent technology allows for "freezing" ultrasound pictures for consecutive inspection. Another reason for special attention to the planning of evaluations is that multi-institutional and international studies should be undertaken. One institution may not be able to accumulate a sufficient amount of data in a reasonable period of time. Methods are also available for controlled randomized trials when several therapies need to be compared in addition to different diagnostic techniques ("n x m factorial design").

Second, the technology matrix, relating the outcomes to inputs, may have to take other forms – or will have to be expanded – when used at the *level of the health care system* and for planning. The penalties for errors made in the clinic are different from the ones made by the health ministry. However, for evaluation at the level of particular patient-groups one has also to take into account that it requires much more than a patient, a physician, and a machine to put the system into effect. First, within a particular hospital where the technology is used, many organizational problems must be dealt with. It is not only the question of how many assistants, how much room, maintenance etc. are contributing to running costs. Interactions with the various departments of the hospital (costs of data transfer, broadening of the indication, waiting times, hospitalization for investigation, etc.), organization of services for inpatients and outpatients, for private patients and for public patients, interactions with neighbouring hospitals, etc., all play important roles in determining utilization and costs, too. New technologies thus affect both structures and processes in the health system.

Rapid technological development and medical specialization, however, force decision-makers to prepare and take decisions within short periods of time. Information on the health care system (structure, organization, capacities and throughput of the delivery system; demography, etc.) is generally available. It needs to be organized into special medical information systems structured and kept up to date such that it becomes useful – in complementing information such as produced by the technology matrix – to planning and decision agencies.

29 Macroeconomic Evaluation of Computerized Tomographic Scanning

J. L. Wagner

The Urban Institute, Washington

A Definition of Macroeconomic Evaluation of Medical Technology

The major reason for conducting an economic evaluation of a medical technology is to support an economic decision. An economic decision is defined here as one involving the allocation of productive and, hence, valuable resources to a particular end. A physician's decision to order (or not to order) a procedure or drug is an economic decision, as is a hospital's decision to invest (or not to invest) in the capital equipment required for a procedure, a government's decision to approve (or disapprove) the marketing of a drug or procedure, or a third-party payer's to pay (or not to pay) for a drug or procedure. Economic evaluation provides evidence on the relative costs and benefits of alternative courses of action open to decision-makers. Though decisions involving the allocation of resources can be and often are made ignoring economic considerations, they remain economic decisions nonetheless.

To define macroeconomic evaluation of medical technology, then, we might first identify macroeconomic decisions. In this paper, macroeconomic decisions are defined as those governing the investment in the capacity to use a technology[1]. In the case of a capital-intensive procedure like computed tomographic (CT) scanning, the macroeconomic questions are: how many and what kinds of scanners are required? Where should they be placed, and in what sequence over time? These decisions are made in different ways and by different parties, depending upon the organization of health care delivery and financing in a region or country. In the United States, for example, CT scanning investment decisions are essentially private, made by hospitals and other providers of medical care, with some direct intercession by state certificate of need agencies and with the indirect influence of third-party payers, whose decisions on coverage and payment levels strongly affect the financial viability of prospective investments in medical technologies. In countries with national health services, such as Great Britain or Sweden, the macroeconomic questions are largely answered by the central, regional, or county authorities that administer the services.

Investment decisions are always made on the basis of economic evaluations though these may be quite informal, and the benefits and costs considered may be those pertaining only to the invester and not to all segments of society. These informal and private evaluations will not be discussed here; rather, the paper will focus

---

1 In contrast, microeconomic decisions are those involving the use of existing capacity in the provision of patient care.

on economic evaluations whose purpose is to inform the public on the appropriate pattern of investment in new technology. This leads to the central questions of this paper. What kinds of information would inform public decision-makers about the optimal number, types, locations, and timing of investments in CT scanners? To what extent do existing studies offer guidance on these issues? Are there methodological and data problems that inhibit the development of truly useful information? Finally, given these limitations, are there analytical methods that are most useful to the macroeconomic technology decisions?

These questions will be addressed in the following order. First, the paper briefly lays out the information requirements for public investment decisions on CT scanning. Second, it categorizes and reviews existing economic evaluations of CT scanning. This review encompasses those studies in which the costs of CT scanning are considered as well as its clinical benefits. The overriding issue of the literature review will be the extent to which the evaluative information produced enhances our understanding of the macroeconomic questions of CT scanning: how many, what kinds, where, and when? Third, this paper summarizes the major conceptual, methodological, and data limitations that stand in the way of useful macroeconomic evaluations of CT scanning and assess the extent to which they can, or should be overcome. Finally, it suggests a method for evaluating the economic impacts of alternative CT scanning investment strategies that bypasses the data and methodological limitations inherent in existing studies but directly addresses the critical investment questions. This method is based on the rapidly emerging analytic technology of multiobjective programming and planning (Cohon 1978). Its application to CT scanning will be illustrated in the final section of this paper.

What Should the Public Know About the Benefits and Costs of CT Scanning for Investment Decisions?

Though it is common to see assertions in the clinical literature that CT scanning as a whole has been shown to be (or not to be) worth its cost, the question of the overall cost-effectiveness of the technology is irrelevant to the macroeconomic investment decision. This generic focus also is not the most relevant one for those practicing medicine. CT scanning is, without doubt, well worth its cost for some kinds of patients and an obvious waste of resources for others. If, on balance, the benefits to some patients outweigh the extra costs associated with treating others, it nevertheless does not follow that the clearly wasteful uses should be tolerated. The ratio of benefit or effectiveness to cost might well be greatly improved by limiting procedures to the subset of patients who clearly benefit from them. Therefore, a more germane question to those who pracice medicine is, or should be: for what kinds of patients, i.e., for what presenting signs, symptoms, and risk factors, is CT scanning most likely to be worth its costs?

Investment decisions about CT scanning occur at a much more aggregate level. Consequently, the type of data needed also is less discrete. Information is needed simultaneously to answer three interdependent questions: (a) how many CT scanners should be available in a region? (b) where should these scanners be located? (c) what kinds of CT equipment are needed at each location? None of these questions can be answered independently of the others. The required number of scanners, for example, clearly depends on the mix of equipment capabilities – scanner speed, head or whole-body, etc. – selected. Conversely, the desirable configuration of equipment types depends on the number of locations of facilities. Finally, the most appropriate locations depend on the number of scanners and the types selected. The techniques of economic evaluation – cost-benefit and cost-effectiveness analysis – should be germane to these questions, since these techniques were originally developed to assess alternative public sector investments such as water projects, airports, and weapons systems. Thus, to the extent that decisions about capital investment in hospitals are considered to be in the domain of the public sector, the principles of economic evaluation should apply.

An ideal economic analysis of alternative CT investment strategies in a region would compute the net benefit, or some common index of effectiveness, of each possible combination of number, location, and equipment type, and would array this measure against the investment cost of the particular alternative. This approach is complicated, however, because there are thousands of alternative strategies possible, each of which would need to be compared. Suppose, for example, that only one kind of equipment were available, that the total number of scanners were already prescribed at ten, and that only 30 possible locations (hospitals) were reasonable candidates for a CT scanner. This would give 211 000 possible separate combinations of ten scanners in the 30 hospitals. When the number of scanners is unspecified and there is more than one kind of equipment, the number of alternative strategies increases in proportion.

To complicate matters even further, calculation of the benefit or effect of any particular investment alternative implies knowledge of both the kinds of patients (defined by presenting signs, symptoms, and risk factors) that are likely to obtain CT scans under a given configuration of locations and equipment types, and the cost-effectiveness of CT scanning in these patients. Also, because the economic evaluation of public sector investments requires that costs borne and benefits accrued by all parties be counted, the cost of patient travel or transfer would need to be included in the analysis, and this implies that the patterns of patient origin can be specified for each alternative investment strategy.

A state of perfect information as outlined above is unachievable. Not only are some kinds of information unobtainable, but even if they could be collected, they might well not be worth the costs. If better information on the costs and benefits of CT scanning were able to improve investment decisions only marginally, then expensive economic evaluation would itself be a waste of resources. It may well be better to rely on less comprehensive and even less reliable analyses that provide broad guidelines for investment decisions than to seek out perfect information. Yet, more modest approaches to economic evaluation make one uneasy about drawing inferences for investment strategies. The next section reviews selected economic studies of CT scanning with particular emphasis on the extent to which different kinds of study provide useful information regarding investment in CT capacity.

Economic Evaluations of CT Scanning

Because of its high capital costs, and perhaps because of its very importance as a new diagnostic modality, CT scanning has been the subject of more economic analysis than any diagnostic technology introduced before or since. This literature is uneven in quality; yet it does represent the spectrum of approaches to economic evaluation that are likely to be possible with limited financial resources for research.

The economic evaluations of CT scanning fall into three general categories: (a) studies of the implications of CT scanning for a country's or region's health care costs; (b) studies of the impact of CT scanning on diagnostic costs or health care costs in particular institutions; (c) studies of the benefits and costs of CT scanning in patients with specific presenting conditions. Each of these areas is presented separately below.

Studies of the Aggregate Diagnostic Cost Impact of CT Scanning

A logical starting point for economic evaluation is to estimate the impact of CT scanning on health care costs or, more narrowly, on the cost of diagnosis. Under some conditions, this narrow approach to evaluation is sufficient for determining whether the use of the technology is justified for a class of patients. If the availability of CT scanning decreases diagnostic costs by reducing the use of other examinations or shortening inpatient hospital stays while at the same time improving, or at least not decreasing, the safety, accuracy, and timeliness of diagnosis compared with all relevant alternative strategies, then the use of the technology is justified in the class of patients studied.

The more homogeneous the class of patients under study, the more useful are the results, for the outcome of a cost study can be extremely sensitive to the criteria (signs, symptoms, and risk factors) defining the class of patients. If, for example, a study of the impact of CT on the cost of diagnosis is based on the universe of patients with neurological complaints, the evaluation would average together the net diagnostic costs associated with widely divergent presenting conditions. At this extreme, the usefulness of the economic analysis as a guide to resource allocation is questionable. A review of two studies that take this aggregate tack will illustrate the problem.

The first study, by Willems et al. (1979), estimated net changes in total US expenditures for diagnosis due to the introduction of CT head scanning in 1976. The performance of a CT scan generated a technical charge, professional fee, and associated hospital room and board charges, all of which totalled between $ 295 million and $ 28 million in 1976. Savings resulting from reductions in pneumoencephalograms (PEGs), radionuclide (RN) brain scans, and arteriograms were deducted from this total, leaving a net estimate of $ 181 million to $ 390 million in increased expenditures due to CT scanning in 1976.

A study by Arthur D. Little, Inc. (1977) was an attempt to estimate the US national impact of both head and body scanning on the cost of diagnosis. The national impact on the utilization of competing diagnostic procedures and exploratory surgery in 1977 and 1980 was estimated by a variety of sources, including consultations with experts in the field. The technical cost of providing each type of procedure was estimated assuming equipment at full utilization and current costs of replacement of equipment. (Except for exploratory surgery, charges were not used to estimate procedure costs.) To arrive at a unit cost for each of the various diagnostic procedures, the national average hospital room and board charge was applied to the additional days of hospitalization required by each type of procedure.

The Arthur D. Little study predicted that the availability of CT head scanning would raise diagnostic costs in the US by about $ 29 million in 1977 and $ 31 million in 1980. These low estimates of net impact contrast with the results of the Willems study but can be explained by different assumptions about the effect of CT scanning on exploratory surgery and skull X-rays.

The predicted impact of CT body scanning is subject to greater speculation since, at the time of the study, body scanning had only just begun to find its way into the diagnostic process. The authors predicted that in 1980, as a result of the use of CT scanning, the estimated cost of diagnosing abdominal and mediastinal disorders would have increased by $ 152 million. This estimate is based on the assumption that the availability of CT body scanning would reduce the number of exploratory surgeries by 50% and that no other diagnostic procedures would be affected by CT scanning.

What do these studies suggest? Both imply that on aggregate, and as it has been applied to diagnosis, CT scanning cannot be expected to reduce diagnostic costs. Even under optimistic assumptions concerning the degree of substitution of CT for other tests the availability of CT appears to have raised the cost of diagnosis. Yet the significance of these findings for decision-making is negligible. Do they imply that there are too many CT scanners in the US, or too few? Are they being applied appropriately? Can the distribution of scanners be improved? Aggregate studies like these simply do not inform.

Studies of the Impact of CT Scanning on Diagnostic Costs in Particular Institutions

A number of investigators have attempted to estimate the net impact of CT on the diagnostic costs of patients in specific hospitals. These studies are often pre-CT: post-CT comparisons of diagnostic costs for inpatients with particular reasons for admission or discharge diagnoses. Although these studies suffer from a lack of generalizability, they often concentrate on a narrow set of signs, symptoms, and risk factors. Such narrow studies are likely to be more informative for clinical decisions than are the broad cost-impact studies, because despite their limited research designs they do provide direct evidence about whether a given class of patients should be considered for CT scanning. These findings can be used in assessing the amount of scanning capacity that might cost-effectively serve a given population.

Unless they are carefully designed, institution-specific studies are unable to control for changes in patient mix over time. It is insufficient to assume that the introduction of CT would have made no difference to the kinds of patients who were hospitalized. For example, some who might normally have been hospitalized could well receive CT scans as outpatients. The resulting changes in case severity, which are difficult to document, can seriously bias the results of a cost-impact study.

The problem is evident in studies by Wortzman and Holgate (1979), Bahr and

Hodges (1978), Enlow et al. (1980), and Thomson (1977) who estimated the impact of the introduction of CT head scanning on the costs of diagnosis for all neurological admissions at their respective hospitals. Using different analytical methodologies, they concluded that the cost of diagnosis was reduced by the introduction of CT. The savings resulted from reductions both in substitute tests such as PEG and cerebral angiograms and in lengths of stay[2].

Regardless of these conclusions, none of the studies contains evidence relevant to the three central questions of CT investment – how many, what kinds, and where? Because the studies make no attempt to follow specific classes of patients[3], they do not even provide information on the kinds of patients for whom CT is likely to be useful.

Three studies of specific patient-groups with relatively unambiguous and homogeneous signs and symptoms were reported by Larson and colleagues at the University of Washington. They analyzed the impact of CT scanning on the utilization and cost of diagnostic services for patients with presenting conditions suggestive of brain tumors (Larsson and Omenn 1977), cerebrovascular disease (Larsson et al. 1978 a), and hydrocephalus (Larsson et al. 1978 b). Admission forms were abstracted for all inpatients admitted to the university-affiliated hospital with signs and symptoms suggesting one of the three diseases during the year prior to and 2 years after the introduction of a CT head scanner. Patterns of service delivery and medical care in the pre-CT and post-CT patient groups were compared, including the utilization of and charges for neurodiagnostic procedures, the length of hospital stay, the time required to reach final diagnosis, the level of detail of the diagnosis, and the type of therapy employed. CT scanning had a major impact on the configuration of diagnostic studies used for each of the three types of patients, but the relative benefits resulting from these changes varied among the three.

In the study of patients with suspected brain tumors, CT scanning significantly reduced the use of RN brain scanning, angiography, and PEG. The length of hospitalization, speed of diagnostic workup, and timing and type of therapy for these patients, though, did not change significantly. The overall detectability of brain tumors increased markedly after CT scanning became available. Total per-patient hospital charges for neurodiagnostic procedures did not change significantly. The authors, therefore, concluded that CT scanning in the form in which it was integrated into the neurodiagnostic process at the study hospital was cost-effective because it permitted reductions in the use of invasive and somewhat risky procedures but did not raise hospital charges or otherwise affect prognosis.

In the case of patients with suspected cerebrovascular disease, the introduction of CT scanning significantly reduced the number of lumbar punctures and RN

2 In a recent reappraisal of their early study, Wortzman and Holgate (1979) revealed discrepancies between their estimates of potential savings and realized effects in subsequent years. Hospital stays and admissions did not decline as predicted in the study. Although the number of angiograms and PEGs did decline, the cost of these procedures, as measured by charges, rose, thus wiping out much of the estimated savings. The procedure charge increases were necessitated by decreases in utilization without concomitant capacity reduction.

3 Bahr and Hodges disaggregated the study population with three diagnostic groups, based on discharge diagnosis not on patients' presenting signs and symptoms. Consequently, the costs or savings cannot be easily related to a set of patients who might present for a CT scan.

brain scans, but the total per capita hospital charge for neurodiagnostic procedures increased about 33%. The length of hospitalization and speed of diagnostic workup did not change, and although the level of detail of the discharge diagnosis was greatly increased, such detail was unnecessary to plan therapy. In the judgment of the authors, CT scan results were not essential to establishing a diagnosis in those patients with suspected cerebrovascular disease, therefore, CT scanning was found to be of questionable value.

The introduction of CT scanning in the diagnostic workup of children with suspected hydrocephalus led to major reductions in RN brain scans and PEGs. CT scanning also reduced the total charges for neurodiagnostic procedures. Speed of diagnosis, length of hospitalization, and kind of therapy did not change. Thus, CT scanning was found to be particularly appropriate for such patients.

A more recent study by the same authors investigated the impact of outpatient CT scans on headache patients (Larsson et al. 1980). Three cohorts of patients were selected for study: one cohort containing patients seen before installation of a CT scanner, a second cohort containing patients seen shortly after installation, and a third cohort containing patients seen 1 year after installation of the CT scanner. The patients in each of these cohorts were selected from a review of electroencephalogram (EEG) records, where headache was the reason for the EEG. Thus, the patient-sample excluded those who may have had CT scans without EEGs. Diagnostic testing charges per patient increased 16% after the introduction of CT scanning. The neuroradiological diagnostic yield of patients with normal neurological workups was low and, in the case of CT, was negligible. This finding led the authors to suggest that abnormal findings on neurological examination should be a screening criterion for performing CT scans and other neuroradiological procedures for patients with headaches.

The fact that diagnostic charges increased after the introduction of CT scanning says very little about the appropriate allocation of resources; the more powerful evidence presented by the authors is the apparent absence of real clinical benefit, even with respect to diagnostic capability, deriving from CT scanning - and, indeed, from most neurodiagnostic procedures. If radiological and other technology-bound procedures are to be performed on patients with no focal findings, then this study has not adequately demonstrated that CT scanning cannot lower the cost of diagnosis if it is appropriately substituted for other tests. A clear cost-reducing option, however, appears to ensue from stopping the diagnostic workup of the patient when the clinical examination reveals no abnormalities. In light of the importance of such a conclusion, it is unfortunate that the sample of patients in this study was chosen by excluding those who may have had CT scans without EEGs. More needs to be done to refine the study of diagnostic procedures for patients with headaches.

Nowhere has CT scanning had a more dramatic effect than in the management of head injuries. Two studies of CT in head injury have documented the impact of CT on the use of other tests and on the rate of exploratory surgery in victims of acute head injury. These impacts on utilization were not converted into dollar savings, however. Ambrose et al. (1976) in Britain studied the impact of CT scanning on the diagnosis of head injuries, but they did not attempt to attach cost estimates to the observed changes in utilization of diagnostic procedures and exploratory surgery. The introduction of CT scanning at the study hospital dramatically reduced the use of arteriography, PEG, and exploratory craniotomy without changing the mortality; however, once CT examinations were available, they were ordered so frequently that net costs may have increased.

In a recent study of CT scanning in acute head trauma at a US teaching hospital, Zimmerman et al. (1978) noted a progressive decrease in utilization of skull X-rays following the introduction of CT scanning, but they also observed that "a certain proportion of the present skull radiographic examinations are done because of the referring physician's adherence to traditional ways of evaluating trauma patients."

Studies of the Benefits and Costs of CT Scanning in Specific Patient Groups

When a new technology increases costs but also yields benefits to patients, the question of its worth must include direct consideration of the magnitude (and sometimes value) of these benefits. Only outcome-oriented studies that attempt to relate incremental patient benefits to costs are useful in determining whether CT is justified in certain classes of patients. Two such studies of CT scanning have been reported.

Knaus and Wagner (to be published) analyzed the effectiveness and costs of two alternative diagnostic pathways for patients presenting with sudden severe headaches but no focal signs; such patients are generally viewed with scepticism as candidates for CT scanning. The analysts in this study compared the outcomes of two diagnostic pathways: (1) performing a CT scan on all such patients referred; and (2) performing a CT scan only on patients presenting additional neurological signs (i.e., depriving the patient of a CT scan unless and until his or her condition deteriorates). Only one possible positive finding was considered – a ruptured intracranial aneurysm resulting in subarachnoid hemorrhage. The authors claim that early diagnosis of this disease significantly improves the prognosis of surgical intervention; consequently, the cost of each life saved by early detection is about \$ 543 000, or \$ 25 000 per life-year saved.

The analysis depended on the attainment of a diagnostic yield at least as high as that obtained at a large teaching hospital: about 1 aneurysm per 125 headache patients. The authors also demonstrated the high degree of sensitivity of cost-effectiveness ratios to small changes in this assumption. It is also possible that finer criteria for offering CT scans to patients with severe headaches could lower the ratio of cost to lives saved by increasing diagnostic yield. For example, since aneurysms peak during distinct age-intervals, age-based criteria might improve the estimates substantially.

Knaus and Wagner observed that the study did not include the cost of errors, i.e., false-positives and false-negatives. In particular, if false-positives lead to additional tests or unnecessary surgery with their attendant morbidity, mortality, and cost, the value of CT scanning as a primary diagnostic tool for severe headaches might be further reduced.

Whether restoring a year of life is worth \$ 25 000 is a question for society. Should it be answered in the positive, the conventional wisdom that CT scanning resources should not be used on headache patients would need revision. More research is needed on the presenting signs, symptoms, and other factors that might improve the cost-effectiveness ratio for headache patients.

A recent study of the cost-effectiveness of CT in radiation therapy represents a credible attempt to obtain reasonable estimates of the value of the procedure in this context (Goitein 1980). Based on clinical evidence that a CT scan changes radiation treatment plans in 38%–50% of patients, the authors made rough but reasonable estimates of the resultant effects on local control (6% of patients) and on improvements in 5-year survival (3½%). These benefits appear large relative to the cost of a CT examination, especially when one considers that society is already paying approximately $ 12 000 for each patient's radiation therapy that otherwise has a 52% chance of achieving local tumor control. The authors also calculated that the enhanced ability to achieve local tumor control would avert over $ 1 000 in additional treatment costs for the cost of a CT scan, about $ 250. Though the estimates are not based on precise data, the order of magnitude of benefits to cost would suggest that CT scanning should be available to those undergoing radiation therapy.

What are the Obstacles to the Use of Economic Evaluation in Macroeconomic Technology Decisions?

The literature cited above, uneven though it is, gives a flavor of the kinds of analysis that are likely to be useful as general guidelines for access to CT scanning. Those patient-groups for whom direct savings in medical care costs can be expected are obviously in the strongest position to claim access to CT scanning. But such inferences are possible only if the class of patients under study is sufficiently homogeneous with respect to signs, symptoms, and risk factors.

There is a major obstacle to the use of these findings to develop estimates of required capacity in a region, however. Data in the form needed to make accurate estimates simply do not exist. Since it is the incidence of presenting signs and symptoms, and not final diagnoses, that will dictate how many CT scans are required in a given population, patient-based data systems would have to be organized in a way that is quite different from today's systems. Good estimates of the incidence of certain presenting conditions are achievable – in particular cancer patients requiring CT-assisted radiation – but for others, there is a wide range of possible rates of incidence of signs and symptoms in relation to the rate at which final disease diagnoses occur. It would appear, then, that even with the best analysis, good estimates of capacity requirements are difficult to come by.

A Suggested Approach to Macroeconomic Analysis of Capital-Intensive Medical Technologies

How can information be organized to explore directly the benefits and costs of alternative investment strategies without running into the critical data limitations described above? Here we describe an innovative approach to analyzing alternative investments in CT scanning. The general approach, referred to here as "Facility Location Analysis" is an application of techniques of multiobjective programing (Cohon 1978). The techniques are basically nothing more than ways to display the important implications of alternative locational choices for those who must decide. These relatively new analytic tools recognize that decisions are often made in the

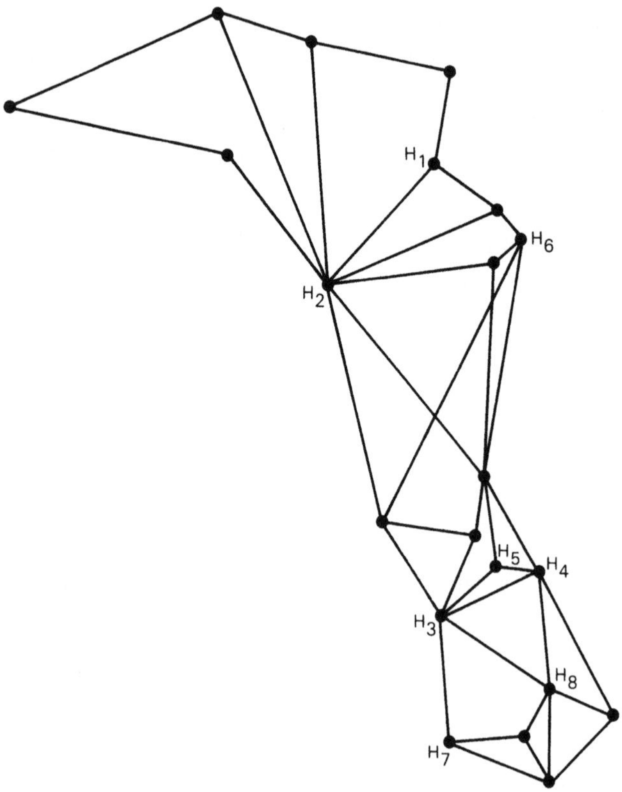

Fig. 29.1. Simple network of a hypothetical region. ●, demand points; H_i, potential supply points (hospitals)

context of multiple and conflicting objectives that cannot be met simultaneously, and that truly "efficient" alternatives are hard to identify. (An "efficient alternative" is one for which there is no other alternative that would do better on all objectives.) Multiobjective programing does not provide a single "best" investment strategy, because such an entity simply does not exist. Rather it can offer information on the trade-offs among access, quality, and costs that are inherent in their choices. It does this by selecting easily measured surrogates of cost and effectiveness and examining the trade-offs among these variables due to different locational configurations.

Locational analysis begins by picturing the region as a set of nodes on a network. Each node constitutes a demand point (a city or town with population) and/or a potential facility supply point (a city or hospital capable of housing a CT scanner). These demand and potential supply points are joined by arcs representing the most efficient method of travel between them. (The arcs may dovetail the major road networks, or they may involve routes that are more circuitous but less congested.) Figure 29.1 shows a simple network. It is assumed that the population at risk for a CT scan at each node is known, as is the travel time or cost between each pair of cities. (This particular example assumes that a scanner would never be placed outside a population center, but the assumption can be relaxed without altering the structure of the problem.) However, the number of population centers and potential facility sites must not be infinite. It is also possible to designate the same node as a potential site for several facilities by treating the site as if it were actually several different sites with the same distance relationships to all other nodes.

The question is – how many and which of the potential sites should be allocated a CT scanner? There is no "best" answer to this question, since different combinations of number and location will have different implications for cost, quality, and access. Therefore, the location analysis approach begins by characterizing measurable objectives related to the three dimensions of performance. Among the possible objectives that might be of interest to the public are the following:

Minimize the total level of investment in CT scanning facilities

Minimize total CT scanning operating costs

Minimize the average waiting time for nonemergency patients to receive a scan

Minimize the maximum distance that any patient would have to travel to obtain a CT scan

Maximize the proportion of full-service oncology centers with CT scanning capability

Maximize the proportion of the population served at hospitals with full-time board-certified radiologists.

Refinements, replacements, or additions to these objectives are possible. One refinement in these objectives might involve further detail on access to head versus whole-body scanning capability. Notice that the objectives are stated so that the question of who "needs" CT scanning procedures is avoided. This is fortunate in light of the inadequacy of the literature available to support claims of efficacy or cost-effectiveness of its current uses.

The objectives compete with one another. If the public were interested solely in minimizing CT scanning costs, for example, it would simply not permit any CT scanners. This is absurd, of course, as reflected in the existence of the objective of minimizing the average appointment lead time. On the other hand, it would not be useful to consider the latter objective in the absence of considerations of cost. The purpose of locational analysis is to explore in an orderly fashion the way in which these objectives are substituted for one another. As it proceeds, locational analysis identifies the set of "noninferior" facility locations – those giving the best performance on one objective for any prespecified levels of performance on the others.

The methods for obtaining and presenting information on noninferior solutions are described in an example below. In brief, one or more of a family of models are used to obtain the best number and locations of CT scanners when the relative importance of one objective versus another is held fixed. The models used to find these solutions are formulated as mathematical programing problems. Solving such models for different relative weights for competing objectives reveals the general shape of the "efficient" trade-off between one objective and others. As an example, consider the following two competing objectives:

Minimize the investment costs of CT scanning equipment for the region

Minimize the proportion of the population residing more than 30-min travel time from a head scanner

The trade-off between these two objectives can be explored by solving a problem in which the second objective is minimized subject to an upper limit on the size

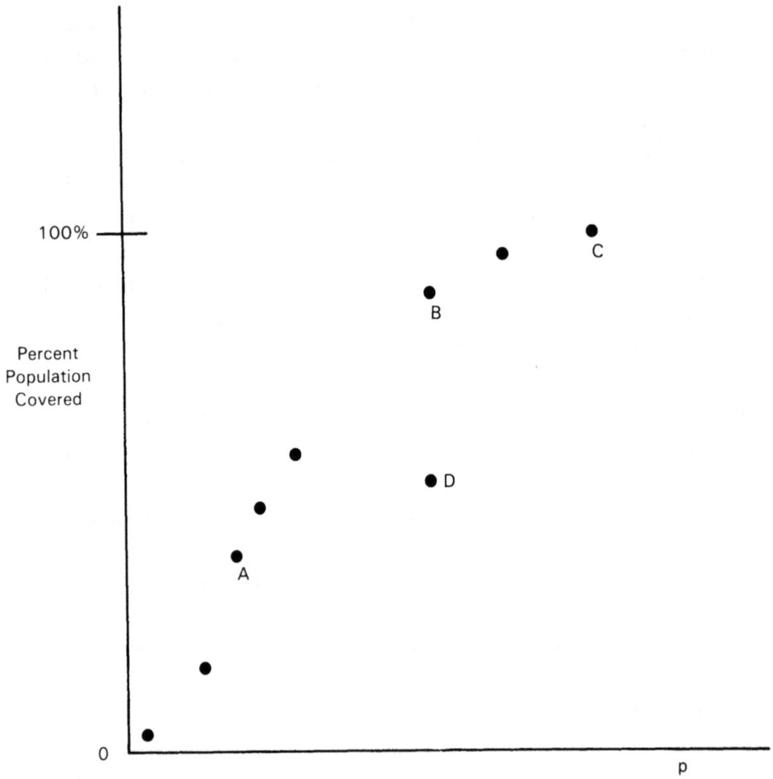

Fig. 29.2. Trade-off between number of facilities and access to CT scanners. **A–D,** see text

of the investment in CT scanning. For the purpose of illustration, we assume that the investment cost of a CT head scanner is the same regardless of its location. Any fixed investment in CT scanning implies that a certain number, p, of such facilities will be acquired. The problem is thus reduced to the maximal covering problem, first formulated and solved by Church and ReVelle (1974). This problem is stated as follows: Locate exactly p facilities among the candidate sites in such a way that the number of people who reside more than 30 min from a CT facility is minimized. The mathematical formulation of this problem is shown in the appendix. Here it suffices to say that quite straightforward methods exist for finding the specific nodes at which the maximal cover of the population will occur for exact facilities.

As p increases, the ability of the facilities to cover more and more cities increases, until at some value of p, all demand points are fully covered within this time. The trade-off between number of facilities and the proportion of the region's population covered within the 30-min time limit can be graphed as shown in Fig. 29.2. Each of the points represents a precise locational configuration based on the solution of the maximization problem defined above.

The addition of a single facility can radically alter the configuration of facility locations. The locations selected when p facilities are constructed may not be the same as those selected when p + 1 facilities are built. Yet some locations may be chosen for a wide range of values of p. Notice also that as p increases, the improvement in coverage decreases. In Fig. 29.2 moving from B to C gains less in the way of coverage than does moving from A to B.

If certain sites not contained in the optimal solution were designated as scanner locations for reasons not explicitly considered in the model, the coverage associated with p facilities would decline as in point D on Fig. 29.2. This is an "inferior" point from the viewpoint of the model, but it may not be inferior when other objectives are considered. In any case, the loss in terms of coverage due to substitution of one location for the other could be demonstrated in the analysis.

The analysis can be readily extended to look at coverage hierarchies for head and whole-body scanners. Moore and ReVelle (to be published) have recently formulated such a problem for planning health facilities in Honduras. The coverage requirements for head and body scanners might be quite different, since head scanning is used so effectively in the diagnosis and management of trauma. Moreover, a whole-body scanner can perform the functions of the head scanner, but the converse is not true. These details can be built into an extension of the model, and the analysis would explore the trade-off between the two kinds of coverage and the investment in various kinds of scanner capability.

The model presented above is one example of locational analysis where only two objectives are considered. Similar methods can be employed with more than two objectives, though the mathematical formulation of the problem might change. Some models recognize explicitly that the capacity of any single CT scanner is limited and would indicate the number of scanners required at each site to meet the demand of each site's covering area. In fact, a family of model formulations is available to support analyses of the trade-offs among competing locations. [See ReVelle et al. (1981) for a concise summary of multiple-objective approaches to location of facilities on networks.]

The major advantage of the locational analysis approach is its ability to present and display information in an orderly fashion on the central trade-offs inherent in a health plan for a service such as CT scanning. It is also a method that allows for specific designations of particular cities or hospitals as sites for a CT facility. Because the approach can be formulated in terms of access versus cost, the question of clinical "need" for CT scanning is largely avoided. Of course, the question of need is implicit in the access objectives, and the public must have some general notion about the reasonableness of 20, 40, or 100 CT scanners in terms of the present and future demands for these services. This is where the results of cost-effectiveness analyses, such as those presented in the earlier section of this paper, would be most helpful. It must be understood, however, that cost-effectiveness and cost-benefit analyses will never be the definitive analytic techniques required for rational allocation of resources.

Appendix: Mathematical Formulation of the Maximal Covering Location Problem (Taken from Church and ReVelle 1974)

The maximal covering location problem finds the locations of a given number of facilities that will serve the maximum population within a stated service distance or time. Let:

I denote the set of demand points
J denote the set of potential facility sites
S denote the maximum distance beyond which a demand point is assumed to be uncovered
d_{ij} denote the shortest distance from node i to node j
A_i denote the population to be served at i
p denote the number of facilities to be established
X_j denote the opening of a facility at j. If $X_j = 1$, a facility is placed at j. If $X_j = 0$, no facility is opened at j
Y_i denote whether demand point i is covered by any open facility ($Y_i = 1$ if point i is covered, 0 otherwise)
N_i denote the set of facility sites eligible to proved "cover" to demand point i. (N_i represents all sites within S units of i.)

The problem can be written as:

$$\text{Maximize } Z = \sum_{i \varepsilon I} A_i Y_i \quad (1)$$

Subject to:

$$\sum_{j \varepsilon N_i} X_j \geqslant Y_i \text{ for all i in I} \quad (2)$$

$$\sum_{j \varepsilon J} X_j = p \quad (3)$$

$$X_j = (0,1) \text{ for all j in J} \quad (4)$$

$$Y_i = (0,1) \text{ for all i in I} \quad (5)$$

This is an integer programing problem, however, Church and ReVelle (1974) found that if solved as a linear program [without imposing constraints (4) and (5), but merely requiring X_j and Y_i to lie between 0 and 1] the optimal solution is all integer about 80% of the time. They also suggest efficient methods to resolve cases of non-integer solutions.

1392

30 Discussion of Paper by Wagner

N. T. Racoveanu

World Health Organization

The paper under discussion is an attempt to offer to health planners a method of reaching decisions related to numbers, types, location, and time of investment for CT scanners, needed in an area (or state) in order to provide adequate medical care to the population with a minimum possible investment. In her approach to this subject Wagner has examined the following four points:

1. The layout of the information requirement for the investment in CT scanners
2. A review of existing data on economic evaluations of CT scanners, looking in particular at studies that can answer:
   a) How many
   b) What types (head or whole-body, or both)
   c) Where (possible locations)
   d) When – the timing of investment
3. A summarized presentation of the conceptual, methodological, or data limitations that interfere with useful macroeconomic evaluation of CT scanners
4. A suggested methodology for evaluation of the economic impact of alternative investment strategies for CT scanners that will bypass the limitations mentioned under point 3; the method proposed is based on the analytic technology of multiobjective programming

In analysing the first point, the author came to the conclusion that the CT scanner is a diagnostic technology with important benefits for some patients and a useless investigation for others. If the category of patients benefiting from the CT scanner can be clearly defined by signs, symptoms, or risk factors, the use of the CT scanner can maximize its cost/benefit ratio and the CT technology would reach a high level of efficiency.

The second point leads the author to review a number of the studies published mainly during 1975–1980 where the CT scanner was analysed either from the viewpoint of diagnostic efficacy or from that of cost savings, both direct and indirect, that this technology can offer. Good examples of such savings are described by a number of authors (Ambrose et al. 1980; Larsson and Omenn 1977, 1978a and b; Thomson 1977; Wortzmann et al. 1975), which have demonstrated that CT scanning could efficiently reduce the number of other diagnostic investigations, in particular those involving intervention, such as pneumoencephalography, cerebral angiography, exploratory surgery, and other tests (plain radiographs, radionuclide scanning, EEG, etc.), as well as reduce the duration of hospitalization, increase the diagnostic accuracy, and influence therefore the therapeutic decision, which may lead to a better end result.

All studies presented, according to the author, were unable to offer adequate data for planning purposes and did not give answers to the defined questions, namely: (a) how many? (b) what types? (c) where? (d) when? Under the third point the major obstacles preventing the use of economic evaluations available in macroeconomic technology decisions are briefly analysed. The major obstacle is the lack of data concerning the incidence of patients presenting signs and/or symptoms indicating the need for CT scanning. Such data would constitute essential information on which CT scanner planning could be made. It seems that for at least a group of patients with certain malignant tumours that are deeply seated, such data can be obtained, but the author seems to be afraid that obtaining similar data for nonmalignant disease would represent a much higher investment than should be envisaged for the planning decision. As a result of the lack of appropriate data on number of patients who will need CT scanning the planning solution has to be found in the absence of such objective information.

The fourth part of the paper deals with the solution proposed by the author, considered as "an innovative approach to analyzing alternative investment in CT scanning". This approach represents an application of the technique of multiobjective programming which, and I quote:

> Recognize that decisions are often made in the context of multiple and conflicting objectives that cannot be met sumultaneously, and that truly "efficient" alternatives are hard to identify. (An "efficient alternative" is one for which there is no other alternative that would do better on all objectives). Multiobjective programing does not provide a single "best" investment strategy, because such an entity simply does not exist. Rather it can offer information on the tradeoffs among access, quality, and costs that are inherent in their choices.

Under this carefully worded description the method proposed consists of a mathematical exercise of locating CT scanners in a given area in such a way that with a minimum of scanners population coverage can be obtained and easy access to the machine given to the maximum number of people. Six objectives are formulated by the author in guiding the mathematical model to be applied. They can be further refined and one suggested refinement is to detail the access to head versus whole-body CT scanner. The paper elaborates further on the proposed method, giving examples and an appendix in which the mathematical formulation that can be used is described.

I have attempted to summarize the content of the paper in an objective way, without introduction of any personal views, to which I now turn. Let me start with the last part of the suggested method for planning CT scanners. This method, which implies an ideal location of the scanners to match the six prerequisite conditions identified by the author, or eventually seven, eight, or ten such conditions, which might be defined by a more ambitious health planner, does not appear to me to be an approach that is acceptable for such a sophisticated diagnostic tool as a CT scanner.

The approach described could be easily accepted for locating public facilities of a general nature, including basic health institutions, health centres, general hospitals, etc. These are institutions used by the whole population with little differentiation in terms of particular groups. For such institutions we do not have too much information on the particular groups that will be using them most frequently, and what is needed is that access should be easy in order not to discourage their use, leading to delay in diagnosis and treatment of the most common diseases. The CT scanner is a device used for diagnosis in a relatively restricted area of human pathology; it cannot be considered yet as a front-line instrument to be planned in a way similar to that for primary health care institutions. The information that the author has defined in her paper as being able to guide the use and therefore the planning of CT scanners is not fully available, but could be obtained if the necessary effort were to be made.

In recent years radiologists have started to become more critical of the use of X-ray procedures and a number of studies on efficacy/efficiency of such procedures and CT scanners represents an area where such studies started very early after the introduction of the technique. An issue of the American Journal of Roentgenology in July 1978 was devoted to this subject. Ideas that are of importance in rationalizing X-ray investigations have started to circulate among radiologists, such as, high- and low-yield criteria, referral criteria, indications, and contraindications. High-yield criteria define such signs, symptoms, or risk factors that if appropriately used in referring patients for a diagnostic investigation will maximize the positive outcome of the given investigation. Referral criteria represent a more complex notion that is aimed at minimizing useless diagnostic investigations. A number of such referral criteria have already been widely accepted in the US for some radiological investigations.

With regard to the indications for X-ray procedures these could be conceived as a method to increase the utility of the radiological investigations and decrease their overutilization. Attempts in this direction are seen in the professional literature and the WHO is planning a Scientific Group that will address this subject later in 1982.

It is interesting to note that the Society for Computer Tomography has published a special report (1979) and that very recently the National Institute of Health (NIH) panel of experts has defined such indications and limitations for head CT scanning. The panel recognizes the utility of CT scanning as a primary diagnosis for the following: suspected brain abscess, intracranial mass lesions, spontaneous intracranial haemorrhage, and severe head injuries. CT scanning is also able to detect and localize more precisely small primary brain tumours, metastatic lesions, and differentiate between ischaemic and haemorrhagic intracranial lesions. A number of other lesions are also considered to be general indications for CT scanning: suspected arteriovenous malformations, hydrocephalus, herpes encephalitis, parasitic infestations, and progressive degenerative brain diseases. For infants and children CT is recommended in the primary diagnosis of intracranial haemorrhage and mass lesions, severe head trauma, increased intracranial pressure, coma, progressively focal neurological signs, and megalocephaly.

At the same time the panel warns against the overutilization of CT in conditions such as: minor head trauma, simple or periodic headache, syncope or dizziness unaccompanied by other neurological signs, and most cerebral vascular events. In children, the contraindications are: diagnosis of the causes of developmental retardation, cerebral palsy, seizure disorders, and headache, as well as intraventricular haemorrhage in infants under 1 year of age (JAMA, December 11, 1981).

I have placed emphasis on the indications and contraindications accepted by the NIH panel as these are very clear and can easily be used to define the group of patients that need head CT scanning in a certain area in a given period of time. Such studies are not difficult to make using the medical records available in hospitals and outpatients clinics and cannot involve the high cost claimed.

Another approach that could be envisaged for the planning of CT scanners is to study the work load and waiting time of existing CT scanners in a defined area. Such studies, although having the disadvantages of retrospective studies, which are influenced by particular local conditions and also by the fact that the machine may belong to an old generation with low patient output, are much more informative than the use of the suggested mathematical model. In the absence of CT scanners in the area for which the planning is undertaken, a careful study of the X-ray investigations made by the most developed radiodiagnostic departments could be used in order to obtain information from which an extrpolation to the potential needs for CT scanning could be obtained.

The two methods suggested here will avoid the mechanical distribution of CT scanners that would result from the application of the mathematical model proposed. Such a distribution considers only the population distribution and the places where a CT scanner can be located but is not adapted to a number of variables that can essentially alter the demand for CT scanning, such as: (a) the particular distribution of diseases in an area, which may lead to a higher or lower need for CT scanning; (b) the presence of a reputed specialist (neurosurgeon, neurologist) or an outstanding radiotherapy centre in one of the hospitals, which might induce a bias in patient referral from neighbouring areas; (c) the presence of some particular risk factors in the area (more frequent traffic or industrial accidents). Such factors are difficult to identify in their entirety and the number of patients referred for CT scanning could be heavily influenced by such unforeseen elements.

Considering the essential fact that real health needs should be the basis for planning health care facilities, especially those of a sophisticated level that are located in places where the referral system offers enough recorded data to enable an adequate evaluation of needs, I strongly support the idea that CT scanners should be planned using such an approach. If the multiobjective programming model suggested by Wagner can include in a rational way the needs instead of the "shortest distance" or other such parameters, then this model might be valuable in solving the issue. In its current form it remains a theoretical approach with no other possibility than offering a theoretically optimal coverage of the population rather than optimally meeting the health requirements of the population.

Having considered the planning issue of the CT scanner, I shall give some thought to other aspects presented in Wagner's paper.

CT Scanner and Economics of Health Care

This is a subject that has already produced a considerable amount of literature, which is only partially quoted by the paper discussed here. There is no doubt that the CT scanner has improved the whole diagnostic imaging technology in a fundamental way. As with all new technologies, the first period of application produced a number of over-enthusiastic results, which have been gradually reviewed and corrected. The review made by the NIH expert panel for the use of head CT scanning, as well as the not so critical review of the indications of body CT scanning, published by the Society of Computing Tomography, are very clear examples of attempts to place this technology in an accurate light.

The major problem in the use of the CT scanner that remains to be solved is to spread the information that is available today only to a number of specialists involved in the efficiency/efficacy or cost/benefit analysis of CT scanning to all users of this machine, as well as to all physicians who are referring patients for CT scanning. Two phases should be envisaged: the first will involve the CT scanner users, who will have to be made aware of the indications and limitations of the method in a very detailed way; the second represents a much larger and more difficult task, namely making all the general practitioners and specialist physicians who refer patients for CT scanning aware of the real utility as well as the limitations of this technology. This approach could increase the economic and, at the same time, the health impact of the CT scanner and reduce the pressure exercised today on some of the available machines. Appropriate patient selection for CT scanning constitutes the most essential economic and public health aspect of the use of this technology and requires more research as well as better strategies to achieve the desired aim.

In the economics of the CT scanner, a factor that was given no attention by the author is the large unevenness in the distribution of CT scanners at the present time. Kolata (1981) mentions that of 4000 CT scanners currently installed throughout the world, one-third are in the United States, one-third in Japan, and the rest are scattered around the world. A simple calculation leads to the figure of one CT scanner per 100000 people in Japan and almost one CT scanner per 200000 people in the US (not 1/60000 as stated by Kolata). If Western Europe has at least half of the remaining CT scanners a distribution of one CT scanner per 300000 people can be assumed. At the same time large areas of the world are not at all covered or have only one CT scanner for several million people. Such a difference in distribution does not seem to be clearly reflected by the major health indicators in those areas where such indicators are currently available.

What Studies Are Needed to Obtain Further Data for the Health and Economic Evaluation of the CT Scanner?

a) Efficacy/efficiency studies, in particular of whole-body scanning, in order to obtain more comprehensive information on the diagnostic accuracy, therapeutic implications, and the end result of this technique in different diseases located in the neck, chest, abdomen, pelvis, etc. Such studies will lead to a better identification of the indications and limitations of whole-body CT scanning.
b) Studies on diagnostic algorithms for various common diseases, attempting to rationalize the diagnostic procedures according to a logical sequence, the signs and symptoms present, and the results obtained by the investigations performed. The role of CT scanning in a rational algorithm represents the essential factor to be mentioned here.
c) The incidence of high-yield criteria in a given population of patients and the val-

ue of such criteria for the diagnostic and therapeutic decision, as well as for the end result.

d) The impact of the CT scanner on the diagnostic, as well as on the treatment planning of malignant tumours, based on an objective evaluation of the tumour evolution, as well as on the classic 5-, 10-, and 15-year survival rates.
e) Comparative studies on the diagnostic and/or therapeutic impact of CT scanning, ultrasound, digital radiology, and other recent imaging technologies with a view to evaluating alternatives for future diagnostic algorithms.
f) Studies on the cost/benefit of CT scanning with a more objective evaluation of both the costs and the savings are still needed in order to justify further the expansion of this technology. A similar approach can be applied to the diagnostic algorithms.

As already mentioned, the foregoing additional research is suggested in order to increase the available quantitative information on the health and economic effects of the CT scanner. This research will offer not only a better understanding of the essential planning aspects, as clearly defined in Wagner's paper, but will also contribute to a better integration of the utilization of the CT scanner in general health care activities.

I cannot end my discussion on the subject of the health economics of the CT scanner without referring to the fact that the CT scanner is still at an artificially inflated price, which is not only the result of the research costs invested in the production of the machine and its continuous improvement, but seems also to be related to the manufacturers' tendency to obtain a large and quick return on their investment. The high initial investment and the relatively high cost of operation of the CT scanner have prevented this machine from being widely used within health care services and have therefore kept the demand for new machines at a very low level, thus creating a vicious circle. While computer and microprocessor technology has continuously decreased in price and has become widely available throughout the world, the CT scanner has remained in a strange position of isolation, used only by a relatively restricted part of the world that can afford the cost, the maintenance, and the qualified personnel able to handle such technology. If this situation is to change in future in order to allow a greater part of the world population to have access to this technology in a rational way then it will be essential for the present manufacturing and price policy of CT scanners to be reconsidered and redefined in a more appropriate way.

Summary of Workshop Discussion

Decision-makers in the health care system, i.e. providers, payers, and government, are in need of information that goes beyond effectiveness and efficiency of medical technology. The method of organizing multisectorial information on trade-offs associated with alternative investment decisions described in the chapter by Wagner may serve as one tool for the preparation of resource-allocation decisions. Clearly, the method does not replace economic analysis, but it allows for presentation and display of complex data in a form useful to planners and decision-makers. The criteria used in multiobjective programming may therefore include such diverse data as access, availability of expertise (e.g. presence of trained neuroradiologists), quality of management of the services provided, quality of technology to be allocated. Economic aspects of these could, in principle, be included.

The method may be especially useful when applied in connection with general regionalized frameworks of planning and resource allocation. For radiological service a three-tier system might be proposed:

1. Basic radiological services: 95%–100% of all procedures are radiographs; work with contrast medium is exceptional; supervised by nonradiologists, serving a population of 10000–100000 people
2. General purpose radiological services: involving 80%–90% radiographic work and 10%–20% special procedures such as fluoroscopy, supervised by qualified radiologists, serving a population of 50000–5000000 people
3. Specialized radiological services: more than 20% special radiological procedures, supervised by specialized radiologists, serving a population of about a million inhabitants.

In Canada, the guidelines for the allocation of specialized services require that (a) need, or potential demand, reaches a certain volume, and (b) that the resulting load (throughput) of the service is at a level that ensures maintained expertise. Provided these conditions are fulfilled it is required that a given minimum of supporting services be available on site. Thus, for CT scanners a guideline of one unit per 300000 people has been issued.

The diffusion of CT scanners in Japan has proceeded at an extraordinary rate. Beginning in 1975, when two to three units came into operation, the numbers increased as follows: 1976 – 100, 1977 – 290, 1978 – 530, 1979 – 930, 1980 – 1316, 1981 – 1686, 1982 (middle) – 1876, amounting now to 15.6 units per million inhabitants. There are no large differences between the densities in urban and rural areas. The reasons for this are unknown.

There are 11 industrial companies competing for the market, together with 25 leasing companies. It is interesting to note the effects on the pricing of the scanners, e.g. one Japanese company sold its head scanner in 1976 for $ 0.6 million but 3 years later for $ 0.3 million. Others have followed this trend. Industry also has attempted to standardize the scanners so that today it does not require special skills to operate a machine.

Until 1978, the charges for a CT investigation in Japan were US $ 200 and had to be covered out-of-pocket. The National Health Insurance then approved the scanners and fixed the reimbursement rate at US $ 60. After the introduction of reimbursement by the National Health Insurance, the number of patients investigated with CT scanning went up fourfold.

The question of using accessibility as a criterion, in terms of say a minimum of travelling time, should be approached with caution. Swedish experience has shown, for example, that – through decentralized regional planning and resource allocation – the density of coronary care units today is such that their catchment areas are larger than theoretical (epidemiology-based) predictions would require. Additional criteria in the economic domain should be taken into account. In particular, the information on optimal organization and staffing of special services employing medical technology is important. These are essential boundary conditions determining costs and thus play important roles in the negotiations on reimbursement rates.

Part V

Envoi

31 The Future of Evaluation

A. Wojtczak

World Health Organization

We are, it seems, in agreement that we have started to develop some new lines of communication – not only at the international level but also between different professions – in an effort to promote cooperation. Of course the development of interprofessional collaboration is a very painful exercise in which we have to learn to be tolerant and that also requires the ability to learn new ways of thinking. These are exercises that certainly involve costs but which also involve benefit if conscientiously done. Thinking about the future, I should like to emphasize three points. The first one was strongly stressed by White in his speech. It is the need for the development of proper teaching, including new teaching methods and tools, both at the international and national levels. During recent years the WHO has put a lot of effort into the development of some form of interregional and regional training activities in such areas as health management, and health evaluation. We have also organized international and national courses in epidemiology and biostatistics, and the time has come when we should urgently develop training activities in health economics. Those of us who are physicians have learned during the past 3 days a good deal about what economics is all about and, indeed, the way in which economists think. There have been a lot of misconceptions about the role of health economics among the medical profession, who have often crudely identified it with accounting or financing. We have a long way to go to change this attitude and can do so only by the development of more training activities and a better understanding of each other, perhaps by starting some joint project that would manifestly demonstrate that interdisciplinary collaboration is worthwhile.

The second area that was underlined in the discussions is research; research that should be interdisciplinary and interprofessional from the very beginning. It is impossible to evaluate anything if, from the planning stage, the representatives of different professions or disciplines are not working together. We have to learn how to develop this sort of joint activity and also define the role to be played by intergovernmental organizations such as the WHO. I do not doubt that the WHO has an important role to play not only in promoting the development of such research but also in promoting and stimulating the interdisciplinary approach within a network of collaborating centres.

The third area of future work relates to our discussions about the need for an international effort in the evaluation (at least) of high technology used in medicine. I mean here the development of a network of collaborating centres – as was mentioned by Kaprio in his introductory paper – that would help at the international level to evaluate the usefulness, effectiveness, and efficiency of certain highly technological procedures used in diagnosis of treatment. One such example is CT scanning.

The European Regional Office of the WHO has, in my opinion, an important role to play in promoting and supporting such developments. I would also like to remind you of what was said by Wahba: that it is of the greatest importance to develop a much broader understanding of these issues within the profession and teach the methodology of evaluation that is needed. We have to start with undergraduate and continue all the way through to postgraduate education to reach this aim.

Finally, a brief personal reflection. It has been fascinating to follow the development of the interprofessional dialogues during these 3 days. I have to say that having an opportunity to observe similar interprofessional discussions between physicians and representatives of behavioural sciences, the dialogues that have taken place here in Wolfsberg prove that economists and physicians can easily take part not only in discussions with another but also in productive cooperation.

32 Medical and Economic Evaluation: A Postscript

A. J. Culyer and B. Horisberger

The preceding papers and discussions offer a rich menu of principles and practice, ideals and practical possibilities, and provide a large number of illustrations of what can be – and cannot be – accomplished given available knowledge and understanding. In this final chapter we shall try to impose some order on an otherwise bewildering complexity. We have imposed the order in the following way: we have taken a set of key issues that arise from a practical point of view in conducting evaluative studies, illustrated the kinds of problem that arise with reference to the work reported and discussed in this book, and indicated how "best" to overcome the problems raised. We have put "best" in quotation marks because there is rarely an unambiguous "best" way of proceeding. In practice, ideal methods are rarely applicable. Moreover, the "best" method will depend on the objective of the work being undertaken. So "best" really means getting as close an approximation as possible to the ideal that is relevant to the purposes in hand, making allowances for the shortfall between what would be ideal and what has to be practicable in any conclusions one draws from one's study.

Evaluative Objectives

Since the aims of studies can vary, it is important, first, to design a study with as clear a statement as possible of its objective. This not only keeps the researcher on the right track, it also avoids the danger of drawing conclusions from the study that are not warranted and minimizes the danger of misplaced criticism, for example, criticism of the form that arises from the possibility that the question of concern to a critic was not that addressed by the study.

In the course of this book we have seen a large number of different types of objective. For example, a study whose objective is to determine which patients to put on short-term cimetidine treatment under conditions where the local resource constraints place a definite limit on the availability of the drug has a quite different aim from one that seeks to find out whether, for a given probability of relapse or of symptomatic recurrence, it is more effective to treat with the drug or by vagotomy with some form of drainage. A further different objective would be to determine whether the one is more *cost*-effective than the other from the point of view of the whole health system in order to decide, for example, whether resources ought to be made more readily available for the one or the other, or whether the insurance companies should in general reimburse only particular types of treatment (others requiring, let us say, a special case to be made).

This is but one way of identifying legitimate differences in the focus of interest – clinical management of specific patients, general guidelines for good practice, or more global investment and financing decisions. The objective will profoundly affect the nature of the study and the results of one type may be quite useless in the context of another. Thus, for example, one technology is rarely a *complete* alternative to another: dialysis patients may subsequently receive a transplant and some patients may be suitable for one treatment but not the other; cimetidine patients may subsequently receive antacid therapy or surgery and, again, some patients may be unsuited to some of the alternatives being considered; computed tomographic (CT) scans can be substituted by other imaging methods. A study whose aim is to work out the expected system cost of a particular technology will have to allow for the possibility of that technology being used in conjunction with other technologies on a system basis, a study whose aim is to determine the relative effectiveness of several procedures at accurately locating a lesion will not.

There are other differences of objective too: is the study designed to evaluate the relative effectiveness of alternative diagnostic procedures in terms of diagnostic accuracy or of eventual health improvement or remission? Is the study concerned with symptomatic relief or with cure? Is the study concerned with short-term or long-term consequences? Is the study concerned with the optimal use of just one technology or with the optimal mix of several technologies through time? Is the study concerned with the ideal amount of resources to embody in a particular technology or with predicting which patients would benefit most from using an existing stock of resources? Is the study concerned to establish provisional results that may be used to provide a part of the basis for policy to control the diffusion of a technology (and accompanied by appropiately designed monitoring and longer-term evaluation studies)? Of the various studies reviewed and reported here, examples of each can be found, and it is plain that a large part of the variation in study design results from these differences in objectives, which themselves transcend the distinction between efficacy, effectiveness, and efficiency that has so often been stressed in the foregoing papers.

There is no uniquely correct objective; they are as varied as the needs of the clients for evaluative studies – practising clinicians, medical researchers, hospital managers, insurance agencies, and public authorities, those needing quick provisional results, and those needing more substantional longer-term appraisals. The list is not, of course, exhaustive. And each potential client may have a need for more than just one kind of information.

What emerges from all this? One simple lesson: a study that purports to be evaluative must be clear and specific about its objective(s). The "right" objective is not a question of *principle* but of who the imagined client is. Since the interests of clients vary, studies done for one purpose may be quite useless for another. It is almost certainly overambitious to attempt to meet the needs of *all* possible clients for information within the scope of a single study (though this does not mean that a study must necessarily have only *one* objective or a *single* client).

Comparators

One type of evaluative study is concerned with the very basic question "what properties does a particular technology have?" These are often termed *efficacy* studies. They relate to what Russell calls the "technology matrix". Examples include the effect of various doses of cimetidine on ulcer healing and/or symptomatic relief, the proportion of false-negatives and false-positives found by CT scanning, or the number of life-years enjoyed (if that is the right word!) by patients on continuous ambulatory peritoneal dialysis.

The essential problem with this type of study is how to be sure that the effects attributed to the technology in question really are due to it rather than to placebo or Hawthorne effects or to other factors. These other factors are implicitly assumed constant but may, in actual fact, systematically vary and hence bias the results in one direction or another. This raises important questions of study design, which are discussed in the next section.

A characteristic of efficacy studies of this sort is that they give no information about the *relative* efficacy of one procedure compared with another (including "doing nothing"). The next stage of sophistication is therefore to compare relative efficacy as between a set of chosen alternatives: is the effect of a given dosage of cimetidine on ulcer healing and/or symptomatic relief greater or smaller than that of, say, doing nothing, prescribing placebos, prescribing antacids. or adopting any one of a set of surgical alternatives? Is the diagnostic accuracy of a CT head scan greater or smaller than that of pneumoencephalography, cerebral angiography, radionuclide brain scanning, echoencephalography, electroencephalography, skull X-ray, or exploratory surgery? Is the number of life-years gained via continuous ambulatory peritoneal dialysis greater or smaller than those gained via transplantation or various forms (and locations) of machine haemodialysis or, indeed, of programmes designed to prevent nephropathy? Again, the sophisticated analyst may have to take account of the fact that one procedure is rarely a complete substitute for another (so one type of efficacy study may, for example, be concerned with the optimal *sequencing* of alternative procedures) and that not all alternatives may be relevant for all imaginable clients for the research results.

Efficacy studies seek, so far as is possible, to identify efficacy in an institution-free, purely "technical" context. Once one brings in the context (for example the fact that not all users of a technology have the same skills, not all populations at risk have the same access to health services) one is in the realm of *effectiveness* studies, which allow for the possibility that what, in principle, is a relatively efficacious procedure may not, in practice, be a relatively effective one. To take an extreme case: arming barefoot medical aides in the third world with a modern technology may be grossly less effective than arming them with the skills to persuade and help people to change harmful life-styles. The same is often true in the developed world. And it applies not only to the technology in question but also to others with which it may be compared: Bardhan reported in discussion, for example, that in the hands of the most skilled surgeons, ulcer recurrence after a highly selective vagotomy is only about 7% but in the hands of surgical trainees it may be as high as 25%. Moreover, most cimetidine is taken by non-duodenal ulcer (DU) patients, which highlights another important factor that effectiveness studies must take into account but which efficacy studies do not. In principle, however, while the complexity of effectiveness studies is inevitably greater, the same general issues arise in them as in efficacy studies – again involving the judicious selection of *prima facie* relevant alternatives (or mixes) whose effectiveness is going to be compared, and designing the study in such a fashion as to allow for the effect of other influential factors.

In the context of *efficiency* studies, whose aim is to identify the least cost method of achieving a clearly specified objective (or set of objectives), or to maximize "achievements" given the resources available, or (more ambitiously) of maximizing the difference between the expected benefits and the expected costs, the idea of absolute efficacy or effectiveness is well-nigh useless. The reason for this is that information about the costs and outcomes (or benefits) of *one* procedure is information that cannot be used for any purpose of *choice*. Efficiency is about the best way of doing something where there are alternatives. Hence *relative* efficacy and *relative* effectiveness are *sine qua nons* of any efficiency analysis. Without the medical and epidemiological information one simply cannot proceed with efficiency evaluation.

It follows, therefore, that economists are crucially dependent on their medical colleagues for information about relative efficacy and effectiveness. Lest this suggests that there is a natural sequencing here (first the efficacy/effectiveness analysis, then the efficiency analysis), it should be emphasized that this is not the case. If the ultimate goal of a study is couched in terms of efficiency, then it is crucial that appropriate concepts of cost and benefit, or gain and loss, be incorporated into the study design from the very beginning. Each of the technologies in this book furnishes examples of economic ad hoc assessments fastened onto the coat-tails of a on-going or already completed medical study. From an effectiveness point of view it may be immaterial to compute, say, the value of earnings lost by sick patients or the value of time given up by family and friends. From an efficiency point of view, however, these may be crucial (whether they are or not depends, of course, on the scope of costs and benefits considered and again brings us back to the study objectives and the ultimate client for whom the information is intended). A sequential approach incurs the grave risk, therefore, that important information may not be gathered at the time when it is easiest to do so (which may be the *only* time). It also has the danger that the relevant skills for identifying, conceptualizing, and measuring data relevant for efficiency analysis will not be applied – even if there is recognition that some information of this sort is needed. Instead a good efficacy or effectiveness study turns into an amateurish efficiency study that brings the *whole* exercise into disrepute. Common pitfalls here include the uncritical use of market prices, the neglect of unpriced resources (like time or capital goods already owned by an agency), the treatment of transfers as costs and benefits, and the neglect, or inappropriate use, of discounting procedures.

Correct Attribution of Consequences

The problem of correct attribution has already been touched upon: it is to do with making the most confident statement one can about causes and effects rather than apparent associations. It has, rather obviously, two strands. First, is there some reason (a theory) for expecting one thing to lead to another? For example, are there biochemical reasons for expecting ingestion of cimetidine to increase ulcer healing, increase the risk of impotence or renal failure? A mere association may be no more than that, rather like the association between the prevalence of dysentery in Scotland and the UK rate of inflation where the correlation coefficient of +0.71 suggests to nobody that either one causes the other. Second, has an appropriate statistical procedure been followed that allows for the possible effects of other variables and the possible interaction of variables? As was seen in the cimetidine case, the frequency of surgery was already falling at the time the drug was introduced so an association between the frequency of use of the drug and the frequency of the operation is not itself sufficient to conclude that the former caused the latter. In this case, as it happens, there are good reasons both for predicting the association and for supposing the use of the drug to have actually reduced the frequency of surgery (at least over the study periods).

Generally, correct attribution of effect to cause requires a careful study design: case-control, cohort or longitudinal, or (ideally) randomized clinical trials so that other variables are either specifically allowed for (which requires a rather comprehensive understanding of the proper specification of the "model" to be tested) or generally allowed for by randomization (which requires a less comprehensive understanding). The papers of Balaban and Goldfarb and of Russell give an exemplary treatment of these issues.

Time

The foregoing papers have, between them, highlighted four major ways in which time must be carefully considered in an evaluative study. Summarily, these are the time-span of the study, the use of time as an input, the use of time as an output, and the effect of distance in time on the calculation of present costs and benefits. The first of these aspects of time requires careful treatment because, as is particularly clear from the cimetidine case, some conditions are self-limiting with some probability distribution over time (and hence the period of benefit attribution due to any technology should not exceed the expected period during which disease or symptoms are present) and because the effects of a technology may both take time to become apparent and last for a limited time period.

The second aspect of time is important because in some cases time inputs are easily overlooked. Time is a valuable resource with alternative uses. This is plain in the case of human resources that receive a salary or wage per unit of time, or of capital goods that are rented at a particular rate per unit of time. It is no less true of unpriced time inputs – like those of patients, families, friends, voluntary workers, and the like. To ignore such time costs is to treat such resources promiscuously. One cost-reducing effect of CT-scanning is the reduced length of time spent by patients as inpatients compared with other investigative procedures. Pedersen showed, with his "treatment-resource profile", that time costs also feature in the evaluation of dialysis, and Weisbrod referred to studies that have also taken explicit account of such time aspects. The involvement of family members in a procedure like home dialysis has also been noted as important in the renal failure cases. Nearly all studies manage to make some allowance for paid time (lost or gained). Relatively few carry the logic of that policy through to the end.

The use of time as an output is exemplified by the life-years gained approach in clinical evaluation and cost-effectiveness analysis, especially in the renal disease analyses. This is an approximation of the more ideal measure "healthy days". But merely to assert this is to indicate the measurement difficulties inherent in either measuring "health" directly or indirectly by adjusting life-years for "quality". Granted that "health" can be validly seen as a kind of ultimate end-objective of medicine (including prevention) there is plainly a large research programme needing to be done to enable usable measures to be available for routine efficacy, effectiveness, and efficiency studies. This research programme has been alluded to several times in the papers and all evaluators are potential clients of such research. By comparison, many of the proximate objectives used (freedom from disease, reduction of symptoms, etc.) are very poor substitutes for the "real thing". They may not even be the best approximations available, so it is encumbent on all evaluators to familiarize themselves with the health measurement literature. This became clear particularly in the treatment of end-stage renal failure, where the efficacy of both dialysis and transplantation has been firmly established for a long time but, despite this, there is very little systematic knowledge of quality of life differences.

The final aspect of time is the discounting of future benefits and costs – whether or not they are cast in monetary terms. Whenever costs and benefits flow over a period that is more than a couple of years there is the possibility that failure to deal satisfactorily with the discounting problem can seriously distort results. Nearly all studies by economists use discounting when appropriate. Hardly any studies by medical experts do, even when they are explicitly economic in their aims. Indeed, one of the most obvious characteristics of most medical and epidemiological evaluations is their failure to deal satisfactorily with at least one of these time aspects. Those that try almost always do restrict themselves to time that is paid for and uncritically accept market prices as the relevant weights to apply to units of time.

Generalizability

The generalizability of the results of any evaluative study depends crucially on the statistical design of the study and its objective. The design question has been ably discussed in several papers (notably Balaban and Goldfarb's and Russell's) and needs no further emphasis here, though it is absolutely crucial. Efficacy studies are not typically generalizable as they are not characteristically conducted in an institutional and human context that would permit this. Compliance by patients varies in different types of study (and practice). So does "misuse" of a technology.

Aside from these points, however, it is worth emphasizing that the objectives of a study may rule out certain types of generalizability. One aspect of this is brought out clearly in Weisbrod's paper: a study designed to answer the question "what are the relative costs of two (or more) alternative procedures?" will not (alone) give an answer to the general systems question "what is the expected reduction in cost per case when a new technology becomes available?" Again, therefore, it is important to have one's aims very clear from the outset so that the questions one is answering are really the ones one *thinks* one is answering and that one *wants* to ask!

Effectiveness and efficiency studies (unlike efficacy studies) may also need to take account (depending on their objective) of "scenarios" or "pathways" of treatment. Patients are not, for example, typically treated *either* by home dialysis *or* transplantation (whose efficacy is roughly the same, with transplantation perhaps having the edge in terms of long-term survival rates), but more between modes of treatment: they may first be in hospital dialysis, go on to home dialysis, receive a transplant, and then revert to home dialysis (Ludbrook 1981). Such dynamic patterns also occur with DU patients and in many other medical areas. Moreover, these patterns may not be independent of the financial and other terms of access for patients and the method of paying physicians and financing hospitals. The issues rapidly widen into questions of the *behavioural* response of various actors on the stage to the various constraints they are confronted with.

Each of the technologies discussed in this book shows a wide international variation in its use. The most comprehensive kind of effectiveness or efficiency study would seek to provide reasons for this variability, which seems to relate far more to planning systems, reimbursement methods, physician payment systems, and industrial policy than to any underlying demographic or morbidity indicators of need. Although it is not much pursued in the papers, it is clear that investigations of this sort may take one into an even more multidisciplinary setting than is represented here and that would include, say, sociological and political modes of enquiry. Effectiveness and efficiency, then, are not independent of the social, economic, and political environment, and one cannot readily generalize *across* political and cultural boundaries. Indeed, the papers that discuss the effectiveness of kidney transplantation explicitly bring out the significance of current limits on the availability of live and cadaver donors. Easing such constraints takes one well beyond the medical and economic fields but is also itself subject to evaluative work: what "harvesting" procedures are, for example, the most cost-effective?

Classifying Gains and Losses, Benefits, and Costs

Suppose one seeks to undertake a *complete* evaluation of a technology. Setting aside some of the wider ramifications just discussed, there are two basic ways in which one can set about devising a matrix whose elements will contain all the relevant quantitative or qualitative information. The first is to categorize all effects into benefits and costs. This, as Williams plainly shows, is a minefield for the inexperienced, for the logically appropriate concept of cost is that of *opportunity cost* (and usually *marginal* opportunity cost at that), which can be very different from the conventional notion of cost (= expenditure) that we all carry in our heads.

The second approach is less of a minefield in the first instance because it uses less specialized concepts as the criteria for classification. This approach entails the identification of *all* parties that are affected by any decision regarding a technology and, for each of these, to identify *gains* and *losses*. This is less of a minefield in the sense that, if it is truly comprehensive, the risk of doublecounting, overcounting, and undercounting will be minimized. To illustrate: economists using the opportunity cost approach are insistent (correctly) that transfer payments not be included. Noneconomists often have difficulty with this. Discussion in the workshops often centred on these difficulties. In the gains/losses approach, however, the difficulty vanishes, for if one counts as a gain to a *sick patient* his receipt of whatever cash welfare payments he may get, this will show up as a loss to the *tax payer* who provides the money. Provided that the system of accounting is sufficiently comprehensive, the gain and the loss will each be picked up – and will, of course, cancel out (as the opportunity cost approach insists they do). But while the comprehensive explicitness of the gains/losses approach is less of a minefield in this respect, it still has abundant snares for the unwary, for the business of assigning (monetary) values to gains and losses is a skilled affair based on sophisticated theory, and it is here probably more than anywhere else that the economists' skills complement those of the experts in the technology and those of the experts in the statistical design of trials.

Incidentally, while the benefit-cost approach in practice tends to commit one to a particular view of the appropriate general objective of efficiency studies (namely the maximization of the difference between *all* benefits and *all* costs) the gains/losses approach is particularly good at identifying *who* gains and loses and can hence be of use in analyses that seek to appraise the efficiency of a procedure from the point of view of various parties. It also may help in understanding *why* some ostensibly globally efficient procedures do not become adopted while other ostensibly globally inefficient procedures do. The answer is most likely that they were not in the interests, or were in the interests, of *particular* parties.

Both types of analysis go, of course, under the general rubric "cost-benefit" or "cost-effectiveness" analysis: the fundamental theoretical precepts are the same, only the manner of presentation is different.

Many of the empirical studies have to date taken a distressingly limited view of benefit. Most medical and economic analysts agree that simple revealed willingness to pay for treatment substantially underestimates true benefit and also introduces discriminatory distortions that depend to much on the prevailing distribution of wealth. The same disquiet is felt about the human-capital approach, which effectively treats people like workhorses and again has distributional distortions. Consequently such approaches can, at best, indicate that a procedure is efficient if the measured benefits exceed costs but the contrary conclusion, that it is inefficient if measured benefits fall short of costs, would not be warranted. Again, therefore, discussion at this symposium has returned repeatedly to the unsatisfactory nature of much current benefit (or outcome) measurement. The obvious alternative is to face up to the development and use of health indexes (even if one does not go so far – and it would indeed almost certainly be premature in the current state of our knowledge – as to place a money value on changes in a measure of health).

On Not Making the Perfect the Enemy of the Merely Good

A collection of papers that seeks to identify good evaluative practice by examining actual practice in three selected areas, and by reflecting on the procedures adopted, runs the risk of counselling perfection. How, then, is one to proceed when perfection is inevitably denied one? The dilemma is starkly posed by *new* technologies, for decision-makers want evaluative results *before* the technologies are adopted and yet evaluation can proceed only when technologies have *already* been adopted. CT scanning is a spectacular example of a very widely diffused technology that was widely implemented before a single evaluation had been performed.

The answer has to lie in *conceptual clarity.* Only if one is as clear as one can be about one's objectives and the appropriate measures of efficacy, effectiveness, and efficiency can one begin to make some assessment of which short cuts, approximations, are likely to be least compromising. Only then can one make a reasoned assessment, moreover, of the validity of the results obtained. To know (approximately) what one has *not* done is often as important as knowing what one (precisely) *has* done. To know (approximately) what the *principal* attributes of a technology are is more important than knowing (precisely) its minor attributes. In short, good evaluation requires good judgement. And good judgement comes from factual knowledge placed in a clear conceptual framework.

In the discussions there was widespread agreement that carefully done "quick and dirty" studies coupled with careful monitoring, so that the diffusion of a technology generated information that could be used at a later decision point, were the appropriate means of achieving a short-term response to the demand for an early evaluation of new technologies. The monitoring aspect of it is helped if those who finance new technologies require those who use them to state what they hope to accomplish by using them and how they propose to measure their accomplishment! It is also, however, worth bearing in mind that most new technologies also become old technologies with the passage of time and that, as White points out in his paper, the vast majority of extant procedures have an *unknown* effectiveness.

There is, therefore, ample scope for a variety of studies in terms of their depth, period of follow-up, and so on. Moreover, the "quick and dirty" studies will usually identify some of the crucial areas for investigation that only more sustained in-depth studies can undertake; they hence have the virtue not only of giving the best answers to immediate questions that cannot be fully or confidently answered at present, they also help to provide the agendas for the in-depth studies. But there is no harm in – and a good ideal to be said for – setting in train major in-depth studies of new technologies when there is the suspicion that they are going to diffuse quickly and also be very costly. This suggests that a good strategy in this regard is to *concentrate* one's currently limited evaluative skills rather than spread them thinly over a set of studies whose ultimate pay-off in terms of changes in effective medical practice, or (preferably) changes in cost-effective medical practice, is likely to be very variable.

Multidisciplinary Studies

Repeatedly in this symposium it has become clear that the conecptual skills of experts in the respective technologies, the conceptual skills of clinical and epidemiological statistical designers of trials, and the conceptual skills of economists are all complementary to one another. In efficiency evaluation any one proceeding without the other two, and any two proceeding without the other one, is to court failure. Indeed, the most general lesson to be drawn from this volume is the evidence it accumulates that multidisciplinary collaboration is the sine qua non of successful evaluation for efficiency.

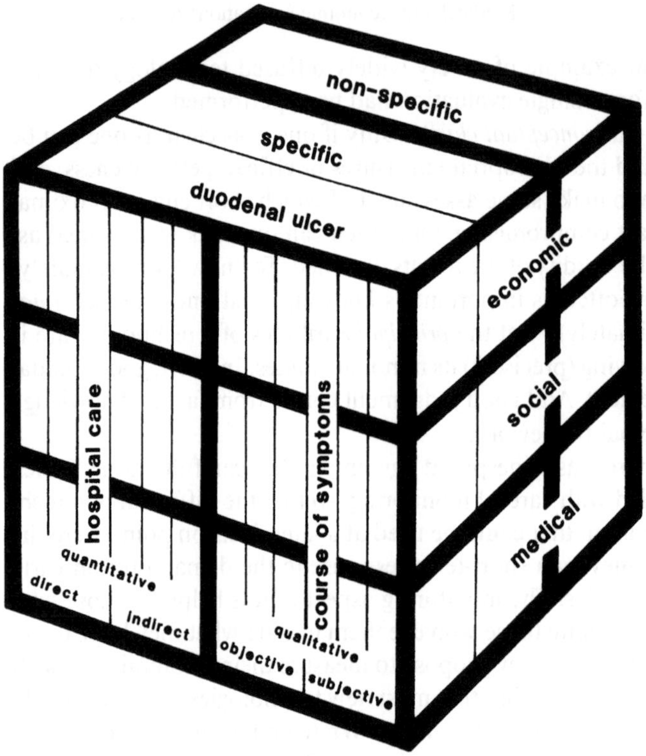

Figure 32.1. Illustration of the multidimensional relation between application of a medical technology (specific/non-specific), the various kinds of effect (quantitative/qualitative) and different scales of evaluation (economic, social, medical).

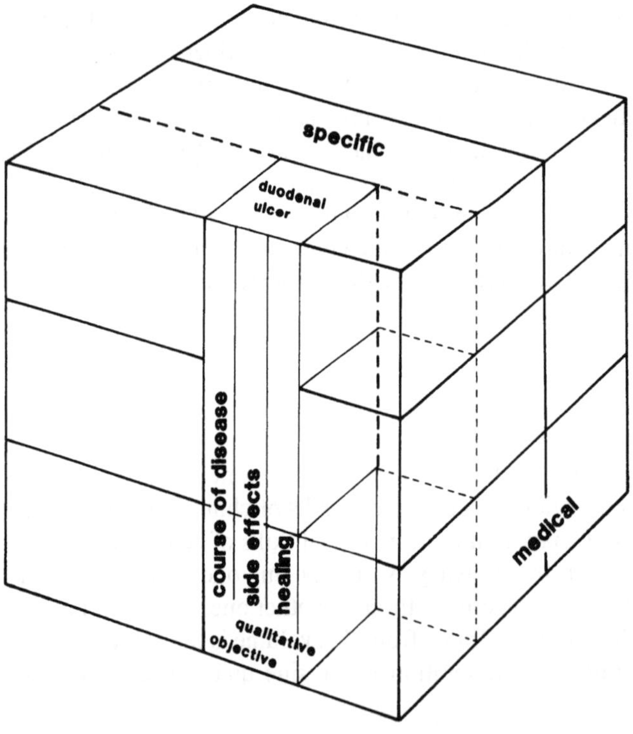

Fig. 32.2. Illustration of the medical perspective in the case of specific application of a medical technology (cimetidine in duodenal ulcer) and objective effects on the healing process

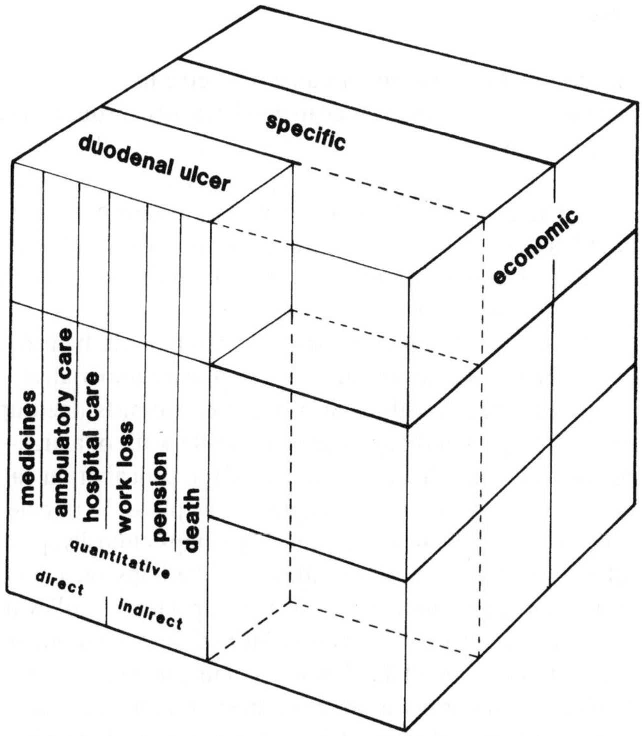

Fig. 32.3. Illustration of the economic perspective in the case of specific application of a medical technology (cimetidine in duodenal ulcer) and a set of factors relevant to measurement of direct and indirect effects

But this is not, of course, to say that it is true at all levels of evaluation. Indeed, there are types of evaluation that do *not* need multidisciplinary collaboration. One may illustrate from the cimetidine case. Figure 32.1 shows "Horisberger's Cube" as applied to cimetidine. On the front face we see the nature of various kinds of effect that the use of the drug may have (the divisions are illustrative rather than exhaustive). On the side face we see these effects classified according to medical, social, and economic levels. On the top face we see an array of technologies some of which are specific (cimetidine in this case) and others nonspecific (e. g. cimetidine in the case of gastritis). The cube may be sliced according to one's focus of interest. In Fig. 32.2, for example, the cube is sliced from a medical perspective, in particular looking at the objective evolution of the illness, where the side effects of the healing process produced by cimetidine in DU cases may be of interest, and we then compare the effectiveness of the drug with that of other preparations or against placebo. Alternatively, as in Fig. 32.3, we may slice the cube from an economic perspective and investigate a set of factors that are relevant in that case.

Envoi

The editors hope that this volume will serve to assist the cause of good evaluation, and perhaps will form a guide to good practice through the combination of the early papers outlining the principles of evaluation and the more specialist papers seeking to apply them in reviewing and reporting on the work on the three selected technologies. The glossary will, we hope, assist those who are unfamiliar with the jargon – or at least some of it. The reference section will, we hope, offer a reasonably comprehensive set of possibilities for those wishing to deepen their knowledge of principles or practice in these three territories.

We hope that, at the very least, the volume will banish fears – as the symposium from which it has come did – of disciplinary imperialism and *amour propre*. If the symposium began with clinicians and economists lined up – as one commentator put it – like girls and boys against opposite walls of a high-school dance hall, it ended with a much fuller appreciation of the contribution each has to make and with the beginnings of genuine dialogue taking place. To pursue the high-school analogy, some were even dancing together – perhaps clumsily, perhaps treading on one another's feet, but nonetheless enjoying it. Perhaps even more telling: it was clear that more than one bashful 'boy' was sizing up a likely 'girl' with a view to making a date privately after the ball was over! More than one commentator, towards the end of the conference, noted that it was becoming increasingly hard, when someone spoke, to identify him or her as an economist or a medical doctor. If this volume furthers that sort of thing, then it will have done its immediate job. And its main job – contributing to the improvement of evaluative studies yet to come – will have got under way.

33 Glossary

Arteriography. See *Angiography.*

Ambulatory care. Care provided to patients who are not confined to bed. The main types of ambulatory care are care as an outpatient or day-patient and care given by a general practitioner.

Angiography. Diagnostic procedure in radiology, using injected contrast media to produce images of blood vessels.

Aneurism. Large local dilation of arteries as a consequence of a degenerative process in the vessel wall (e.g. arteriosclerosis). Rupture can occur; surgical excision of the aneurisms is the treatment of choice.

Alkalosis. Clinical term signifying a decrease of acid in the body fluids. May be a result of respiratory abnormality, persistent vomiting (with loss of hydrochloric acid), or excessive ingestion of buffer substances like sodium bicarbonate (so-called antacids).

Biopsy. Excision of a tissue specimen for subsequent analysis, usually under microscopic inspection. (Specimens are sometimes obtained by puncture, i.e. by "needle biopsy".)

Cerebral angiography. See *Angiography,* angiography of cerebral blood vessels.

Cerebrovascular disease. Disease of cerebral blood vessels. Arteriosclerosis accounts for most forms.

Chronic (disease, illness). An impairment or bodily structure or function that necessitates a modification of the patient's normal life and has persisted or may be expected to persist over an extended period of time.

Continuous ambulatory peritoneal dialysis (CAPD). See *dialysis* for general description of the method. CAPD is a variant of *intermittent peritoneal dialysis* (q.v.) involving, however, a constant process of gradual exchange with the dialysate fluid introduced into the peritoneal cavity, with drainage into a portable bottle or bag that can be periodically detached and emptied.

Cost-benefit analysis (CBA). A method of comparing the costs and benefits of various alternative courses of action usually (though not necessarily) measured in monetary terms and *present values* (q.v.). It entails the systematic comparison of all the costs and benefits of proposed alternative schemes with a view to determining (a) which scheme or combination of schemes maximizes the difference between benefits and costs, or (b) the magnitude of the benefit that can result from schemes having various costs. The concept of cost or benefit employed is usually that of *social cost or benefit* (q. v.). However, in some cases the scope of the cost and benefit concepts is defined by the interests of the clients for whom the analysis is conducted after extensive discussion between clients and analysts about the options to be considered and the objectives to be sought. See also *cost-effectiveness analysis.*

Cost-effectiveness analysis (CEA). A method of comparing the costs of various alternative courses of action having the same benefit or in terms of a common unit of output, outcome, or other measure of accomplishment. This procedure is used when benefits are difficult to value or when those that are measurable are not commensurable. It is similar to *cost-benefit analysis* (q. v.) except that benefit, instead of being expressed in monetary terms or in terms of several noncommensurable benefits, is expressed in terms of a homogeneous index of results achieved, e. g. number of lives saved or number of days free from disease.

Craniotomy. Operative opening of the skull.

Computerized tomographic (CT) or computerized axial tomographic (CAT) scanner. An X-ray technology producing images of selected planes through the body as though sliced by a knife. The computer-produced images contain structural information depending on X-ray absorption of the various tissues. Sequences of slices (scans) can be used to reconstruct three-dimensional images of regions of the body.

Dalton. Unit of relative molecular (or atomic) mass.

Dialysis. The term derives from the Greek "to separate" and "to dissolve". Thus haemodialysis is literally "blood separation". Dialysis involves selective separation of small molecules and ions (so-called crystalloids such as electrolytes, metabolic waste products, toxic substances) from large molecules or particles (proteins, blood corpuscles, etc.). This is achieved by interposing a semipermeable membrane between the blood and a suitable fluid (i. e. the dialysate), in the machine called artificial kidney.

Discount factor. See *discounting* for general description. The discount factor for year t is given by $1/(1+r)^t$ where r is the annual discount rate. Thus, if $r=0.1$, the discount factor for $t=1$ is 0.909 and for $t=5$ it is 0.620.

Discounting. A procedure for reducing flows of cost or benefits occurring at different dates into a common measure by use of an appropriate discount rate. Thus, with an annual discount rate r (expressed as a decimal fraction) the present value (PV) of a cost (C) in 1 year's time is $PV=C/(1+r)$ and that of a cost in 5 years' time is $PV=C/(1+r)^5$.

Double-blind trial. Used to describe a trial in which the nature of the treatment received by a subject at any time is unknown to both subject and observer.

Duodenum. The first section of the small intestine, about 28 cm in length, extending from the pylorus, i. e. the stomach exit, to the junction of the jejunum (the midsection of the small intestines) at the level of the first or second lumbar vertebra of the left side.

Echoencephalography. Imaging process of brain and skull structures using ultrasound as a source of energy.

Effectiveness. A measure similar to *efficacy* (q.v.) except that it refers to the effect of a particular medical technology or of a procedure and its effects or outcomes when used in actual practice. It thus differs from efficacy in that efficacy concerns only the technical relationship between the procedure and its effects under "ideal" conditions.

Efficacy. Benefit or utility to the individual of the service, treatment regimen, drug, preventive or control measure advocated or applied. The probability of benefit to individuals in a defined population from a medical technology under ideal conditions of use. More generally, the effect of a particular medical action in altering the *natural history* (q.v.) of a particular disease for the better.

Efficiency. In a restrictive sense defined either as minimizing the *opportunity cost* (q.v.) of attaining a given output or as maximizing the output for a given opportunity cost. The general term used by economists is known as "Pareto-efficiency". This is an allocation of resources such that it is not possible to reallocate them without imposing uncompensated losses on some individual. A variant is "potential Pareto-efficiency", where it is not possible to reallocate resources without imposing uncompensatable losses on someone.

Epidemiology. The study of the distribution and determinants of disease and disability in human populations, of the factors influencing that distribution, and of the impact of intervention on it.

Electroencephalography. Mapping of bioelectrical activity of the brain by multichannel recordings of signals on the scalp.

Endoscope. Optical instrument used to examine internal organs.

Glomerulonephritis. A form of kidney inflammation (i.e. inflammatory changes of structures within the kidney called glomeruli). The most common form of primary disease in Europe amongst those treated for end-stage renal failure. Disease may continue for many years, death from uremia is the usual outcome, but the cause is variable and patient may live a reasonably normal life for 20–30 years.

H_2-receptor antagonists. Inhibitors of basal acid secretion and secreting responses to feeding, gastric, histamine, and vagal stimulation. They block the access of histamine to sensitive cells.

Haematoma. A local collection of blood in the tissues (outside blood vessels) after injury or in association with degeneration of blood vessels.

Health care technology. The drugs, devices, and medical and surgical procedures used in medical care and the organizational and supportive system within which such care is provided.

Heparin. A complex anticoagulent (first isolated from canine liver and subsequently found to be a constituent of several types of tissues, especially the liver and lung).

Histamine. Powerful stimulant of gastric secretion and constrictor of bronchial smooth muscle.

Histocompatability. State of immunological similarity or identity of tissues sufficient to permit successful homograft transplantation. Means identity of tissue antigen patterns in donor and recipient.

Human capital. The stock of human skills embodied in an individual or group. In value terms it is usually measured as the present value (see *discounting*) of the flow of marketed skills (for example, the present value of expected earnings over a period of time). It is determined by basic ability, educational attainment, and health status, among other things.

Hydrocephalus. Excessive accumulation of cerebrospinal fluid in the brain.

Iatrogenic disease. Disease caused by actions of the physician ("iatros" = physician).

Incidence. The number of instances of illness commencing, or of persons falling ill, during a given period of time in a specified population.

Intermittent peritoneal dialysis (IPD). See *dialysis* for general description of the method. In IPD, fluid is introduced into the peritoneal cavity. After the equilibration period – to allow diffusion and filtration to take place across the peritoneal membrane – the dialysate is drained from the peritoneal cavity. The usual dialysis lasts 24–72 h. During that period the cycle of inflow, equilibrating period, outflow is repeated many times.

Internal rate of return. That discount rate (see *discounting*) that makes the net present value of costs and benefits equal to zero. Thus, with B_t and C_t representing costs and benefits in year t, the annual internal rate of return is r* in the formula:

$$0=\sum_{t=0}^{n}\frac{B_t-C_t}{(1+r^*)^t}$$

Kidney. The kidney excretes urine into the ureters and so to the bladder. Urine contains a variety of toxic waste materials. The kidneys are two bean-shaped organs, which in man are about 12 cm long, 5 cm wide, and 4 cm thick. They lie on either side of the spine, behind the peritoneum, opposite the 12th thoracic and first three lumbar vertebrae.

Marginal cost or benefit. The additional cost or benefit from increasing the rate or volume of an activity. Mathematically it is the first derivative of cost or benefit with respect to the (continuous) variable in question.

Morbidity. See *prevalence.*

Mortality. The ratio of the total number of deaths from a particular cause in a year in a given population to that of the total population. Age-specific mortality – the number of deaths that occur in a year to 1000 persons of a particular age or age-group.

Natural history of disease. A description of the course of a disease in a patient or group of the population as it proceeds over time without medical intervention.

Needs, health needs. The scientifically (biologically, epidemiologically, etc.) determined deficiencies in health that call for preventive, curative, and, where appropriate, control or eradication measures. Whereas the deficiencies may be scientifically established, the preventive or remedial actions that may follow cannot be said to be "needed" without an ethical judgement or judgements.

Nomogram. A graphical representation, allowing for the numerical evaluation of (functional) relationships among three or more variables.

Nuclear magnetic resonance (NMR). A phenomenon in which atomic nuclei respond to discrete radiowave frequencies when acted upon by magnetic fields. NMR is exhibited only by nuclei with odd numbers of protons or neutrons, i.e. with a net spin. NMR spectroscopy is used in analytical chemistry to elucidate the conformation of organic molecules. Special apparatus, i.e. NMR scanners, produce images of structures and the distribution of certain nuclei (of hydrogen, of phosphorus isotope ^{31}P etc.) in selected sections of the body.

Oligosymptomatic (disease). A disease showing few symptoms.

Opportunity cost. The value of a resource in its most highly valued alternative use. In a world of competitive markets in which *all* goods are traded, opportunity cost is revealed by the prices of resources. Where these stringent conditions are not met opportunity cost and market prices may diverge, and "shadow prices" may be estimated to measure the former.

Peptic ulcer. An ulcer of the alimentary mucosa, usually in the stomach or duodenum.

Perforated ulcer. Ulcer extending through the wall of an organ.

Pneumoencephalography. Encephalography is an X-ray imaging technique of the brain. Pneumoencephalography is a technique whereby air is injected into the ventricles to demonstrate, by X-ray, the size and configuration of the ventricular system.

Present value. See *discounting.*

Prevalence. The number of instances of illness or of persons falling ill, or of any other event such as accidents, in a specified population (e.g. 100000 people of a certain age), without any distinction between new and old cases.

Pulmonary embolism. Obstruction of a pulmonary artery by a clot of blood (or other emboli).

Pyloric stenosis. Narrowing of the gastric pylorus (a muscular ring controlling the outlet of the stomach) especially by congenital muscular hypertrophy and scarring resulting from a peptic ulcer.

Radionuclide brain scanning. A technique in nuclear medicine producing images of the distribution in the brain of injected radionuclides, i.e. radioactive isotopes.

Receiver operating curve (ROC). A locus of points showing the relationship between the proportions of true-positives and true-negatives (false-positives and false-negatives) from a diagnostic test, obtained when shifting the threshold between "positive" and "negative".

Sensitivity. The ability of a test to detect a disease when it is really present, expressed as the number of true-positives as a proportion of all those tested who actually have the disease.

Social cost or benefit. Social costs and benefits include private costs and benefits plus any other effects that may create costs or benefits for other members of the community. Social costs are all *opportunity costs* (q.v.). Thus the social value of the *human capital* (q.v.) of an individual will include any income tax paid, whereas the value of private human capital will not, and the social cost of a medical procedure will include its effects on household and other sectors and not just the costs that are private to a hospital or clinic.

Specificity. The ability of a test to identify correctly the absence of disease, expressed as the number of true-negative test results as a proportion of all those tested who do not actually have the disease.

Subarachnoid haemorrhage. Haemorrhage within the meninges. Meninges are membranes enveloping the brain and spinal cord.

Tomograph. A device for taking sectional roentgenograms. By giving the X-ray tube a curvilinear motion during exposure synchronous with the recording plate but in the opposite direction, the shadow of the selected plane remains stationary on the moving film while the shadows of all other planes have a relative displacement on the film and are therefore obliterated or blurred. Computerized axial tomography is a sophistication of this earlier technique, involving computer reconstruction of a cross-sectional image; see *computerized tomographic scanner.*

Trauma. Morbid condition of body produced by injury, wound, or external violence; emotional shock.

Ulcer. A lesion on the surface of the skin or mucous surface caused by (superficial) loss of tissue, usually with inflammation. (A wound with superficial loss of tissue from trauma is not primarily an ulcer, but may become ulcerated if infection occurs.)

Vagotomy. Operation in which nerve fibres of the vagus (or pneumogastric) nerve leading to the stomach are cut (to reduce production of digestive acid).

X-ray. A form of electromagnetic radiation with a wavelength shorter than visible light. Produced by electrons accelerated by high electric voltages, which bombard a target, normally made of a metal with a large atomic number. The target emits X-rays, which penetrate the body, but are thus used to produce X-ray pictures on (special) photographic films. In the *CT scanner* (q.v.) the X-ray intensity is measured quantitatively upon traversing the body.

Zollinger-Ellison syndrome. Peptic ulceration involving gastric hypersecretion of acid and a particular tumour in the pancreatic islets.

34 References

Aaron H (1981) Economic aspects of the role of government in health care. In: van der Gaag J, Pearlman M (eds) Health, economics and health economics. North Holland Publishing Company, Amsterdam

Abel-Smith B (1980) The rising cost of health care. In: Sharing health care costs. NCHSR Research Proceedings Series. DHEW Pub. No. (PHS) 79-3256, Springfield, Virginia

Abt CC (1977) The issue of social costs in cost-benefit analysis of surgery. In: Bunker JR, Barnes BA, Mosteller F (eds) Costs, risks, and benefits of surgery. Oxford University Press New York, pp 40–55

Abrams HL, McNeil BJ (1978a) Medical implications of computed tomography. N Engl J Med 298: 255–261, 310–318

Abrams HL, McNeil BJ (1978b) Computed tomography: cost and efficacy implications. A J R 131: 81–87

Albano O et al. (1978) Short-term treatment of duodenal ulcer with Cimetidine: results from a controlled multicenter trial. In: Luchelli PE (ed) Proceedings of the 1977 Taormina Cimetine Symposium, Smith Kline and French, Philadelphia

Almy TP (1979) Report of the workgroup on the socioeconomic impact of digestive diseases. In: Report to the Congress of the US of the National Commission on Digestive Diseases: 4, part 4. DHEW Pub. No (NIH) 79-1885. National Institutes of Health, Bethesda

Alstedt G (1953) The incidence of peptic ulcers in Denmark. Danish Sciences Press, Copenhagen

Altman SH, Blendon R (eds) (1979) Medical technology: The culprit behind health care costs? In: Proceedings of the 1977 Sun Valley Forum on National Health. DHEW (DHS) 79-3216: 1–9

Ambrose J, Gooding MR, Uttley D (1980) EMI scan in the management of head injuries. Lancet I: 847–848

American Hospital Association (1977) CT scanners: a technical report. AHA, Chicago

Anonymous (1978) Selection of patients for dialysis and transplantation. Br Med J 2: 1449–50

Armitage P (1972) History of randomized controlled trials. Lancet I: 1388

Armitage P (1975) Sequential medical trials, 2nd edn. Blackwell, Oxford

Arnstein SR (1977) Technology assessment: opportunities and obstacles. In: IEEE Transactions on Systems, Man and Cybernetics SMC-7 No 8: 571–582

Bahr AL, Hodges FJ (1978) Efficacy of computed tomography of the head in changing patient care and health costs: a retrospective study. A J R 131: 45–49

Baker C, Way LW (1978) Clinical utility of CAT body scans. Am J Surg 136: 37–44

Baker HL (1975) The impact of computed tomography on neuroradiologic practice. Radiology 116: 637–640

Balaban DJ, Stolley PJ (1979) Cancer epidemiology. In: Cassileth B, Saunders (ed) Spring

Balaban DJ, Goldfarb NG et al. (1980) Chronic care study: a randomized trial of patients with chronic disease on a special treatment unit. Final report to the Robert Wood Johnson Foundation

Balinsky W, Berger R (1975) A review of research on general health status indexes. Med Care 13 (4): 283–293

Bank S et al. (1976) Histamine H_2-receptor antagonists in the treatment of duodenal ulcers. S Afr Med J 50: 1781–5

Banta D (1979) International workshop on the evaluation of medical technology, Stockholm, Sept. 18–19. SPRI Report, p. 156

Banta D (1980) Computed tomography: cost containment misdirected. Am J Public Health 70: 215–216

Banta D, Bekney C et al. (1978) Assessing medical technologies. Bull NY Acad Med 54 (1): 113–123
Banta HD, McNeil BJ (1978) Evaluation of the CAT scanner and other diagnostic technologies. Health Care Manage Rev 3: 7–19
Bapst L, Horisberger B (1980) Field studies in private medical practice in the Federal Republic of Germany, autumn 1978: 150 ulcer patients, autumn 1979: 103 ulcer patients. Interdisciplinary Research Centre for Public Health, St. Gallen
Bapst L, Horisberger B (1981 a) Analysis of data of the diagnosis and therapy index (DTI). Survey performed by Infratest Gesundheitsforschung Munich, 1974–1981
Bapst L, Horisberger B (1981 b) Analysis of a 101 interviews with physicians in private practice in the Federal Republic of Germany. Interdisciplinary Research Centre for Public Health, St. Gallen (unpublished)
Barakat M et al. (1979) Cimetidine in the treatment of active duodenal ulcer disease: a double-blind controlled trial. J Kuwait Med Assoc 13: 21–6
Bardhan KD (1979) Comparison two doses of cimetidine and placebo in the treatment of duodenal ulcer: a multi-centre trial. Gut 20: 68–74
Bardhan KD (1981) Long-term management of duodenal ulcer – a physician's view. In: Baron JH (ed) Cimetidine in the 80's. Churchill Livingstone, Edinburgh
Bardhan KD et al. (1979) Double-blind comparison of cimetidine and placebo in the maintenance of healing of chronic duodenal ulceration. Gut 20: 158–62
Barnes BA (1977 a) An overview of the treatment of end-stage renal disease and a consideration of some of the consequences. In: Bunker JR, Barnes BA, Mosteller F (eds) Costs, risks, and benefits of surgery. New York, pp 325–341
Barnes BA (1977 b) Cost-benefit analysis of surgery. Am J Surgery 133: 439–446
Barral V (1980) Tomodensitometrie cerebrale et economie de la sante. Dissertation Univ. Renee Descartes
Bartlett JR, Neil-Dwyer G (1978) A clinical study of the EMI scanner: implications for provision of neuroradiological services. Br Med J 2: 813–815
Bartlett JR, Neil-Dwyer G, Banham JMM, Cruickshank DG (1978) Evaluating cost-effectiveness of diagnostic equipment: the brain scanner case. Br Med J 2: 815–820
Bazzato G et al. (1980) Continuous ambulatory peritoneal dialysis without wearing a bag: complete freedom of patients and significant reduction of Peritonitis. Proc Eur Dial Transplant Assoc 17: 266–275
Beecher KK (1955) Powerful placebo. JAMA 159: 1602–1606
Belloc N, Breslow B (1973) Relationship of health practices and mortality. Prev Med 2: 67–81
Bergner M, Bobbitt RA et al. (1976) The sickness impact profile: conceptual formulation and methodology for the development of a health status measure. Int J Health Serv 6 (3): 393–415
Bergner M, Bobbitt RA et al. (1981) The sickness impact profile: development and final revision of a health status measure. Med Care 19 (8): 787–805
Berstad A et al. (1979) Maintenance treatment of duodenal ulcer patients with a single bedtime dose of cimetidine. Scand J Gastroenterol 14: 827
Bice TW (1980) Social science and health services research: contributions to public policy. Health and society. Milbank Mem Fund Q 58 (2): 173–200
Bice TW, Bernstein MJ (1977) Methodological perspectives on health status indexes. In: Elinson J et al. (eds) Health goals and health indicators: policy, planning and evaluation. AAAS Selected Symposium 2, Westview Press, Boulder, Colorado
Black DAH, Pole JD (1975) Priorities in biomedical research. Br J Prev Social Med 29: 222–227
Blackwood WS et al. (1976) Cimetidine in duodenal ulcer: controlled trial. Lancet II: 174–6
Blackwood WS et al. (1978) Prevention by bedtime cimetidine of duodenal ulcer relapse. Lancet I: 621 a
Blagg CR (1979 a) Peritoneal dialysis and the Medicare ESRD Program. Dialysis and Transplantation 8 (11): 1081–1085
Blagg CR (1979 b) Cui Bono? Dialysis and Transplantation 8 (5): 501–2, 513
Blumenthal IS (1959) Research and the ulcer problem. Rand Corporation, Santa Monica
Blumenthal IS (1968) Digestive disease as a national problem. Gastroenterology 54 (1): 86–92
Bodemar G, Walan A (1976) Cimetidine in the treatment of active duodenal and prepyloric ulcers. Lancet II: 161–4

Bodemar G, Walan A (1978) Maintenance treatment of recurrent peptic ulcer by Cimetidine. Lancet: 403–406

Bodemar G, Gotthard R, Strom M, Walan A, Jönsson B, Bjurulf P (1979) Socioeconomic aspects of treatment with cimetidine in peptic ulcer disease. In: Proceedings of the Symposium held at Capri, Oct 18–20. Further experience with H_2-receptor antagonists in peptic ulcer disease and progress in histamine research. Exerpta Medica, Amsterdam, pp 59–67

Bonnevie O (1975) Incidence of duodenal ulcer in Copenhagen County. Scand J Gastroenterol 10: 385–393

Booth T (1978) CAT Screening for neurological disease: an abuse? Med J Aust 2: 248–250

Box GEP, Tiao GC (1965) A change in level of a non-stationary time series. Biometrika 52: 181–192

Bracht GH, Glass BV (1968) The external validity of experiments. Am Educ Res J 5: 437–474

Broman T, Pedersen LE (1975) Effectiveness of CT-scanning of the head at the Sahlgrenska Hospital (in Swedish) two reports. Sahlgrenska Hospital, Gothenburg

Brook RH (1977) Mechanisms for assuring quality of US medical care services: past present and future. Prepared under a grant from the US Department of Health Education and Welfare, August

Brook RH, Williams KN (1976) Effect of medical care review on the use of injections: a study of the New Mexico experimental medical care review organization. Ann Intern Med 85 (4): 509–515

Brook RH, Avery AD, Greenfield S et al. (1977) Assessing the quality of medical care using outcome measures: an overview of the method. Med Care 15: supplement

Bryan FA, Evans RW (1979) Dialysis where? Dialysis and Transplantation 8 (3): 264–272

Bryan FA, Evans RW (1980a) The renal dialysis study: I. An overview of the method. Dialysis and Transplantation 9 (11): 1065–1068

Bryan FA, Evans RW (1980b) The renal dialysis study: II. Demographic description for the patient sample. Dialysis and Transplantation 9 (12): 1173–1178

Bulthius R (1980) Cimetidine related findings by Netherland Economic Institute. NEI March

Bulthius R (1981) Cimetidine, surgery trends and the cost of peptic ulcer disease, Amsterdam, March 1981

Bundesverband der Ortskrankenkassen (1957–1981) Statistik der Ortskrankenkassen, Krankheitsarten-, Krankheitsursachen- und Sterblichkeitsstatistik 1956–1979. Bonn

Bunker JP, Fowles J et al. (1982) Evaluation of medical technology strategies. An article in two parts. N Engl J Med 306 (10): 620–624, 306 (11): 687–692

Bureau D'Informations et de Previsions Economiques (BIPE) (1978) The economics of ulcers in France. Neuilly, Seine Cedex

Burland WL, Hawkins BW, Beresford J (1980) Cimetidine treatment for the prevention of recurrence of duodenal ulcer: an international study. Postgrad Med J 56: 173–6

Burton BT (1969) Kidney disease program analysis: a report to the Surgeon General. HEW, Washington D.C.

Burton C (1979) Computed tomographic scanning and the lumbar spine, part I. Economic and historic review. Spine 4 (4): 353–55 July/August

Bush JW, Anderson JP et al. (1981) Negative preferences in the quality of well-being. Med Care

Buxton MJ, West RR (1975a) The cost of death. Lancet: 38

Buxton MJ, West RR (1975b) Cost-benefit analysis of long-term hämodialysis for chronic renal failure. Br Med J 7: 376–379

Byar DP, Simon RM et al. (1976) Randomized clinical trials: perspectives on some recent ideas. N Engl J Med 295 (2): 74–80

Campbell DT (1969) Reforms as experiments. Am Psychol 24 (4): 409–429

Campbell DT, Ross HL (1968) The Connecticut crackdown on speeding: time-series data in quasi-experimental analysis. Law Soc Rev 3: 33–53

Campbell JD, Campbell AR (1978) The social and economic costs of end-stage renal disease. N Engl J Med 299 (8): 386–392

Carrera GF, Gerson DE, Shnur J, McNeil BJ (1977) Computed tomography of the brain in patients with headache or temporal lobe epilepsy: findings and cost-effectiveness. J Comput Assist Tomogr 1 (2): 200–203

Chalmers TC (1974) Impact of controlled trials on the practice of medicine. Mt Sinai J Med (NY) 41: 753–759

Chalmers TC (1981) The clinical trial. Millbank Mem Fund Q 59 (3): 324–339
Chen MK (1976) The K Index: a proxy measure of health care quality. Health Serv Res 11 (4): 452–463
Chen MM, Bush JW (1979) Health status measures, policy, and biomedical research. In: Mushkin SJ, Dunlop DW (eds) Health: what is it worth? Measures of health benefits, Pergamon, New York, pp 15–42
Chiang CL (1965) An index of health: mathematical models. National Center for Health Statistics, Series 2, No 5
Church R, ReVelle C (1974) The maximal covering location problem. Papers of the Regional Science Association, vol 32: 101–118
Clade H (1977) Finanzielle Grenzen des Dialyseprogramms. Dtsch Ärzteblatt 74 (50): 2967–72
Clade H (1980) Kosten-Nutzen-Analyse des Dialyseprogramms. Ersatzkasse 60 (8): 342–346
Coates J (1974) Some methods and techniques for comprehensive impact assessments. Tech Forecasting and Soc Change 6: 341–357
Cochran WG, Cox GM (1957) Experimental designs, 2nd edn. Wiley, New York
Cochrane AL (1972) Effectiveness and efficiency: random reflections on health services. Nuffield Provincial Hospitals Trust, London
Codman EA (1914) The product of a hospital. Surg Gynec Obstet 18: 491–496
Cohon J (1978) Multiobjective programming and planning. Academic, New York
Cole P (1979) The evolving case-control study. J Chronic Dis 32: 15
Cook TD, Campbell DT (1979) Quasi-experimentation: design and analysis issues for field settings. Rand McNally, Chicago
Cooper BS, Rice DP (1976) The economic cost of illness revisited. Social Security Bulletin, US Department of Health, Education and Welfare, Washington
Crichton E, Woods F, Uldall K (1981) Two years' experience with self-care hemodialysis at Toronto Western Hospital. Dialysis and Transplantation 10 (3): 194–198
Culyer AJ (1978) Measuring health: lessons for Ontario. University of Toronto Press, Toronto
Culyer AJ (ed) (1983) Health indicators. Martin Robertson, Oxford
Culyer AJ, Maynard AK (1981) Cost-effectiveness of duodenal ulcer treatment. Soc Sci Med 15C (1): 3–11
Darby SC, Kendall GM, Rae S, Wall BF (1980) The genetically significant dose from diagnostic radiology in Great Britain in 1977. National Radiological Protection Board Report 106, HMSO, London
Darby SC, Reissland JA (1981) Low levels of ionising radiation and cancer – are we underestimating the risk? J R Stat Soc Series A 144: 298–331
Davis CE (1976) The effect of regression to the mean in epidemiologic and clinical studies. Am J Epidemiol 104: 493–498
Dawber TR, Kannel WB et al. (1972) An approach to longitudinal studies in a community: the Framingham study. Ann NY Acad Sci 107: 539–556
Diaz-Buxo JA, Chandler JT (1980) Home dialysis – the best alternative. Dialysis and Transplantation 9 (9): 812–814
Dixon AK, Fry IK, Kingham JGC et al. (1981) Computed tomography in patients with an abdominal mass: effective and efficient? – a controlled trial. Lancet I: 1199–1201
Dobrilla G et al. (1978) Cimetidine in the treatment of duodenal ulcer: clinical endoscope study on 76 patients. Munich Med Wochenschr 120 (24): 839–42
Docherty P (1971) Uremivardens Kostnadsproblem. Lakartidningen 68 (42): 4757–4764
Dössel DP (1978) An economic analysis of end-stage-renal disease. Research Report Series Monograph no 2, Hospital and Health Services Commission, Canberra
Doll R, Hill AB (1950) Smoking and carcinoma of the lung. Br Med J: 739–747
Dollery C (1978) The end of an age of optimism. Nuffield Provincial Hospitals Trust, London
Donabedian A (1966) Evaluating the quality of medical care. Milbank Mem Fund Q 44: 166–206
Donabedian A (1969) Evaluating the quality of medical care. In: Program Evaluation in the Health Field. Behavioral Publications, New York
Donabedian A (1980) Explorations in quality assessment and monitoring, vol 1. The definition of quality and approaches to its assessment. Health Administration Press, Ann Arbor
Donaldson SW, Wagner CC (1973) A unified ADL evaluation form. Arch Phys Med Rehabil 54: 175–185

Doyle FH, Gore JC, Pennock JM et al. (1981) Imaging of the brain by nuclear magnetic resonance. Lancet II: 53–57

Dronfield MW, McIllmurray MB, Ferguson R et al. (1977) A prospective randomised study of endoscopy and radiology in acute upper-gastrointestinal-tract bleeding. Lancet I: 1167–1169

Dronfield MW et al. (1979) Controlled trial of maintenance cimetidine treatment in healed duodenal ulcer: short and long term effects. Gut 20: 526–30

Drucker PR (1974) Management: tasks, responsibilities practices. Harper and Row, New York

Drummond MF (1980) Principles of economic appraisal in health care. Oxford University Press, Oxford

Drummond MF (1981 a) Studies in economic appraisal in health care. Oxford Univ Press

Drummond MF (1981) Welfare economics and cost benefit analysis in health care. Scott J Pol Econ 28 (2): 125–143

du Boulay GH, Radue EW (1978) Comparison of computerised tomography with other neuroradiological methods: a plea for a different kind of analysis. Neuroradiology 16: 474–476

Dunlop JM (1968) Peptic ulcer in Central Scotland. Scot Med J 13: 192–201

Egdahl RH, Chapman Walsh D (1979) Industry's voice in health policy. Springer Berlin Heidelberg New York

Ekbom K, Marke L-A (1975) Economic implications of CT-scanning of the head of South Hospital (in Swedish). The County Council of Stockholm

Emami B, Melo A, Carter BL et al. (1978) Value of computed tomography in radiotherapy of lung cancer. A J R 131: 63–67

Enlow RA, Ehlert K, Glenn W, Hodak J, Rall K, Wilson WJ (1979) Utilization of computed tomography scanners and the health planning issue: a process data summary. J Comput Assist Tomogr 3 (2): 256–260

Enlow RA, Hodak JA, Pullen KW, Bedworth DD, Moor WC, Reahard TM, Milligan VA (1980) The effect of the computed tomographic scanner on utilization and charges for alternative diagnostic procedures. Radiology 136 (2): 13–417

European Dialysis and Transplant Association (various years) Combined report on regular dialysis and transplantation in Europe

Eurotransplant (1980) Annual Report. Leiden

Evens RG (1981) Economic implications of a new technology installation: a CT model. A J R 136: 673–677

Evens RG, Jost RG (1976) Economic analysis of computed tomography units. A J R 127: 191–198

Evens RG, Jost RG (1977) The clinical efficacy and cost analysis of cranial computed tomography and the radionuclide brain scan. Semin Nucl Med 5 [2]

Evens RG, Jost RG (1979) Utilization of head computed tomography units. Radiology 131: 691–693

Evens RG, Rujanavech N, Mikhael MA (1977) Utilization reliability, and cost effectiveness of cranial computed tomography in evaluating pseudotumor cerebri. A J R 129: 263–265

Evens RG, Blagg CR, Bryan FA (1981) Implications for health care policy, a social and demographic profile of hemodialysis patients in the United States. JAMA 245[5]: 487–491

Farrington JF, Felch WC et al. (1980) Quality assessment and quality assurance: the performance-review alternative. N Engl J Med 303 (3): 154–156

Farrow SC, Fisher DJH, Johnson DB (1971) Statistical approach to planning an integrated hämodialysis/transplantation programme. Br Med J 3: 671–676

Feinstein AR (1976) 'Compliance bias' and the interpretation of therapeutic trials. In: Sackett DL, Hays RB (eds) Compliance with therapeutic regimens. Johns Hopkins University Press, Baltimore, pp 152–166

Feinstein AR (1977) Clinical biostatistics. St. Louis, Mosby

Figueroa RB et al. (1979) Cimetidine in active duodenal ulcer. Curr Ther Res 25 (1): 16–24

Fineberg H (1979) Medical technology policies and computed tomography. Ann Intern Med 90 (1): 114–15

Fineberg HV, Bauman R, Sosman M (1977 a) Computerized cranial tomography: effect on diagnostic and therapeutic plans. JAMA 238: 224–227

Fineberg HV, Hiatt HH (1979) Evaluation of medical practices: the case for technology assessment. N Engl J Med 301 (20): 1086–1091

Fineberg HV, Pearlman LA (1981 a) Benefit and cost analysis of medical interventions: the case of

cimetidine and peptic ulcer disease. Case study II, Background paper 2: Case studies of medical technologies, O T A, Washington DC
Fineberg HV, Pearlman LA (1981b) Surgical treatment of peptic ulcer in the United States: trends before and after the introduction of cimetidine. Lancet I: 1305–1307
Fineberg HV, Parker G, Pearlman L (1977b) CT scanners: distribution and planning status in the United States. N Engl J Med 297 (4): 216–218
Fisher DJ (1975) Indications for home dialysis. In: Lindholm T (ed) The Gamro Symposium on home dialysis. Brugge, Lund
Fisher RA (1966) The design of experiments, 8th edn. Oliver and Boyd, Edinburgh
Flagle CD (1963) Operational research in the Health Services. Ann NY Acad Sci 107: 748–759
Forsyth G (1963) An inquiry into the drug bill. Med Care 1: 10–16
Freeman HE, Rossi PH (1981) Social experiments. Milbank Mem Fund Q 59: 346–373
Freeman H, Sherwood CC (1969) Program evaluation in the health fields. In: Schulberg HC et al. (ed)
Friedson E (1970) Profession of medicine. Dodd, Mead and Co, New York
Fries JF, Spitz P (1980) Measurement of patient outcome in arthritis. Arthritis a. Rheum 23 (2): 137–145
Fry I (1964) Peptic ulcer: a profile. Br Med J 2: 809
von Fuchs C (1979) Zur Technik der Dauer-Peritonealdialyse Theorie, Trainingsmethoden, Indikationen und Kosten. Nieren- und Hochdruckkrankheiten 8 (5): 183–187
Gaus CR (1976) Biomedical research and health care costs. Testimony of the Social Security Administration before the Presidents Medical Research Panel
Gehan EA, Freireich EJ (1974) Non-randomized controls in cancer clinical trials. N Engl J Med 290 (4): 198–203
Gempel PA, Harris GH, Evens RG (1977) Comparative cost analysis: computed tomography vs alternative diagnostic procedures, 1977–1978. Little Cambridge, Mass.
George RO, Wagner HN Jr (1975) Ten years of brain tumor scanning at Johns Hopkins: 1962–1972. In: De Blanc HJ Jr, Sorensen JA (eds) Noninvasive brain imaging, computed tomography and radionuclides. The Society of Nuclear Medicine, New York, pp 3–16
Geweke J, Weisbrod B (1981) Some economic consequences of technological advance in medical care: the case of a new drug. In: Heluis RB (ed) Drugs and Health. American Enterprise Institute, Washington DC
Geweke J, Weisbrod B (1982a) Clinical evaluation vs economic evaluation: the case of a new drug. Med Care
Geweke J, Weisbrod B (1982b) Assessing technological change: the case of a new drug. University of Wisconsin, Madison
Gilsanz V et al. (1979) Cimetidine for duodenal ulcer. Lancet I: 151
Glass N (1975) The cumulative cost of death. Lancet: 1341–1342
Goddeeris J, Weisbrod B (1980) Medical progress and health care expenditures: the uneasy marriage. In: Viewpoints. Hoffmann-LaRoche, Nuttey, N. 5.
Godden JO (1979) National symposium on diagnostic imaging review value and economics of imaging modalities. Car Med Assoc J 120: 219–228
Goitein M (1979) The utility of computed tomography in radiation therapy: an estimate of outcome. Int J Radiat Oncol Biol Phys 5: 1799–1807
Goitein M (1980) Benefits and costs of computerized tomography in radiation therapy. JAMA 244: 1347–50
Goitein M, Wittenberg J, Mendiondo M et al. (1979) The value of CT scanning in radiation therapy treatment planning: a prospective study. Int J Radiat Oncol Biol Phys 5: 1787–1798
Gottschalk CW (1967) Report of the Committee on chronic kidney disease. B O B, Washington DC
Gray GR et al. (1977) Oral cimetidine in severe duodenal ulceration: a double-blind controlled trial. Lancet I: 4–7
Gray GR et al. (1978) Long term cimetidine in the management of severe duodenal ulcer dyspepsia. Gastroenterology 74: 397–401
Green LW, Lewis FM (1979) Issues in relating evaluation to theory, practice and policy in health education.
Greenland S, Watson E et al. (1981) The case-control method in medical care evaluation. Med Care 19 (8): 872–878

Greenwood M (1948) Medical statistics from Graunt to Farr. Cambridge University press, Cambridge
Greibe J et al. (1977) Long term prognosis of duodenal ulcer: follow-up study and survey of doctor's estimates. Br Med J 2: 1572–4
Grosse RN (1970) Problems of resource allocation in health. In: Haveman RH, Margolis J (eds) Public expenditures and policy analysis. Merkham Chicago, pp 518–548
Gudmand-Høyer E et al. (1977) A pragmatic trial of cimetidine in duodenal ulcer patients. Scan J Gastroenterol 12: 611–3
Gudmand-Høyer E et al. (1978) Prophylactic affect of cimetidine in duodenal ulcer disease. Br Med J I: 1095–7
Hafter E (1978) Praktische Gastroenterologie vol 6. Georg (ed) Thieme, Stuttgart
Hallan JB, Harris BSH (1968) The economic cost of end-stage uremia. Inquiry 5 (4): 20–25
Hallinan JM (1979) CT and nuclear medicine in screening for neurological disease. Med J Aust 1: 451–452
Hammond EC, Horn D (1958) Smoking and death rates. JAMA 166: 1294–1308
Hampers CL, Hager EB (1979) The delivery of dialysis services on a nationwide basis – can we afford the non-profit system. Dialysis and Transplantation 8 (4): 417–423/442
Hanley JA, McNeil BJ (to be published a) Comparing two ROC curves from the same sample of subjects. Radiology
Hanley JA, McNeil BJ (1982a) The meaning and use of the area under a receiter operating characteristic (ROC) curve. Radiology 143: 29–36
Hanley JA, McNeil BJ (1982b) Maximum attainable discrimination and the utilization of radiologic examinations. J Chonic Dis 35: 601–11
Hansky J et al. (1980) Relapse rate of duodenal ulcer after healing with cimetidine or Mylanta II. Gastroenterology 2: 1179 (abstract)
Harberger AC (1971) Three basic postulates for applied welfare economics. J Ec Lit 9: 785–797
Harrington JC, Brener ER (1973) Patient care in renal failure. Philadelphia
Hart D (1972) History of randomized controlled trials. Lancet I: 965
Hartunian NS, Smart CN, Thompson MS (1981) The incidence and economic costs of major health impairments. Lexington Books, Lexington
Harvey M (1981) Risk-benefit estimates for invasive procedures: how adequate are the data? Paper presented to Third Annual Meeting of Society for Medical Decision-Making
Hayden GF, Kramer MS et al. (1982) The case-control study: a practical review for the clinician. JAMA 247 (3): 326–331
Health Services and Protection Branch (1980) Guidelines for establishing standards for special services in hospitals: Computed tomography. Canada
Heinonen OP (1973) DES in pregnancy: frequency of exposure and usage patterns. Cancer 31: 573–577
Heller S (1980) How many CT scanners do you need? Hospitals 55–57
Hentschel E et al. (1979) Treatment and propyloric ulcer with cimetidine. Wien Klin Wochenschr 81 (2): 53–7
Hertzman P, Jönsson B, Lindgren B (1976) The economic costs of ulcer disease. IHE The Swedish Institute for Health Economics, Report 1979: 6, Lund
Hertzman P, Jönsson B, Silverberg R (1981) Magsårssjukdomens kostnader i Danmark (The economic costs of ulcer disease in Denmark). IHE The Swedish Institute for Health Economics, Report 1981: 4, Lund
Hetzel DJ et al. (1978) Cimetidine in the treatment of duodenal ulcer. Med J Aust I: 317–9
Hiatt HH (1975) Protecting the medical commons: who is responsible? N Engl J Med 293 (5): 235–241
Hill AB (1952) The clinical trial. New Eng J Med 247: 114–119
Hill AB (1977) A short textbook of medical statistics. Hodder and Stroughton, London
Hill JD et al. (1978) A randomized trial of home vs hospital. Lancet: 837–841
Hillier L, Baker IR (1976) Computed tomography and neuroradiology: a fortunate primary union. AJR 127: 101–110
Hobday P, Hodson NJ, Husband J et al. (1979) Computed tomography applied to radiotherapy treatment planning: techniques and results. Radiology 113: 477–483
Hoffstein PA, Drueger KK, Wineman RJ (1976) Dialysis costs: results of a diverse sample study. Kidney Int 9: 286–293

Holgate RC, Wortzman G (1978) The medical and financial impact of computed tomography scanning: effects of inertia. J Belge Radiol 61: 427–37
Holland WW et al. (eds) (1979) Measurement of levels of health. WHO European Regional Study No 7, WHO Copenhagen
Hoult DI (1981) An overview of NMR in medicine. National Center for Health Care Technology (NCHCT) Monograph Series, US Dept of Health and Human Services, Hyattsville, Maryland
Houston TP (1972) The behavioral impact – effectiveness model. In: Rossi PH, William W (eds) Evaluating social programs. Seminar Press, New York, pp 51–65
Husband JE et al. (1982) Computed tomography of the body: when should it be used? Br Med J 284: 4–8
Institute of Medicine (1977) A policy statement: computed tomographic scanning. National Academy of Sciences, Washington DC
Institute of Studies in Political Economy (ISPE) (1978a) The determination of the social costs of peptic ulcer in Italy, University of Pavia
Institute of Studies in Political Economy (ISPE) (1978b) Assessment of the social benefits deriving from the introduction of cimetidine. University of Pavia
International Commission on Radiological Protection (1977) Recommendations of the ICRP. Pergamon, Oxford
Jacobsen II, Kragsholm M, Holm C (1975) On the economics of CT-scanning (in Danish). Rikshospitalet, Copenhagen
Jenkins PG, Gutmann FD, Rieselbach RE (1976) Self-hemodialysis – the optimal mode of dialytic therapy. Arch Intern Med 136: 357–361
Jensen K et al. (1979) Prophylactic effect of cimetidine in gastric ulcer patients. Scand J Gastroenterol 14: 175–6
Jones-Lee MW (1976) The value of life: An economic analysis. University of Chicago Press, Chicago
Jönsson B, Lindgren B (1980) Five common fallacies in estimating the economic gains of early discharge. Soc Sci Med [C] 14
Jönsson B, Silverberg R (1982) Variations between and within countries in hospital care for peptic ulcer – A comparison between Denmark and Sweden. Scand J Soc Med 10: 63–69
Jonsson E (1980) Economic evaluation of medical technology: The case of CT-scanning of the head. In: Jonsson E (ed) Studies in health economics. The Economic Research Institute, Stockholm School of Economics, Stockholm
Jonsson E, Marké LA (1981) Computerized tomography in Sweden: An analysis of cost-effectiveness (in Swedish). SPRI Report 73. SPRI, Stockholm
Jonsson E et al. (1976) Economic evaluation of CT in Sweden. SPRI, Stockholm
Kahneman D, Tversky A (1982) The psychology of preferences. Sci Am 246: 160–173
Kang JY et al. (1979) The use of long-term cimetidine in the prevention of gastric ulcer relapse: double-blind trial. In: Proceedings of the annual scientific meeting of the Gastroenterological Society of Australia, Brisbane
Kaplan RM, Bush JW et al. (1976) Health status: Types of validity and the index of well being. Health Serv Res 11 (4): 478–507
Kaplan RM, Bush JW et al. (1979) Health status index: Category rating versus magnitude estimation for measuring levels of well being. Med Care 17 (5): 501–525
Karnofsky DA, Burchenal JH (1946) The clinical evaluation of chemotherapeutic agents in cancer. In: McLeod C (ed) Evaluation of chemotherapeutic agents. Columbia University Press, New York, pp 191–205
Karstaedt N, Maynard CD (eds) (1982) Nuclear magnetic resonance symposium abstracts. Radiology 142: 243–247
Katz S, Ford AB et al. (1963) Studies of illness in the aged. The index of ADL. A standardized measure of biological and psychosocial function. JAMA 185: 914–919
Kemp E, Kristiansen J et al. (1974) Nitten maneders erfaring med hjemmedialyse i Danmark. Ugeskr Laeger 136 (3): 136–141
Kendall GM, Darby SC, Harries SV, Rae S (1980) A frequency survey of radiological examinations carried out in national health service hospitals in Great Britain in 1977 for diagnostic purposes. National Radiological Protection Board Report 104, HMSO, London
Kjellstrand CM (1980) Current problems in long-term hemodialysis. Dial Transplant 9 (4): 295–299

Klarman HE (1974) Application of cost-benefit analysis to health systems technology. J Occup Med 16 (3): 172–186
Klarman HE, Francis JO'S, Rosenthal GD (1968) Efficient treatment of patients with kidney failure. Med Care 6: 48–54
Knaus WA, Davis DO (1978) Utilization and cost-effectiveness of cranial computed tomography at a university hospital. J Comput Assist Tomogr 2 (2): 209–14
Knaus WA, Schroeder SA, Davis DO (1977) Impact of new technology: the CT scanner. Med Care 15: 533–542
Knaus WA, Wagner DP (to be published) CT scanning patients with headache: A cost-benefit calculation. Am J Neurol
Knaus WA, Wagner DP, Davis DO (1980) CT for headache: cost-benefit for subarachnoid haemorrhage. Am J Neuroradiol 1: 567–572
Kohn R, White KL (eds) (1976) Health care: An international study. Oxford University Press, London
Kolata G (1981) The consensus on CT scanners. Science, V: 214, 1327–1328
Krause U (1963) Long-term results of medical and surgical treatments of peptic ulcer. Acta Chir Scand [Suppl] 310: 1–111
Lambert EC (1978) Modern medical mistakes. Indiana University Press, Bloomington
Lambert Y (1980) Trend in ulcer surgery, gastrointestinal hemmorrhages, appendectomies and cholecystectomies 1976–79. (Updated Oct 1981)
Larsson EB, Omenn GS (1977) The impact of computed tomography on the care of patients with suspected brain tumor. Med Care 15: 543–551
Larsson EB, Omenn GS, Margolis MT, Loop JW (1977) Impact of computed tomography on utilization of cerebral angiograms. AJR 129: 1–3
Larsson EB, Omenn GS, Loop JW (1978a) Computed tomography in patients cerebrovascular disease: impact of a new technology on patient care. A J R 131: 35–40
Larsson EB, Omenn GS, Magno J (1978b) Impact of computed tomography on the care of patients with suspected hydrocephalus. A J R 131: 41–44
Larsson EB, Omenn GS, Lewis H (1980) Diagnostic evaluation of headache: impact of computerized tomography and cost-effectiveness. JAMA 243: 359–362
Lecomte TH (1977) La concentration des dépenses medicales, les 10% plus forts consommateurs de soins. CREDOC, Paris
LeSourd DA, Fogel ME, Johnston DR (1968) Benefit-cost analysis of kidney disease programs. DHEW, Public Health Services Publication No 1941. Government printing office Washington DC
Levene RJ, Cohen ED (1974) The Hawthorne effect. Clin Res 22: 111–112
Leveson I (1978) Policy issues in evaluation of health technology. In: Egdahl RH, Gertman PM (eds) Technology and the quality of health care. Aspen Systems Corporation, Germantown, Maryland
Levy NB, Schribner BH (eds) (1974) Living or dying – adaption to hemodialysis. Springfield I 11
Levy NB, Wynbrandt GD (1975) The quality of life on maintenance haemodialysis. Lancet I: 1328–1330
Lille K, McCullough G (1977) CT scanners: A technical report. American Hospital Association, Chicago
Little AD (1977) Comparative cost analysis: Computed tomography vs alternative diagnostic procedures 1977–1980. Little Cambridge, Mass
Litton A, Murdoch WR (1963) Peptic ulcer in South West Scotland. Gut 4: 360–366
Lloyd Johnson Associates (1976) The demand for computed tomography and its impact on diagnostic imaging market. Lloyd Johnson Associates, Northfield 1: 11.
Lohr KN, Winkler JD, et al. (1981) Peer review and technology assessment in medicine. R-2820-OTA prepared for the Office of Technology Assessment, Rand Corporation, California
Longmore DB, Rehahn M (1975) The cumulative cost of death. Lancet I: 1023–1025
Lowrie EC, Hampers CL (1981) The success of Medicare's ESRD-program, The case for profits and the private Marketplace. N Engl J Med 305 (8): 434–438
Ludbrook A (1981) A cost-effectiveness analysis of the treatment of chronic renal failure. Appl Econ 13: 337–50
Machell RJ, et al. (1979) Cimetidine in the prevention of gastric ulcer relapse. Postgrad Med J 155: 393–5

McKeown T (1976) The role of medicine: dream, mirage or nemesis? Nuffield Provincial Hospitals Trust, London
McKinlay JB (1981) From "promising report" to "standard procedure": Seven stages in the career of medical innovation. Milbank Mem Fund Q 59 (3):
McKinlay JB, McKinlay SM (1977) The questionable contribution of medical measures to the decline of mortality in the United States in the twentieth century. Millbank Mem Fund Q 405–428
McNeil BJ (1979) Pitfalls in and requirements for evaluations of diagnostic technologies. In: Wagner JL (ed) Medical technology: proceedings of Urban Institute conference. National Center for Health Services Research (NCHSR) Research Proceeding Series, US Department of Health, Education and Welfare, DHEW publications. (DHS) 79–3254: 33–39, Hyattsville, Maryland
McNeil BJ (1982) Decision making in radiology: ROC curves. In: Benson ES et al (eds) Clinical decisions and laboratory use. University of Minnesota Press, Minneapolis
McNeil BJ, Collins JJ, Adelstein SJ (1977) Rationale for seeking occult metastases in patients with bronchial carcinoma. Surg Gynecol Obstet 144: 389–393
McNeil BJ, Hanley JA (1983) Statistical approaches to the analysis of receiver operating characteristic (ROC) curves. Med Dec Mak (in press)
McNeil BJ, Hanley JA, Funkenstein HH, Rumbaugh C (1981) Utilization of computed tomography of the head in a tertiary care hospital. Radiology 139: 113–118
McNeil BJ, Weichselbaum R, Pauker SC (1978) Fallacy of the five-year survival in lung cancer. N Engl J Med 299 (25): 1397–1401
Marcus H (1974) Die faule Gesellschaft – Wie die Deutschen arbeiten (6th edn). Droste, Düsseldorf
Mather HG, Morgan DC et al. (1976) Myocardial infarction: A comparison between home and hospital care for patients. Br Med J 1: 925–929
Mazure PA, et al. (1980) Cimetidine in the treatment of active duodenal ulcer. Acta Gastroenterol Latinoam 8: 17–28
Mechanic D (1968) Medical sociology: A selective view. Free Press, New York
Mehta D, Mehta S, Drake F (1981) A medical audit of the use of CAT scan in a CMHC inpatient unit. Hosp Community Psychiatry 32: 345–347
Meier P (1975) Statistics and medical experimentation. Biometrics 31: 511–529
Mekel RCPM (1978) Long term treatment with cimetidine. Afr Med J 54: 1089
Menz FG (1971) Economics of disease prevention: Infectious kidney disease. Inquiry 8 (4): 3–18
Menz FC (1975) The costs of detection and treatment programs for infectious kidney disease. Am J Public Health 65 (4): 401–407
Metz CE, Kronman HB (1980) Statistical significance tests for binormal curves. J Math Psychol 22 (3): 218–243
Miettinen OS (1970) Matching and design efficiency in retrospective studies. Am J Epidemiology 91 (2): 111–118
Mishan E (1971) Evaluation of life and limb: A theoretical approach. J Polit Econ 79: 687–705
Mishan EJ (1981) Economic efficiency and social welfare. Allen and Unwin, London, chaps 14, 16
Monheit AC (1978) Issues in the allocation of resources to health technology. In: Egdahl RH, Gertman PM (eds) Technology and the quality of health care. Germantown, pp 53–70
Moore G, ReVelle C (to be published) The hierarchical service location problem. Management Science
Moseley I (1982) Recent developments in imaging techniques. Br Med J 284: 1141–1144
Moser CA, Kalton G (1971) Survey methods in social investigation. Heinemann, London
Murphy EA (1976) The logic of medicine. Johns Hopkins University Press, Baltimore
Musgrave R, Musgrave P (1980) Public finance in theory and practice. McGraw-Hill, New York
National Institutes of Health (1980) Consensus development conference summaries 3. National Institutes fo Health
Neiss (1980) Investigation on 3312 ulcer episodes in the Federal Republic of Germany (unpublished)
Netherlands Economic Institute (1977) Present cost of peptic ulceration to the Dutch economy and possible impact of cimetidine on their cost. Netherlands Economic Inst Rotterdam
Neuhauser D (1979) International workshop on the evaluation of medical technology, Stockholm, Sept. 18–19. SPRI Report, pp 13–16
Neuhauser D, Lewicki AM (1975) What do we gain from the sixth stool guaiac? N Engl J Med 293 (5): 226–228

Nightingale F (1859) Notes on hospitals. Parker, London

Odum HT (1971) Environment power and society. Wiley Interscience, New York

Office of Health Economics (1978) Renal failure: a priority in health? Office of Health Economics, London

Office of Health Economics (1980) End stage renal failure. Office of Health Economics, London

Office of Technology Assessment (1978a) Assessing the efficiency and safety of medical technologies. Government Printing Office, Washington DC

Office of Technology Assessment (1978b) Policy implications of the computed tomography (CT) scanner. Congress of the United States. Government Printing Office, Washington DC

Office of Technology Assessment (1980a) The implications of cost-effectiveness analysis of medical technology. Background paper 1, Methodological issues and literature review. Congress of the United States, Government Printing Office, Washington DC

Office of Technology Assessment (1980b) The implications of cost-effectiveness analysis of medical technology. Background paper no 4; The management of health care technology in ten countries. Government Printing Office, Washington DC

Office of Technology Assessment (1981a) Policy implications of the computed tomography (CT) scanner: an update. Congress of the United States, Government Printing Office, Washington DC

Office of Technology Assessment (1981b) Case study no 11: Benefit-and-cost analysis of medical interventions: The case of cimetidine and peptic ulcer disease. Government Printing Office, Washington DC

Ogden DA, Kopec C, Guy AD (1981) Cost-effectiveness of multiple dialyzer use. Dial Transplant 10 (5): 407–411

Oreopoulos DG, et al. (1980) Continuous ambulatory peritoneal dialysis in Canada. Dial Transplant 9 (3): 224–226

Palmore E, Luikart C (1972) Health and social factors related to life satisfaction. J Health Soc Behav 68

Parkin DM (1978) Chronic renal failure: the economics of treatment. Community Health 9: 134–141

Pearson DA, Stranova TJ, Thompson JD (1976) Patient and program costs associated with chronic hemodialysis care. Inquiry 13: 23–38

Piachaud D, Weddell JM (1972) Cost of treating varicose veins. Lancet II: 1191–2

Pliskin JS, Beck CH (1976a) Decision analysis in individual decision making: A real-world application in treatment of renal disease. Methods Inf Med 15: 43–46

Pliskin JS, Beck CH (1976b) A health index for patient selection: A value function with application to chronic renal failure patients. Management Sci 22: 1009–1021

Pliskin JS, Steinman TI, Lowne EG, Bech CH (1976) Hemodialysis – projecting future bed needs. Deterministic and probabilistic forecasting. Compu Biomed Res 9: 317–336

Pliskin JS, Shepard DS, Weinstein MC (1980) Utility functions for life years and health status. Oper Res 28 (1): 106–224

Popovich RP, Moncrief JW, et al. (1978) Continuous ambulatory peritoneal dialysis. Ann Intern Med 88: 449–456

Prasad SC, Pilepich MV, Perez CA (1981) Contribution of CT to quantitative radiation therapy planning. A J R 136: 123–128

Pulvertaft CN (1968) Comments on the incidences and natural history of gastric and duodenal ulcers. Postgrad Med J 44: 597–602

Ragan DP, Perez CA (1978) Efficacy of CT-assisted two-dimensional treatment planning: analysis of 45 patients. A J R 131: 75–79

Raiffa H (1968) Decision analysis.

Reiser SJ (1978) Medicine and the reign of technology. Cambridge University Press, Cambridge

Relman AS (1979) Cat scanners – "Coinferring the greatest benefit on mankind". N Engl J Med 301 (19): 1063–1063

Relman AS (1980) Assessment of medical practices: A simple proposal. N Engl J Med 303 (3): 153–154

Relman AS (1982) An institute for health care evaluation. N Engl J Med 306 (11): 669–670

Rettig RA (1976) Valuing lives: The policy debate on patient care financing for victims of end-stage renal disease. RAND, p 5672. Rand Corporation, Santa Monica

Rettig RA (1977) End-stage renal disease and the 'costs' of medical technology. RAND, p 6029. Rand Corporation, Santa Monica
Rettig RA (1978) Lessons learned from the end-stage renal disease experience. In: Egdahl RH, Gertman PM (eds) Technology and the quality of health care. Germantown pp 153–173
Rettig RA (1980) The federal government and medical technology. Policy Sci 11: 343–356
Rettig RA (1981) The implications of cost-effectiveness analysis of medical technology, Case study 1, Background paper 2. Office of technology assessment, congress of the United States, Washington DC
Rettig RA, Marks EL, Baier M (1981) Implementing the ESRD-program of medicare. HCFA, Office of Research, Demonstrations and Statistics
Rettig RA, Webster TC (1975) Implementation of the end-stage renal disease program: A mixed pattern of subsidizing and regulating the delivery of medical services. RAND, p 5555. Rand Corporation, Santa Monica, CA
Revelle C, Cohon J, Shokrup D (1981) Multiple objectives in facility location. Paper 81-01, Operations Research Report. Johns Hopkins University, Baltimore, Maryland
Rhode Island Health Services Research Inc (1981) The effect of cimetidine on peptic ulcer disease in Rhode Island. Rhode Island Health Services Research Inc
Ricardo-Campbell R (1980) Risk-benefit/cost-benefit: Improving government regulation of approval of new drugs. Presented at the world congress on health and economics, Leyden University, Netherlands, 9. Sept. 1980, p 13 (mimeo)
Ricardo-Campbell R, Eisman M, Wardell WW, Crossley R (1980) Preliminary methodology for controlled cost-benefit study of drug impact: the effect of cimetidine on days of work lost in a short-term trial in duodenal ulcer. J Clin Gastroenterol 2: 37–41
Rice DP (1966) Estimating the cost of illness. Health Economics Series no 6, US Public Health Service, Government Printing Office, Washington DC
Rice DP, Feldman JJ, White KL (1976) The current burden of illness in the United States. National Academy of Sciences, Institute of Medicine, Washington DC
Riecken HW (1977) Principal components of the evaluation process. Prof Psychol 392–410
Riecken HW, Boruch R (eds) (1974) Social experimentation: A method for planning and evaluation of social interventions. Academic, New York
Rimm AA, Lemann J, Hussey JL (1978) A model for planning health care in patients with end-stage renal disease. Arch Intern Med 138: 1783–1786
Robbins AH, Pugatch RD, Gerzof SG et al. (1978) Observations on the medical efficacy of computed tomography of the chest and abdomen. A J R 131: 15–19
Roberts D, Maxwell DR, Gross TL (1980) Cost-effective care of end-stage renal disease: A billion dollar question. Ann Intern Med 92: 243–48
Roberts EB et al. (eds) (1981) Biomedical innovation. MIT Press, p 268
Robinson Associates (1978) The impact of cimetidine on the national cost of duodenal ulcers. Robinson Associates, Bryn Mawr, Pennsylvania
Robson MD, Oreopopoulos (1978) Continuous ambulatory peritoneal dialysis – a revolution in the treatment of chronic renal failure. Dial Transplant 7 (10): 999–1003
Roethlisberger FJ, Dickson WJ (1939) Management and the worker. Harvard University Press, Cambridge, MA
Rosenthal G (1979) Anticipating the costs and benefits of new technology: A typology for policy. In: Altman SH, Blendon R (eds) q. v. pp 77–87
Rosser R, Kind P (1978) A scale of valuations of states of illness: is there a social consensus? Int J Epidemiol 7: 347–358
Rudnick MR, Bastl CP, et al. (1982) Cimetidine-induced acute renal failure. Ann Intern Med 96 (2): 180–182
Russell IT, Devlin HB, Fell M et al. (1977) Day-case surgery for hernias and haemorrhoids: a clinical, social and economic evaluation. Lancet I: 844–847
Russell LB (1979) Technology in hospitals: Medical advances and their diffusion. Brookings Institution, Washington DC
Ryan A (1977) Diagnostic technology and medical care costs, part 2. Postgrad Med 61 (3): 14–16
Sackett DL, Chambers LW (1977) The development and application of indices of health: General methods and a summary of results. Am J Pub Health 67 (5): 423–428
Sackett DL, Haynes RB (eds) (1976) Compliance with therapeutic regimens. Johns Hopkins University Press, Baltimore

Sackett DL, Torrance GW (1978) The utility of different health states as perceived by the general public. J Chronic Dis 31: 697–704

Sartwell PE (1974) Retrospective studies: A review for the clinician. Internal Medicine 81: 381–386

Sartwell PE, Masi AT et al. (1963) Thromboembolism and oral contraceptives: An epidemiologic case-control study. Am J of Epidemiol 90 (5): 365–380

Schanke K (1946) Behaviour of gastric and duodenal ulcer in a fishing district in the North of Norway. Acta Chir Scand [Suppl 115] 94: 1–157

Schippers HMA, Kalff MW (1976) Cost comparison – Hämodialysis and renal transplantation. Tissue Antigens 7: 86–90

Schlesselman JJ, Stolley PD (1982) Case control studies. Oxford University Press, New York

Schmoranz I (1980) Kosten-Nutzen Analyse fur Cimetidine (A cost-benefit analysis of cimetidine). Endbericht, Band I–III. Institut fur höhere Studien, Vienna

Schröder SA, Showstack JA (1911) The dynamics of medical technology use: Analysis and policy options. In: Altmann SH, Blendon R (eds) q. v.

Schwartz D, Lellouch J (1967) Explanatory and pragmatic attitudes in clinical trials. J Chronic Dis 20: 637–648

Schwartz D, Flamant R, Lellouch J (1980) Clinical trials. Academic Press, London

Schwartz WB, Joskow P (1978) Medical efficacy versus economic efficiency: A conflict of values. N Engl J Med 299: 1462–1464

Semb LS, et al. (1976) A double-blind multicenter comparative study of cimetidine and placebo in short term treatment of active duodenal ulceration. In: Buland WL, M Alison (eds) Cimetidine: Scandinavian international symposium on histamine H_2-receptors antagonists. Royal College of Physicians, London

Shapiro AK (1960) A contribution to a history of the placebo effect. Behav Sci 5: 109–135

Shepard DS, Thompson MS (1979) First principles of cost-effectiveness analysis in health. Public Health Rep 94 (6): 535–543

Shepard DS, Zeckhauser RJ (1980) Long-term effects of interventions to improve survival in mixed populations. J Chronic Dis 33: 413–433

Siemsen AW, et al. (1980) Economic impact of an integrated approach to hemodialysis and dialyzer reuse. Dial Transplant 9 (10): 933–936

Silverberg RV (1981) The prevalence and social costs of ulcer disease in Norway. Report 6. IHE Swedish Institute for Health Economics, Lund, Report 1981: 6

Simler S (1979) Body CT purchases may be halted. Mod Health Care 9: 43

Slater P (1971) The pursuit of loneliness: American culture at the breaking point. Beacon, Boston

Society for Computer Tomography (1979) New indications for computed body tomography, American Journal of Radiology, 113, 115–9

Sonnenberg A, Blum AL (1982) The cost of knowing the truth: cost-benefit analysis of upper G.I. endoscopy. J Clin Gastroenterol 4: 109–114

Sonnenberg A, Hefti ML (1979) The cost of postsurgical syndroms. Clin Gastroenterol 8: 235–248

Sonnenberg A, et al. (1981) Predictors of duodenal ulcer healing and relapse. Gastroenterology 81: 1061–1067

Sonnenberg A, et al. (1982a) Was kostet ein Ulkus? In: Blum AL, Siewert JR (eds) Ulkus Therapie. Springer, Berlin Heidelberg New York, pp. 138–150

Sonnenberg A, et al. (1982b) Erwartungskosten bei der konservativen und chirurgischen Behandlung der unkomplizierten Cholezystolithiasis. Z Gastroenterol 20: 66–71

Sonnenberg et al. (1982c) Epidemiologie und Genetik der Ulkuskrankheit. In: Blum AL, Siewert JR (eds) Ulkus Therapie. Springer, Berlin Heidelberg New York, pp. 3–22

Spitzer WO, Feinstein AR, Sackett DL (1976) What is a health care trial? JAMA 233 (2): 161–163

Spitzer WO, Starfield B (1977) Health services research can make a difference. N Engl J Med 1046

Sponheim N (1960) Incidences and prevalence of peptic ulcer in a part of the country. Nord Med 63: 377–385

Stange PV, Summers AT (1978) Predicting treatment costs and life expectancy for end-stage renal disease. N Engl J Med 298 (7): 372–378

Statens Medicinska Forskningsrad (1976) Njurforskning – ett underlag for langsiktig planering av forskningen inom de medicinska njursjukdomarnas omrade. Stockholm

Starfield B (1973) Health services research: A working model. N Engl J Med 289: 132–136

Sterman AB, et al. (1980) The role of cranial CT scan in municipal hospital. Am J Public Health 70: 268–270

Stewart JH, Topp WD, et al. (1973) The cost of domicilliary maintenance haemodialysis: A comparison with alternative replacement regimes. Med J Aust 1 (1): 156–159

Stocking BS, Morrison SL (1982) The image and the reality: a case-study of the impacts of medical technology. Oxford University Press for the Nuffield Provincial Hospitals Trust, London

Suchman EA (1967) Evaluative research: Principles and practice in public service and social action programme. Russell Sage Foundation, New York, pp 75–77

Sugden R, Williams A (1978) The principles of practical cost benefit analysis. Oxford University Press, London, p 234

Sullivan DF (1971) A single index of mortality and morbidity. HSMHA Health Rep 86: 347

Swartz R, Des Harnais S (1977) Computed tomography: The cost-benefit dilemma. Radiology 125: 251–253

Swets JA (1979) ROC analysis applied to the evaluation of medical imaging techniques. Invest Radiol 14: 109–121

Swets JA, Pickett RM, Whitehead AF, et al. (1979) Assessment of diagnostic technologies. Science 205: 753–759

Thomson JLG (1977) Cost-effectiveness of an EMI brain scanner: a review of a two-year experience. Health Trends 9: 16–19

Thomson JLG (1979) Cost-effectiveness of an EMI brain scanner: an updated review, 1977–78. Health Trends 11: 46–48

Thorne MC, et al. (1968) Chronic disease in former college students. Am J Epidemise 87 (3)

Torrance GW (1976) Towards a utility theory foundation of health status index models. Health Serv Res 11: 349–369

Torrance GW, Thomas WH, Sackett DL (1972) A utility maximization model for evaluation of health care programs. Health Serv Res 7 (2): 118–133

Torrance GW, Sackett DL, Thomas WH (1973) Utility maximization model for program evaluation: A demonstration application. In: Berg RL (ed) Health status indexes. Hospital Research and Educational Trust, Chicago, pp 156–165

Ubilluz R (1979) Cimetidine in the treatment of active duodenal ulcer: a double-blind study. Curr Ther Res Clin Exp 25 (2): 243–50

UK Transplant (1981) UK transplant service review 1981. UK Transplant Service, Bristol

US Department of Health Education and Welfare, Office of the Assistant Secretary for Program Coordination (1966) Selected disease control programs. DHEW U.S. Government Printing Office, Washington DC, p 9

Venables CW (1981) Surgery and hospitalization trends in the UK before and after Cimetidine. Freeman Hospital, Newcastle-upon-Tyne (mimeo)

Vogt TM, Johnson RE (1980) Recent changes in the incidence of duodenal and gastric ulcer. Am J Epidemiol 111 (6): 713

von Haunalter G, Chandler VV (1977) Cost of ulcer disease in the United States. Stanford Research Institute, Menlo Park, CA

Wagner JL (1981) Case study no 2: the feasibility of economic evaluation of diagnostic procedures: the case of CT scanning. In: The implications of cost-effectiveness analysis of medical technology. Background paper No 2: Case studies of medical technologies. Office of Technology Assessment, Congress of the United States, Government Printing Office Washington DC

Wai L, Richard J, Burton H, Lindsay RM (1981)

Wall BF, Fisher ES, Shrimpton PC, Rae S (1980) Current levels of gonadal irradiation from a selection of routine diagnostic X-ray examinations in Great Britain. National Radiological Protection Board Report 105, HMSO, London

Ware JE (1976) The reliability and validity of general health ratings. Rand paper. The Rand Corporation, CA, p 5720

Warner JD, Kalff WJ (1976) Cost of home dialysis versus institutional dialysis. J Dial 1 (1): 67–73

Webster EW (1981) On the question of cancer induction by small X-ray doses. A J R 137: 647–666

Weinman EJ et al. (1980) Continuous ambulatory peritoneal dialysis: Initial experience as a home training and in-hospital procedure. Dial Transplant 9 (8): 749–750

Weinstein MC (1979) Economic evaluation of medical procedures and technologies: progress, problems and prospects. In: Wagner JL (ed) Medical technology: Research priorities. Working paper 1262-1. Urban Institute, Washington DC

Weinstein MC, Stason WB (1977) Foundations of cost-effectiveness Analysis for health and medical practices. N Engl J Med 296 (13): 716–21

Weinstein M, et al. (1976) Computed tomography versus skull radiography. A J R 127: 873
Weisbrod BA (1961) Economics of public health. University J Pennsylvanien Press, Philadelphia
Weisbrod B (1969) Collective action and the distribution of income: conceptual approach, the analysis and evaluation of public expenditures: the PPB system. Joint economic committee, US Congress GPO, Washington DC pp 177–198 (reprinted in: Haveman R, Margolis J (eds) Public expenditures and policy analysis. Markham, Chicago)
Weisbrod B (1978) Public interest law. University of California Press, Berkeley
Weisbrod B (1981) Benefit-cost analysis of a controlled experiment: Treating the mentally ill. J Hum Resour 16: 523–548
West RR, Crosby DL, Jones MJ (1974) A mathematical model of an integrated haemodialysis and renal transplantation programme. Br J Prev Soc Med 28: 149–155
White KL (1974) Contemporary epidemiology. Int J Epidemiol 3 (4): 295–303
White KL (1980) Health information systems: an epidemiological perspective. Inquiry 17: 296–312
White KL, Williams TF (1961) The ecology of medical care. N Engl J Med 265 (18): 885–892
White KL, Anderson DO, Purola T, et al. (1977) Health services: Concepts and information for national planning and management. Public health papers 67. World Health Organization, Geneva
Willems J, et al. (1979) The computed tomography (CCT) scanner, Medical technology: The culprit behind health care costs? In: Altman SH, Blendon R (eds) Proceedings of the 1977 sun valley forum on national health. DHEW publication no (PHS) 79-3216. Government printing office, Washington DC
Williams A (1974) Measuring the effectiveness of health care systems. In: Perlman M (ed) The economics of health and medical care. Macmillan, London
Williams A (1979) One economist's view of social medicine. J Epidemiol Community Health 33: 3–7
Williams A (1981) Welfare economics and health status measurement. In: Van der Gaag J, Perlman M (eds) Health economics and health economics. North Holland, Amsterdam
Williamson JW (1971) Evaluating quality of patient care: a strategy relating outcome and process assessment. JAMA 218 (4): 564–569
Wing AJ, Brunner FP, Brunger HOA, et al. (1978) Mortality of and morbidity of reusing dialysers. Br Med J 853–855
Winston KR (1978) Neurodiagnostic tests in children with brain tumors: Changing patterns of use and impact on cost. Pediatrics 61 (6): 847–852
Winter J (1978) Efficiency of utilization of a computed tomography scanner. Am J Radiol 131 (1): 89–93
Wittenberg J, Fineberg HV, Black EB et al. (1978) Clinical efficacy of computed body tomography. A J R 131: 5014
Wittenberg J, Fineberg HV, Ferrucci JT et al. (1980) Clinical efficacy of computed body tomography II. A J R 134: 1111–1120
Wolff C Jr (1979) A theory of nonmarket failure: Framework for implementation analysis. J Law Econ 22: 107–139
World Health Organization (1980) National medical technologies assessment programmes. H4/48/12, Regional Office for Europe, WHO, Copenhagen
Wortzman G, Holgate R (1979) Reappraisal of the cost-effectiveness of computed tomography in a government-sponsored health care system. Radiology 130 (1): 257–61
Wortzman G, Morgate RC, Morgan PP (1975) Cranial computed tomography: and evaluation of cost effectiveness. Radiology 117: 75–77
Wylie JH, Alexander-Williams J, Kennedy TL, Clarke CG, Bell PRF, Kirk RM, MacKay C (1981) Effect of cimetidine on surgery for duodenal ulcer. Lancet I: 1307–1308
Young IR, Hall AS, Pallis CA et al. (1981) Nuclear magnetic resonance imaging of the brain in multiple sclerosis. Lancet II: 1063–1066
Zeckhauser R (1975) Procedures for valuing lives. Public Policy 23: 419–464
Zelen M (1969) Play the winner rule and the controlled clinical trial. J Am Stat Assoc 64: 131–146
Zelen M (1979) A new design for randomised clinical trials. N Engl J Med 300: 1242–1245
Zimmerman RA, Bilaniuk LT, Genarelli T et al. (1978) Cranial computed tomography in diagnosis and management of acute head trauma. A J R 131: 27–34

Appendix

List of Members of Health Economists' Study Group

Abel-Smith, Professor B., Department of Social Science and Administration, London School of Economics, Houghton Street, Aldwych, London WC2A 2AE.

Akehurst, R. L., Institute of Social and Economic Research, University of York, Heslington, York, Y01 5DD.

Allen, D., Health Services Management Unit, Booth Street West, Manchester 50.

Ament, Dr. A. J. A., Rijksuniversiteit Limburg, Postbus 616, 6200 MD Maastricht, The Netherlands.

Appleby, J., South Birmingham Health Authority, Oak Tree Lane, Selly Oak, Birmingham, B29 6JF.

Artelles-Herrero, J., c/sta Amelia; 22; exB, e°1ª, Barcelona 34, Spain.

Baigent, N., Department of Economics, University College Swansea, Singleton Park Swansea SA2 8PP.

Bailey, J. M., Transport Studies Unit, Oxford University, 11 Bevington Road, Oxford, OX2 6NB.

Bally, Ms. Y., Koningin Julianastr. 35, 2825 BJ Berkenwonde, The Netherlands.

Barer, Dr. M. L., Associate Director, Division of Health Services Research and Development, University of British Columbia, Vancouver, B.C., Canada, V6T 1Z6.

Barnard, K., The Nuffield Centre for Health Services Studies, Clarendon Road, Leeds LS2 9PL.

Barnett, J. A., Science Policy Research Unit, Mantell Building, University of Sussex, Falmer, Brighton BN1 9RF.

Barnoon, Dr. S., Ben-Gurion University of the Negev, New Campus, Beer Sheva 84 120, P. O. Box 653, Israel.

Backhouse, M., 65 Nunnery Lane, York, N. Yorks.

Beesley, Professor M., London Business School, Sussex Place, Regent's Park, London, NW1 4SA.

Benham, Professor L., Box 1208, Economics, Washington University, St. Louis, Missouri 63130, USA.

Benson, T. J., Flat 4, 55 Mablethorpe Rd, London SW 6.

Bentkover, Dr. J. D., Arthur D Little, Inc., Acorn Park, Cambridge, Mass. 02140, USA.

Best, G., King Edward's Hospital Fund for London, King's Fund College, 2 Palace Court, London W2 4HS.

Bilheimer, Mrs. L., University of Arkansas Medical School, 324 West Fourteen Street, Little Rock, Arkansas 72202, USA.

Binkley, Dr. H. L., Director, Institute for Health Service Policy, HOPE Center, Millwood, VA 22646, USA.

Blades, Miss C. A., Institute of Social & Economic Research, University of York, Heslington, York, Y01 5DD.

Boan, Professor J., Department of Economics, University of Regina, Regina, Saskatchewan, Canada.

Bohigas, L., Paseo Del Rio 20, Manresa (Barcelona) Spain.

Borgonovi, Professor E., Direttore C.E.R.G.A.S., Universita Bocconi, Via R. Sarfatti, 20136 Milano, Italy.

Bosanquet, N. R. G., Department of Economics, The City University, Northampton Square, London, EC1V OHB.

Bowles, R. A., Department of Humanities and Social Sciences, University of Bath, Claverton Down, Bath, BA2 7AY.

Brenna, A., Instituto per la recerca di Economia Sanitaria, 20123 Milano, C.so Magenta 42, Italy.

Bridge, J., Department of Industrial Relations & Management Studies, University College, P. O. Box 78, Cardiff, CF1 1XL.

Brittain, Dr. R.D., District Medical Officer, North Warwickshire Health Authority, Newtown Road, Nuneaton, CV11 4HW.

Brittan, Ms. Y., Centre for Socio-Legal Studies, University of Oxford, Wolfson College, Oxford.

Brooks, R.G., Department of Economics, University of Strathclyde, Stenhouse Building, 173 Cathedral Street, Glasgow G4 ORQ.

Broome, J.R., The Cottage, Tucking Mill, Midford, Bath.

Brown, Professor M.G., Department of Preventive Medicine & Department of Economics, Dalhousie University, Halifax, Nova Scotia B3H 4H7, Canada.

Brus-Ramer, Ms. H., Manager, Economic Analysis, Smith Kline & French Overseas Co., 1500 Spring Garden Street, P.O. Box 7929, Philadelphia, PA 19101, USA.

Burchell, A., Economic Advisors Office, Room 720 Friars House, 157–168 Blackfriars Road, London, SE1 8EV.

Buxton, M., Department of Economics, Brunel University, Uxbridge, Middlesex, UB8 3PH.

Cabases, J.C., San. Miguel 7–3°, Pamplona, Spain.

Cairns, J., Department of Political Economy, Edward Wright Building, Dunbar Street, Old Aberdeen AB9 2TY.

Callingham, M., District Treasurer, Southampton and South West Hampshire Health District, 119 Tremona Road, Southampton, SO1 6HU.

Chamberlain, Miss A., Information Services Division, Trinity Park House, South Trinity Road, Edinburgh

Chapalain, Mlle. M.T., Chef du Bureau des Etudes et du Plan, Director Générale de la Santé, Ministère de la Santé et de la Sécurité Sociale, 1 Place Fontenoy, Paris 75007, France.

Charles, Miss S., Department of Economics, University of Loughborough, Loughborough.

Chernichovsky, Dr. D., Ben-Gurion University of the Negev, Beer Sheva 84, P.O.B. 653, Israel.

Clarke, Ms. R., Department of Economics, Faculty of Commerce and Social Science, The University of Birmingham, P.O. Box 363, Birmingham B15 2TT.

Cohen, D., Health Economics Research Unit, Department of Community Medicine, University Medical Buildings, Foresterhill, Aberdeen, AB9 2ZD.

Collard, Professor D.A., School of Humanities and Social Sciences, University of Bath, Claverton Down, Bath, BA2 7AY.

Cook, B.V., 12 Riverside Court, Nine Elms Lane, London, SW8 5DB.

Cook, H.G., 66 White Street, Martham, Gt. Yarmouth, Norfolk.

Cooke, A., Department of Industrial Economics, University of Nottingham, University Park, Nottingham, NG7 2RD.

Cooper, Professor M.H., Department of Economics, University of Otago, Dunedin, New Zealand.

Costas, E., Calle de Ian Blas 5, Madrid 14, Spain.

Cox, H., USHP Dept. of Community Medicine, Guy's Hospital, St. Thomas Street, London, SE1.

Coulson, Mrs. A., West Midlands Regional Health Authority, Arthur Thomson House, 146 Hagley Road, Birmingham, B16 9PA.

Creese, A.L., Centre for Development Studies, University College Swansea, Singleton Park, Swansea SA2 8PP.

Crossley, Professor J.R., School of Economics Studies, University of Leeds, Leeds LS2 9JT.

Cullis, J.G., School of Humanities and Social Sciences, University of Bath, Claverton Down, Bath BA2 7AY.

Culyer, Professor A.J., Department of Economics, University of York, Heslington, York YO1 5DD.

Cumper, Dr. G.E., Evaluation and Planning Centre, Ross Institute, London School of Hygiene and Tropical Medicine, Gower Street, London WC1.

Cunningham, R.L., Room B717, DHSS, Alexander Fleming House, Elephant & Castle, London, SE1 6BY.

Dale, Dr. J.W., Specialist in Community Medicine, South East Thames RHA, Randolph House, 46–48 Wellesley Road, Croydon CR 9 30A.

Davies, Dr. B., Personal Social Services Research Unit, Cornwallis Building, University of Kent, Canterbury CT2 7NS.

Davis, C., Centre for Russian and East European Studies, The University of Birmingham, P.O. Box 363, Birmingham B15 2TT.

de Campos, A.C., Escola Nacional de Saude Publica, Av. Padre Cruz, 1699 – Lisboa – Codex, Portugal.

de Kadt, Professor E. J., Institute of Development Studies, University of Sussex, Falmer, Brighton, BN1 3RH.
De Kok, Dr. H. J. G., Central Council for Health Care, Postbus 226, 2280 AE Rijswijk, The Netherlands.
Deeble, Dr. J. S., Director, Health Research Project, Australia National University, Canberra, Australia.
Dennerlein, Dr. R., BASYS, 8900 Augsburg 1, Calmberg Straße 5, West Germany.
D'Intagno, Professor B. M., Universite de Clermont 1, 19 rue Paul Delong, 75002 Paris, France.
Dorland, J., The Policy Development and Research Branch, Ontario Ministry of Health, 15 Overlea Boulevard, Toronto, Ontario, Canada M4H 1A9.
Dowie, Dr. J. A., Social Sciences, Open University, Milton Keynes MK7 6AA.
Dowie, R. F., 14 Lisburne Road, London NW3 2NR.
Doyle, J., 173 Withington Road, Manchester, M16 8EF.
Drummond, M. F., Health Services Management Centre, 40 Edgbaston Park Road, Birmingham 15.
Dunlop, Dr. D., Dartmouth Medical School, 1800 R. St. N.W. # 609, Washington D.C. 20009, USA.
England, R., C/O Tibbalds Partnership, 39 Charing Cross Road, London, WC2H OAW.
Engleman, Dr. S. R., Department of Community Medicine, Usher Institute, Warrender Park Road, Edinburgh EH9 1DW.
Erickson, P., Clearinghouse on Health Indexes, Division of Analysis, Department of Health, Education and Welfare, Public Health Service, Health Resources Administration, Rockville, Maryland 20852, USA.
Evans, Professor R. G., Department of Economics, University of British Columbia, 997–1873 East Mall, Vancouver, B.C., Canada, V6T 1Y2.
Fallick, J. L., Department of Economics, Faculty of Economics and Social Studies, University of Manchester, Dover Street, Manchester.
Fein, Professor R., School of Public Health, 642 Huntington Avenue, Harvard University, Boston, Massachusetts 02015, USA.
Feldstein, Professor P. J., Department of Economics and School of Public Health, University of Michigan, Ann Arbor, Michigan 48104, USA.
Fenn, P., Centre for Socio-Legal Studies, University of Oxford, Wolfson College, Oxford.
Fethke, Professor C., Department of Economics, Queen Mary College, Mile End Road, London EC1.
Fitton, Mrs. F., Department of General Practice, 2908 Stopford Building, University of Manchester, Oxford Road, Manchester.
Fleishman, A. B., National Radiological Protection Board, Harwell, Didcot, Oxon, OX11 ORQ.
Forbes, J. F., Social Paediatric and Obstetric Research Unit, University of Glasgow, 64 Oakfield Avenue, Glasgow, G12 8LS.
Forster, Dr. D. P., Dept. of Community Medicine, University of Newcastle, Claremont Road, Newcastle.
Forsyth, Professor G., Health Services Management Unit, Booth Street West, Manchester 50.
Fraser, N., Dept. of Social Administration, University of Edinburgh, Adam Ferguson Building, George Square, Edinburgh, EH8 9LL.
Frost, C. E. B., Division of Economic Studies, University of Sheffield, Sheffield S10 2TN.
Gaag, J. van der, World Bank, DED, I.8-135, 1818 H. Street N.W., Washington D.C. 20433, USA.
Ginsberg, G., Operational Research Department, Room 411, Ministry of Health, Ben Tbai 2, San Simone, Jerusalem, Israel.
Gravelle, H.S. E., Economics Department, Queen Mary College, University of London, Mile End Road, London E1.
Gray, A. M., Department of Community Medicine, University Medical Buildings, University of Aberdeen, Foresterhill, Aberdeen.
Green, A. T., Longrigg, Thornton Rust, Leyburn, N. Yorks.
Griffiths, D. A. T., Sandoz Institute for Health and Socio-Economic Studies, 5 Route de Florissant, CH 1206, Geneva, Switzerland.
Groot, Professor L., University of Maastricht, Roerzicht 22, Roermund, The Netherlands.
Grund, J., The Health Services of Norway, AKERSGT 42, Oslo-Dep., Oslo 1, Norway.

Gunnarsson, D. A., Managing Director, National Hospital System Administration Office, Eiriksgata 5–101 Reykjavik, Iceland.
Gustavsson, Professor G., Department of Economics, University of Gothenburg, Fack 400 10, Goteborg 3, Sweden.
Hagard, Dr. S., Cambridgeshire Area Health Authority (Teaching), Purbeck House, Purbeck Road, Cambridge CB2 2PF.
Hagen, Dr. J. H., Stichting Hogere School voor Gezondheidszorg, Leidseweg 83, 3531 B G Utrecht, The Netherlands.
Hammond, T. R., Central Marketing, Glaxo Operations UK Ltd., Greenford, Middlesex, UB6 OHE.
Hardie, M. A., International Hospital Federation, 126 Albert Street, London NW1 7NX.
Haycox, A., I.S.E.R., University of York, Heslington, York, YO1 5DD.
Heasell, S., Department of Economics & Public Administration, Trent Polytechnic, Burton Street, Nottingham, NG1 4BU.
Henderson, J., Health Economics Research Unit, Department of Community Medicine, University Medical Buildings, Foresterhill, Aberdeen, AB9 2ZD.
Heras, Alumedena Duran, Ministerio de Sanidad y Sequridad Social, Instituto de Estudios de Sandidad Y Seguridad Social, Madrid, 7, Spain.
Hersh, Professor M., Texas Woman's University, Department of Business and Economics, Denton, Texas 76204, USA.
Hertzman, Dr. P., The Swedish Institute for Health Economics, Stora Sodergatan 3, 22223 Lund, Sweden.
Hewitt, S., Oxford Regional Health Authority, Planning Services Division, Old Road, Headington, Oxford.
Hodkinson, S., Policy and Planning Department, Northern Health and Social Services Board, County Hall, Galgorm Road, Ballymena, Northern Ireland.
Holtermann, Ms. S., Department of Health and Social Security, 151 Great Titchfield Street, London W1P 8AD.
Hooijmans, Ms. E., COEPS, University of Leiden, Hugo de Grootstraat 32, 2311 XK Leiden, The Netherlands.
Hoskins, M., Public Sector Economic Research Centre, Department of Economics, University of Leicester, Leicester LE1 7RH.
Huppertz, Dr. P. H., Seminar für Finanzwissenschaft, Universität Za Köln, 5 Köln 41 (Lindenthal), Albertus-Magnus-Platz, Germany.
Hurst, J., Department of Health and Social Security, Friar's House, 157–168 Blackfriars Road, London, SE1 8EU.
Hutt, Mrs. R., Institute of Manpower Studies, University of Sussex, Mantell Building, Falmer, Brighton BN1 9RF.
Hutton, J., ISER, University of York, Heslington, York, YO1 5DD.
Hyman, Dr. S. Dean, Regional Management Centre, School of Management Studies, Portsmouth Polytechnic, High Street, Old Portsmouth.
Jackson, Professor P. M., Director, Public Sector Economics Research Centre, Leicester University, Leicester, LE1 7RH.
Jamesen, R. M. K., Department of Health Care Administration, University of Kuopio, P.O. Box 138, 70101 Kuopio 10, Finland.
Jones-Lee, Professor M., Department of Economics, University of Newcastle-Upon-Tyne, Newcastle-upon-Tyne NE1 7RU.
Jonsson, Professor B., Department of Economics, Fack S 22005 Lund 5, Sweden.
Judge, K., Personal Social Services Research Unit, Cornwallis Building, University of Kent, Canterbury, CT2 7NS.
Jung, H. Abt. Wirtschaftswissenschaft, Osteuropa-Institut, Freie Universität Berlin, Z1 1; 1000 Berlin 33, Garystraße 55, Germany.
Kaewsonthi, Professor S., Faculty of Economics, Chulalongkorn University, Bangkok 5, Thailand.
Kaser, Dr. M. C., St. Antony's College, Oxford OX2 6JP.
Kiesling, Professor H. J., Department of Economics, Indiana University, Ballantine Hall, Bloomington, Indiana 47405, USA.
Kind, Mr. P., Department of Psychiatry, Charing Cross Hospital Medical School, Fulham Palace Road, London W6 8RF.

Knapp, Dr. M.R.J., Personal Social Services Research Unit, Cornwallis Building, University of Kent, Canterbury.

Knappe, Professor E., Universität Trier, Fakultät für Volkswirtschaftslehre und Soziopolitik, D-5500 Trier, W. Germany.

Knight, Ms. Rose, Research Fellow, Health Services Research Unit, Cornwallis Building, University of Kent, Canterbury CT2 7NF.

Koskiniemi, Mrs. H., Finnish Medical Association, Ruoholahdenkatu 4, 00180 Helsinki 18, Finland.

Kuh, Mrs. D.J.L., Institute of Biometry and Community Medicine, University of Exeter, Barrack Road, Exeter, Devon EX2 5DW.

Lagas, Dr. A.F., Tongersestraat 53, Maastricht, Netherlands.

Laing, W., 62 Croftdown Road, London, NW5 1EN.

Launois, Professor R.J.R., 7 Place Hoche, 35000 Rennes, France.

Lavers, R.J., Institute of Social and Economic Research, University of York, Heslington, York YO1 5DD.

Lebrun, Ms. T., Centre de Recherches Economiques et de Gestion, 1 Rue Francois Baes, 59046 Lille Cedex, France.

Lee, K., Nuffield Centre for Health Services Studies, University of Leeds, Clarendon Road, Leeds LS2 9PL.

Lee, Michael, Lee Donaldson Associates, 21–24 Bury Street, London SW1Y 6AL.

Leenders, J., Assistent, Centrum voor Ziekenhuiswetenschap, Vital Decosterstr. 102, B-3000 Leuven, Belgium.

Lees, Profesor D.S., Department of Industrial Economics, University of Nottingham, University Park, Nottingham NG7 2RD.

LeGrand, Dr. J., Department of Economics, London School of Economics, Houghton Street, Aldwych, London WC2A 2AE.

Letouze, D., Faculty of Administration, University of Ottawa, 550 Cumberland Street, 017 Ottawa, KIN 6N5, Canada.

Leu, Dr. R.E., Institut für Sozialwissenschaften, Petersgraben 29, 4051 Basel, Switzerland.

Lindgren, Dr. B., The Swedish Institute for Health Economics, Stora Sodergatan 3, 22223 Lund, Sweden.

Lloyd, J., Polytechnic of the Southbank, Borough Road, London, SE1 OAA.

Lowson Ms. K. Or Unit, West Midlands Regional Health Authority, 326 High Street, Harborne, Birmingham, B17 9PX.

Ludbrook, Ms. A., HERU, Dept. of Community Medicine, University of Aberdeen, Foresterhill, Aberdeen, AB9 2ZD.

Luoma, K., 16 McHugh Court, Heslington, York, YO1 5ET.

Machnes, Dr. Y., Bar-Illan University, Department of Economics, Ramat-Gan, Israel.

MacKay, A., Department of Health, P.O. Box No. 100, Woden, A.C.T. 2606, Australia.

Mancini, P.V., Department of Health and Social Security, Friar's House, 157–168 Blackfriars Road, London, SE1 8EU.

Marsden, J., 37 Main Avenue, York.

Martin, Ms. A.L., 182 West Hill, Putney, London, SW15 3SH.

Martini, Professor C.J.M., Divison of Community Health, School of Medicine, University of Colorado, Medical Center, Box 2582, 4200 East 9th Avenue, Denver, Colorado 80262, USA.

Maxwell, G.D.G., Hoppingwood Farm, Robin Hood Way, London, SW20 OAB.

Maynard, A.K., Department of Economics, University of York, Heslington, York YO1 5DD.

McCarthy, D., Secretary, Social Policy Committee, National Economic and Social Council, Oisin House, Pearse Street, Dublin 2, Ireland.

McDonnell, Ms. R., 120 Hull Road, York, YO1 3LQ.

McGuire, A., Department of Community Medicine, University Medical Buildings, University of Aberdeen, Foresterhill, Aberdeen, AB9 2ZD.

McGuire, Professor M.C., Department of Economics, University of Maryland, College Park, Maryland 20742, USA.

McPherson, Dr. K., Department of Community Medicine & General Practice, University of Oxford, 8 Keble Road, Oxford, OX1 3QN.

de Meester, Professor J.-Cl., Faculte des Sciences Economiques & Sociales, Rempart de la Vierge, 8, B-5000 Namur, Belgium.

Melen, C-G., Department of Economics, University of Uppsala, Uppsala, Sweden.
Melinek, S., Fire Research Station, Melrose Avenue, Borham Wood, Herts, WD6 2BL.
Mills, Ms. A., Centre for Epidemiology and Evaluation of Basic Health Planning, Ross Institute, London School of Hygiene and Tropical Medicine, Keppel Street, London WC1E 7HT.
Mills, M.H., World Bank, 9927 Brixton Lane, Bethesda, Maryland 20817, USA.
Milne, R.G., Department of Political Economy, University of Glasgow, Glasgow W2.
Montfort, G. van, National Zeikenhuisinstituut, Zeikenhuiscentrum, Oudean 4, Utrecht, The Netherlands.
Mooney, G., Department of Community Medicine, University of Aberdeen, Foresterhill, Aberdeen AB9 2ZD.
Morris, Ms. S., Department of Community Medicine, Fenner's, Gresham Road, Cambridge.
Mugford, Mrs. M., National Perinatal Epidemiology Unit, Radcliffe Infirmary, Oxford, OX2 6HE.
Mullen, Mrs. P., The University of Birmingham Health Management Centre, 'Park House', 40 Edgbaston Park Road, Birmingham B15 2RT.
Murphy, T., Mitchell College of Advanced Education, Department of Administrative and Political Sciences, Bathurst, New South Wales 2795, Australia.
Muurinen, Ms. J.M., c/o Alcuin College, University of York.
Muvaro, Professor G., Via dei Garari 13, Padova 35100, Italy.
McCarthy, Dr. M., 6 Melrose Gardens, London W6.
Nabri, Dr. H.I., R.U. Jean Sarrailh, 39 Av. Georges Bernanos, 75005 Paris, France.
Nadeau, Ms. N., 37 Charleville Road, London, W14.
Newns, Mrs. B., 15 Stokesay Way, Stretton Court, Telford, Shropshire.
Newton, M., Department of Accountancy, Faculty of Business and Management Studies, Liverpool Polytechnic, Tithebarn Street, Liverpool L2 2ER.
Nonneman, Professor W., University of Antwerp, St.-Ignatious Faculties, Center of Economics & Social Research, Prinsstraat 13, B2000 Antwerp, Belgium.
Nord, Dr. D., Medizinisch Pharmazeutische Studiengesellschaft, Bilhildisstraße 2, 65 Mainz, West Germany.
Normand, C., Dept. of Finance & Personnel, Policy Planning & Research Unit, Stormont, Belfast, BT4 3SW.
O'Brien, B., Department of Economics, Brunel University, Uxbridge, Middlesex, UB8 8PH.
Ohlsson, Dr. O.G.F., Department of Economics, University of Gothenburg, Box 3091, S-40010 Gothenburg, Sweden.
Over, Professor A.M., Department of Economics, Boston University, 125 Bay State Road, Boston, MA 02215, USA.
Ovi, Professor A., Co direttore C.E.R.G.A.S., Universita Bocconi, Via R. Sarfatti, 20136 Milano, Italy.
Palmer, Professor H.C., Department of Economics, Pomona College, Claremont, California 91711, USA.
Parkin, D., Department of Community Medicine, University Medical Buildings, University of Aberdeen, Foresterhill, Aberdeen, AB9 2ZD.
Parsonage, M., Economic Advisors Office, Room 634 Friars House, 157–168 Blackfriars Road, London, SF1 8FU.
Parsons, D., Institute of Manpower Studies, University of Sussex, Mantell Building, Falmer, Brighton BN1 9RF.
Partridge, J., USHP, Department of Community Medicine, Guy's Hospital, St. Thomas Street, London SE1.
Patel, Mr. Mahesh, Department of Community Medicine, University of Manchester, Stopford Building, Oxford Road, Manchester, M13 9PT.
Paul, Mrs. M.E., Lady Margaret Hall, Oxford.
Pearce, Professor D.W., Department of Political Economy, University of Aberdeen, Foresterhill, Aberdeen.
Pearson, R., Institute of Manpower Studies, University of Sussex, Mantell Building, Falmer, Brighton BN1 9RF.
Pedersen, Professor K.M., Institute of Social Sciences, Odense University, Campusvej 55, DK-5230 Odense M, Denmark.
Pentol, Ms. A., Dept. of Psychiatry, University of Manchester, University Hospital of South Manchester, West Didsbury, Manchester, M20 8LR.

Philips, T., The University of New South Wales, P.O. Box 1, Kensington, New South Wales, Australia 2033.

Phillips, Ms. Jenny, Prices Bureau, Glaxo (Holdings) Ltd., Graham Street, London N1.

Piachaud, D., Department of Social Science and Administration, London School of Economics, Houghton Street, Aldwych, London WC2 2AE.

Pole, J.D., Department of Health and Social Security, Friar's House, 157–168 Blackfriars Road, London, SE1 8EU.

Poullier, J., OCDE, 2, rue Andre-Pascal, 75775 Paris, France.

Prescott, N.M., Magdalen College, Oxford University, Oxford OX1 4AU.

Pritchard, Dr. H., 'Yorath', Upper Hartfield, East Sussex.

Ragnarsdottir, L.M., 14 Stevens Street, Winchester M.A. 01890, USA.

Randall, E., Social Science and Administration Department, Goldsmiths College, University of London, New Cross, London SE14 6NW.

Ransom, Ms. E., Social Affairs Committee, Social Science Research Council, 1 Temple Avenue, London, EC4Y OBD.

Reid, Ms. N., School of Physical Sciences, The New University of Ulster, Coleraine, Northern Ireland.

Reynolds, Ms. J., Social Services Committee, Committee Office, House of Commons, London, SW1A OAA.

Richardson, J., Health Research Project, The Australian National University, Box 4, P.O., Canberra, A.C.T., Australia, 2600.

Risan, Dr. A., Institute of Social & Economic Research, University of York, Heslington, York, YO1 5DD.

Roberts, Dr. J.L., Regional General Administrator, West Midlands Regional Health Authority, Arthur Thomson House, 146 Hagley Road, Birmingham B16 9PA.

Roberts, Miss J.A., London School of Hygiene, Keppel Street, London WC1.

Rochaix, Ms. L., 56 Farrar Street, York.

Rosenfield, Dr. P.L., Special Programme for Research and Training in Tropical Diseases, World Health Organisation, 1211 Geneva 27, Switzerland.

Rosenthal, Dr. G., Director, National Center for Health Services Research, Office of Health Policy, Research and Statistics. 3700 East West Highway, Hyattsville, Maryland 20782, USA.

Russell, I., Medical Care Research Unit, The University of Newcastle-upon-Tyne, 21 Claremont Place, Newcastle-upon-Tyne NE2 4AA.

Sailly, J-C., Centre de Recherches Economiques et de Gestion, 1 Rue Francois Baes, 59046 Lille Cedex, France.

Sandesan, C., Centre for Extension Training in Community Medicine, 31 Bedford Square, London WC1B 3EL.

Schicke, Professor R.K., Medical School Hannover, Angerstr.59, 3000 Hannover 72, West Germany.

Schneider, Dr. M., BASYS, 8900 Augsburg 1, Colmberg Straße 5, West Germany.

Schrijvers, Drs. A.J.P., Health Services Research Institute, University of Utrecht, Bijlhouwer Straat 6, 3511 ZC Utrecht, The Netherlands.

Scott, G., 75 Waipapa Road, Hataitai, Wellington 3, New Zealand.

Scotton, Dr. R.B., Director, Planning and Research, Health Commission of Victoria, G.P.O. Box 4057, Melbourne, 3001, Australia.

Scrivens, Ms. E., St. Thomas's Hospital Medical School, Dept. of Community Medicine, London, SE1 7EH.

Semkow, B.W., 902, 75 Eastdale Avenue, Toronto, Ontario, Canada, M4C 5N3.

Shannon, J.R., Medical Care Research Unit, University of Newcastle-upon-Tyne, 21 Claremont Place, Newcastle-upon-Tyne, NE2 4AA.

Sharp, Professor Ansel M., Economics Department, College of Business Administration, Oklahoma State University, Stillwater, Oklahoma, 74074.

Sharpe, D., Thomas Coram Research Unit, University of London Institute of Education, 41 Brunswick Square, London WC1N 1AZ.

Simpson, P.R., Department of Economics, The Queen's University of Belfast, Belfast BT7 1NN, Northern Ireland.

Sintonen, H., Research Department, Ministry of Social Affairs and Health, Box 303, SF-00171, Helsinki 17, Finland.

Slattery, D. G., Economics Division, Policy Planning & Research Unit, Stormont, Belfast, BT4 3SW.

Smith, Dr. R. P., Department of Economics, Birkbeck College, University of London, Gresse Street, London W1P 1PA.

Smulders, Dr. A. F. M., Teaching Hospital of the Free University, De Boelelaan 1117, 1007 MB Amsterdam, The Netherlands.

Soderstrom, L., Department of Economics, Lund University, Fack 22005, Lund 5, Sweden.

Spackman, M. J., Treasury Chambers, Parliament Street, London SW1P 3AG.

Spek, Professor Jan-Erik, c/o Professor G. Gustavsson, Department of Economics, University of Gothenburg, Fack 40010, Goteborg 3, Sweden.

Stafford, Dr. G. B., Department of Economics, University of York, Heslington, York YO1 5DD.

Stahl, Professor I., Department of Economics, Fack 22005, Lund 5, Sweden.

Steele, R., Health Service Management Unit, Department of Social Administration, University of Manchester, Booth Street, Manchester, M15 6PB.

Stehlin, Dr. M.-B., F. Hoffmann-La Roche & Co., CH-4002 Basle, Switzerland.

Stilwell, J., Health Services Research Centre Medical School, University of Birmingham, Birmingham B15 2TT.

Stoddart, Dr. G. L., Department of Clinical Epidemiology & Biostatistics, McMaster University, 1200 Main Street West, Hamilton, Ontario L8N 3Z5, Canada.

Stone, Ms. C., Project Manager, Policy Analysis Inc, 1577 Beacon Street, Brookline, Massachusetts 02146, USA.

Sugden, R., University of Newcastle-upon-Tyne, Department of Economics, The University, Newcastle-upon-Tyne NE1 7RU.

Tatchell, M., Health Research Project, Australia National University, Canberra, Australia.

Taylor, D., Office of Health Economics, 12 Whitehall, London, SW1A 2DY.

Taylor, S. H., Management Services Division, Wiltshire Health Authority, Rowden Hill House, Chippenham, Wilts, SN15 2AN.

Teeling-Smith, Prof. G., Office of Health Economics, 12 Whitehall, London, SW1A 2DY.

Temple, Mrs. B., Department of General Practice, 2908 Stopford Building, University of Manchester, Oxford Road, Manchester.

Thompson, S. O., Department of Economics, University of Karlstad, Box 9501, S-65009 Karlstad, Sweden.

Thunhurst, C. P., Department of Mathematics and Statistics, Sheffield Polytechnic, Pond Street, Sheffield S1 1WB.

Townsend, J. L., MRC Epidemiology & Medical Care Unit, Northwick Park Hospital, Watford Road, Harrow, Middlesex, HA1 3UJ.

Turpin, P., Planning Unit, Department of Health, Custom House, Dublin 1.

Tussing, Professor A. D., Syracuse University, Health Studies Program, 723 University Avenue, Syracuse, New York 13210, USA.

Van Doorslaer, E., Jules Draeyersstraat 5, B-2610 Wilrijk, Belgium.

Van de Kar, Dr. H. M., Erasmus University Rotterdam, Eur Room H5-25, P. O. Box 173P, 3000 DR Rotterdam.

Van der Star, Dr. Th., Center for Research in Public Economics, Hugo de Grootstraat 32, 2311XK Leyden, The Netherlands.

Varley, Mrs. R., Health Services Management Unit, Booth Street West, Manchester 50.

Ven, Wynand van der, Fac. Studierichting Algemene Gezondheidszorg, Postbus 1738, 3000 DR Rotterdam, The Netherlands.

Verwayen, H., Social Indicators Section, OECD, 2 Rue Andre Pascal, 75775, Paris, Cedex 16, France.

Vinten, G., Toynbee Hall, 28 Commercial Street, London, E1 6LS.

Walker, Dr. A., 27 Hargill Drive, Washington 13, Tyne & Wear.

Ward, H., Allied Medical Group Limited, P. O. Box No. 2816, Riyadh, Kingdom of Saudi Arabia.

Ward, P., Institute of Biometry and Community Medicine, University of Exeter, Bowmoor House, Exe Vale Hospital, Dryden Road, Exeter EX2 5AE.

Waterton, R. Head, Department of Economics, Leicester Polytechnic, P. O Box 143, Leicester LE1 9BH.

Wells, N., Office of Health Economics, 12 Whitehall, London, SW1A 2DY.
Werff, A. van der, Ministry of Public Health and Environment, Dokter Reijersstraat 12, Leidschendam, The Netherlands.
West, Dr. P. A., Department of Community Medicine, St. Thomas's Hospital Medical School, London SE1 7EH.
Westcott, Ms. G., Nuffield Centre for Health Services Studies, The University of Leeds, 71–75 Clarendon Road, Leeds, LS2 9PL.
Wheeler, M., Deputy Course Director, Project Planning Centre, University of Bradford, Bradford BD7 1DP.
Whynes, D., Department of Economics, University of Nottingham, University Park, Nottingham NG7 2RD.
Wilde, Ms. Jayne, Trent Regional Health Authority, Manpower Planning Section, Fulwood House, Old Fulwood Road, Sheffield.
Wilkinson, R., Avon AHA, Greyfriars, Lewin's Mead, Bristol.
Williams, Professor A. H., Department of Economics, University of York, Heslington, York YO1 5DD.
Wiseman, Professor J., Institute of Social and Economic Research, University of York, Heslington, York YO1 5DD.
Wolfson, Dr. A., Department of Health Administration, Faculty of Medicine, Community Health, Fitzgerald Building, University of Toronto, Toronto, Ontario, Canada.
Wolfson, Professor D. J., Erasmus University Rotterdam, Institute for Fiscal Studies, Burgemeester Oudlaan 50, Rotterdam 3016, The Netherlands.
Wood, P., Department of Political Economy, University of Aberdeen, Edward Wright Building, Old Aberdeen.
Wood, R., 118 Moira Terrace, Edinburgh EH7 6TG.
Wright, K. G., Institute of Social and Economic Research, University of York, Heslington, York YO1 5DD.
Yett, Professor D. E., Director, Human Resources Research Center, University of Southern California, Los Angeles, California 90007, USA.
Yfantopoulos, Dr. Y., 12 Sachtour, Chalandri, Athens, Greece.
Yule, B., Department of Community Medicine, University Medical Buildings, University of Aberdeen, Foresterhill, Aberdeen, AB9 2ZD.
Zöllner, Dr. H. G. K., Health Planning and Evaluation Officer, World Health Organisation, Regional Office for Europe, 8 Scherfigsvej, DK-2100 Copenhagen, Denmark.
Zweifel, Dr. P. Institute of Empirical Research in Economics, Kleinstrasse 15, CH-8008 Zurich, Switzerland.

Index of Authors

Subject Index

Tables and Figures are indicated by "T." and "F." respectively, following the page number.

MIX
Papier aus verantwortungsvollen Quellen
Paper from responsible sources
FSC® C105338

FSC
www.fsc.org

If you have any concerns about our products,
you can contact us on
ProductSafety@springernature.com

In case Publisher is established outside the EU,
the EU authorized representative is:
Springer Nature Customer Service Center GmbH
Europaplatz 3, 69115 Heidelberg, Germany

Printed by Libri Plureos GmbH
in Hamburg, Germany